Clinical Applications
of Functional Brain MRI

Clinical Applications of Functional Brain MRI

Edited by

Serge A.R.B. Rombouts

Department of Physics and Medical Technology
VU University Medical Centre
Amsterdam, The Netherlands

and

Leiden Institute for Brain and Cognition (LIBC)
Institute for Psychological Research, Leiden University
Department of Radiology, Leiden University Medical Centre
Leiden, The Netherlands

Frederik Barkhof

Department of Radiology
VU University Medical Centre
Amsterdam, The Netherlands

Philip Scheltens

Department of Neurology/Alzheimer Centre
VU University Medical Centre
Amsterdam, The Netherlands

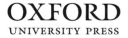

OXFORD
UNIVERSITY PRESS

OXFORD
UNIVERSITY PRESS

Great Clarendon Street, Oxford OX2 6DP

Oxford University Press is a department of the University of Oxford.
It furthers the University's objective of excellence in research, scholarship,
and education by publishing worldwide in

Oxford New York

Auckland Cape Town Dar es Salaam Hong Kong Karachi
Kuala Lumpur Madrid Melbourne Mexico City Nairobi
New Delhi Shanghai Taipei Toronto

With offices in

Argentina Austria Brazil Chile Czech Republic France Greece
Guatemala Hungary Italy Japan Poland Portugal Singapore
South Korea Switzerland Thailand Turkey Ukraine Vietnam

Oxford is a registered trade mark of Oxford University Press
in the UK and in certain other countries

Published in the United States
by Oxford University Press Inc., New York

© Oxford University Press 2007

The moral rights of the authors have been asserted

Database right Oxford University Press (maker)

First published 2007

British Library Cataloguing in Publication Data
Data available

Library of Congress Cataloging-in-Publication Data
Data available

Typeset by Cepha Imaging Private Ltd., Bangalore, India
Printed in Spain
on acid-free paper by
Cayfosa Quebecor, Barcelona, Spain

ISBN 978–0–19–856629–8

10 9 8 7 6 5 4 3 2 1

Whilst every effort has been made to ensure that the contents of this book are as
complete, accurate and up-to-date as possible at the date of writing, Oxford University
Press is not able to give any guarantee or assurance that such is the case. Readers are
urged to take appropriately qualified medical advice in all cases. The information in this
book is intended to be useful to the general reader, but should not be used as a means of
self-diagnosis or for the prescription of medication.

Contents

Contributors *vii*

Preface *ix*

1 An introduction to clinical functional magnetic resonance imaging of the brain *1*

2 Preoperative assessment: motor function *39*

3 Preoperative assessment: language *71*

4 Ageing: age-related changes in episodic and working memory *115*

5 Dementia: mild cognitive impairment and Alzheimer's disease *149*

6 Dementia: visualizing the metabolic changes of early Alzheimer's disease *173*

7 Schizophrenia *185*

8 Depression and anxiety disorders *209*

9 Stroke *265*

10 Parkinson's disease *285*

11 Multiple sclerosis *311*

12 fMRI and pharmacology: what role in clinical practice? *343*

Index *381*

Contributors

Edward T. Bullmore
Brain Mapping Unit, Department of
Psychiatry, University of Cambridge,
Cambridge, UK

Roberto Cabeza
Department of Psychology and
Neuroscience,
Center for Cognitive Neuroscience,
Duke University, Durham, NC, USA

Steven C. Cramer
Departments of Neurology and Anatomy
and Neurobiology, University of
California, Irvine, CA, USA

Sander Daselaar
Psychological and Brain Sciences,
Center for Cognitive Neuroscience,
Duke University, Durham, NC, USA

Nancy Dennis
Department of Psychology and
Neuroscience,
Center for Cognitive Neuroscience,
Duke University, Durham, NC, USA

Bradford C. Dickerson
Department of Neurology and
the Athinoula A. Martinos Center for
Biomedical Imaging, Massachusetts
General Hospital; Memory Disorders Unit,
Division of Cognitive and Behavioral
Neurology, Department of Neurology,
Brigham & Women's Hospital;
Department of Neurology, Harvard
Medical School, Boston MA, USA

Thomas Eckert
Center for Neurosciences, North Shore;
LIJ Research Institute, New York
University School of Medicine,
Manhasset, NY, USA

David Eidelberg
Center for Neurosciences, North Shore;
LIJ Research Institute, New York
University School of Medicine,
Manhasset, NY, USA

Gunther Fesl
Department of Neuroradiology,
University of Munich,
Munich, Germany

Massimo Filippi
Neuroimaging Research Unit,
Department of Neurology, Scientific
Institute and University Ospedale
San Raffaele, Milan, Italy

Garry D. Honey
Brain Mapping Unit, Department of
Psychiatry, University of Cambridge,
Cambridge, UK

René S. Kahn
Rudolf Magnus Institute of
Neuroscience;
University Medical Center Utrecht,
Division of Neuroscience,
Department of Psychiatry,
Utrecht, The Netherlands

Nick F. Ramsey
Rudolf Magnus Institute of
Neuroscience;
University Medical Center Utrecht,
Division of Neuroscience,
Department of Psychiatry
Utrecht, The Netherlands

Maria A. Rocca
Neuroimaging Research Unit,
Department of Neurology, Scientific
Institute and University Ospedale
San Raffaele, Milan, Italy

Franck–Emmanuel Roux
Institut National de la Santé et de la
Recherche Médicale, Unité 455;
Federation de Neurochirurgie,
Centres Hospitalo-Universitaires,
Toulouse, France

Geert–Jan Rutten
Department of Neurosurgery,
University Medical Center Utrecht,
Utrecht, The Netherlands

Scott A. Small
Taub Institute for Research on Alzheimer's
Disease and the Aging Brain, New York;
Department of Neurology and
Department of Pathology, Center for
Neurobiology and Behavior, Columbia
University College of Physicians and
Surgeons, New York, NY, USA

Reisa A. Sperling
Department of Neurology and the
Athinoula A. Martinos Center for
Biomedical Imaging, Massachusetts
General Hospital; Memory Disorders
Unit, Division of Cognitive and
Behavioral Neurology, Department
of Neurology, Brigham & Women's
Hospital; Department of Neurology,
Harvard Medical School,
Boston MA, USA

Stefan Sunaert
Department of Radiology, University
Hospital of the Catholic University of
Leuven, Leuven, Belgium

Bejoy Thomas
Department of Radiology, Sree Chitra
Tirunal Institute for Medical Sciences and
Technology, Trivandrum, Kerala, India

Dick J. Veltman
Department of Psychiatry,
VU University Medical Center and
UvA Academic Medical Center,
Amsterdam, The Netherlands

William Wu
Taub Institute for Research on Alzheimer's
Disease and the Aging Brain, New York;
Department of Neurology and
Department of Pathology, Center for
Neurobiology and Behavior,
Columbia University College of Physicians
and Surgeons, New York, NY, USA

Tarek A. Yousry
Institute of Neurology, Queen Square,
London, UK

Dennis Zgaljardic
Center for Neurosciences, North Shore;
LIJ Research Institute, New York
University School of Medicine,
Manhasset, NY, USA

Preface

In less than 15 years, MRI has matured rapidly as a tool for studying brain function. In particular, the fast development of methods for data acquisition, paradigm design, and data analysis techniques of blood oxygenation level dependent (BOLD) functional MRI (FMRI) have enabled a multidisciplinary community of researchers to study normal brain function. In just a few years, FMRI has become the most widely used method for imaging brain function, leading to impressive accomplishments in the studies of normal brain function.

Developments in the use of FMRI in clinically related research have been slower. Yet FMRI has, by now, also become a valuable tool in the study of many neurological and psychiatric disorders. The motivation for starting this book came from the notion that FMRI is increasingly being applied clinically, yet no overview as to its ability and potential had seen the light. Our goal, therefore, was to provide an overview of the current status of clinically related FMRI research of a selection of neurological and psychiatric disorders.

Each of Chapters 2–11 covers a specific disorder, with the exception of Chapter 4, which deals with normal ageing. The reason for including ageing is that it has been widely studied with FMRI, and understanding ageing and brain function is very important in relation to studies of disorders in elderly populations, such as dementia. These chapters are preceded by a general introduction to clinical FMRI in Chapter 1, and followed by Chapter 12 on pharmacological FMRI (phMRI). This is a method to study the effects of medication on brain function, which can be applied in a variety of diseases.

This book is not meant to explain brain physiology, offer understanding of the physics of MRI, or to provide an introduction on how to set up an FMRI study. Instead, it is meant to explain the status of current clinical applications and, especially, clinically oriented research using FMRI in preoperative evaluation, diagnosis, and discrimination of pathology and understanding recovery, therapeutics, and rehabilitation. The target audience is of a multidisciplinary nature: both the novice FMRI researcher and the expert FMRI scientist with an interest in clinical FMRI, as well as clinicians.

This book does not offer a complete description of clinical FMRI of all disorders studied with FMRI. The choice of topics was dictated by the potential and expected impact of FMRI as related to a particular disease and whether the accomplishments, so far, were significant enough to justify a chapter in this book.

The reader will also note that clinical FMRI has developed further in some diseases than in others. The speed with which these developments occur depends on the amount of attention a disease has received in the field of functional brain imaging, as well as on the specific, sometimes unique, difficulties that some studies of a particular disorder are facing.

We are extremely fortunate that all chapters have been written by colleagues who are all leading researchers around the globe in their respective fields of expertise. Our utmost gratitude goes to these contributors. We also thank Oxford University Press for their help and patience.

Serge Rombouts   *Amsterdam, October 2007*
Frederik Barkhof
Philip Scheltens

An introduction to clinical functional magnetic resonance imaging of the brain

Stefan Sunaert and Bejoy Thomas

1. Introduction

The first papers on functional magnetic resonance imaging (FMRI) were published just fifteen years ago, and in the relative short time since, FMRI has assumed a major role in mapping human brain functions. A search of the term "FMRI" in the medline database reveals that more than 5000 peer reviewed original articles have been produced world-wide, a number which has increased exponentially, since last year alone more than one FMRI article a day was published. Almost nine out of ten publications cover either technical aspects of FMRI or the neurophysiological research concerned with the function of the human brain in normal subjects. The latter field is undergoing an explosive growth due to several distinctly advantageous characteristics of FMRI. These include total non-invasiveness, relatively high spatial and temporal resolution, and the ease of imaging the underlying anatomy. In addition, state-of-the-art whole brain FMRI can now be performed on almost all recently installed clinical MR scanners, and online analysis tools allow the visualization of neuronal activity at the level of the single subject (or patient) in real time. The non-invasive character means that subjects can be studied repeatedly, without harm, allowing for longitudinal studies. These benefits have thus led to a considerable growth of neurophysiological data of the human brain — normal and pathological.

The development of applications of FMRI for diagnostic and therapeutic purposes in patients with neurological, neurosurgical, or psychiatric diseases forms about ten per cent of the total number of publications since the beginning of the FMRI era, and this field is growing almost as fast as that of 'neurophysiological FMRI'. This (at first view) limited share of clinical FMRI is actually a tremendous achievement, considering the fact that clinical FMRI is much more difficult to perform than non-clinical FMRI. The reasons for this are multiple and pertain to all aspects of functional imaging. First, at the design stage of a FMRI experiment, compared to the paradigms or stimuli employed in the neurophysiological study of volunteers, those that will be used to elucidate neuronal activity in patients will have to be adapted to their pathology. Second, at the stage of acquiring the functional scans, acquisition time will often be much more limited than in young healthy volunteers. Third, the post-processing of the FMRI data will often have to be altered or improved due to the presence of 'unexpected' signals from the brain abnormalities that may be present. The results that are obtained from functional mapping experiments in patients are often more difficult to understand and, most importantly, will have to be validated by comparison with the present gold-standard techniques, such as intra-operative recordings. Nonetheless, a vast body of present clinically valuable studies, as well as pre-liminary work on potential future clinical applications has been published.

This chapter will introduce the reader of this book to the different aspects of clinical FMRI. The blood oxygen level dependent (BOLD) contrast that forms the basis of FMRI will be introduced, as well as the possible alterations of this contrast in pathological conditions. Second, the specific challenges of FMRI experiments intended at visualizing activity in patients, at the design, scanning, and post-processing stages, will be discussed. Next, a brief overview of clinical applications will be given. And, last but not least, the future directions of clinical FMRI, such as the combined use of FMRI and diffusion tensor imaging, will be addressed.

2. FMRI basics: principles of the blood oxygen level dependent (BOLD) contrast

2.1 Brain activation and cerebrovascular physiology: neurovascular (un)coupling

Activation of a brain area (Fig. 1.1) produces an increase in the metabolism of its neuronal and glial cell populations, accompanied by an increase in blood flow (rCBF) and blood vol-ume (rCBV) in that area. This coupling between rCBF, rCBV, and neuronal metabolism has been under investigation ever since Roy and Sherrington introduced the concept of neu-rovascular coupling in 1890 (for a review, see[1]). The fact that rCBF varies with local neu-ronal activity has allowed the study of brain function in vivo, via the measurement of rCBF by PET and SPECT techniques. The function of this activation-dependent coupling seems logical: it has to maintain an adequate supply of oxygen and glucose to the brain for vary-ing levels of neuronal metabolism. The reality, however, is more complicated than this. The amount of supplied oxygen does not seem to follow the actual consumption. As expected, the oxygen level of the blood initially slightly drops during the first second(s) of brain acti-vation (the 'early response'), indicating an increase in cerebral metabolic rate of oxygen (CMR_{O2}). However, this event is followed by a huge increase in the oxygen concentration (the 'late' response) since the increase in blood flow overcompensates the metabolic demand for oxygen (Fig. 1c). An uncoupling between rCBF and oxidative metabolism thus takes place and leads to a local increase of blood oxygenation during brain activation. This late response reaches its maximum 3 to 9 seconds after onset of the neuronal activation. Researches have found that the 'early response' corresponds to the neuronal activity both temporally and spatially, but it is more difficult to measure in clinical settings[2].

2.2 Blood oxygen level dependent (BOLD) image contrast

The described neurovascular (un)coupling between brain activation and cerebrovascular physiology leads to three effects that can contribute to the FMRI signal: an increase in the blood flow velocity, an increase in the blood flow volume, and an increase in the blood

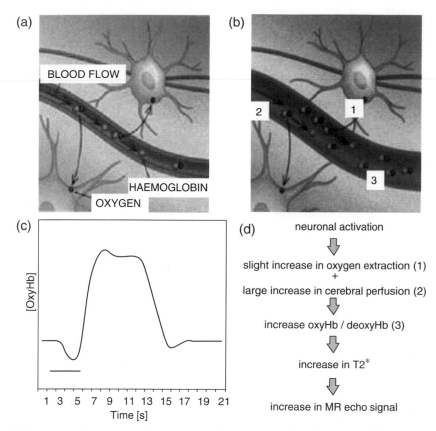

Fig. 1.1 Brain activation and cerebrovascular (un)coupling: (**a**) situation at rest; (**b**) during neuronal activation; (**c**) time course of the change of oxyhaemoglobin concentration upon regional neuronal activation (during horizontal bar); (**d**) sequence of cerebrovascular changes leading to increased T2* and MR signal.

oxygenation level. Using carefully chosen MR imaging parameters, the contribution of blood flow velocity and blood flow volume can be minimized, while maximizing the blood oxygenation dependency of the FMRI signal. The FMRI contrast thus obtained was therefore called 'blood oxygenation level dependent (BOLD) contrast'.

The first MR images which were sensitive to the level of blood oxygenation were presented by Ogawa and coworkers[3]. Dark lines, coinciding with blood vessels, could be seen in gradient-echo images of anoxic rat brain, but not when the rat was breathing 100% oxygen. Initial FMRI experiments[4–6] confirmed the possibility of mapping brain function following sensory stimulation. The BOLD imaging contrast finds its basis in the observation of Thulborn *et al.*[7] who observed that the transverse relaxation time of water protons in the blood provides information about the oxygenation state of the blood. The magnetic state of the iron contained in the oxygen-carrying molecule haemoglobin (Hb) is dependent on the amount of oxygen that is present in Hb: it is paramagnetic when Hb is depleted of oxygen (deoxyhaemoglobin), while it is diamagnetic when the Hb molecule is saturated (oxyhaemoglobin). Therefore, susceptibility weighted sequences — T2*w images — are very suited to measure the change in BOLD contrast upon neuronal activation.

The most widely used FMRI scan technique is ultrafast echo-planar imaging (EPI)[8]. This technically challenging method makes it possible to form a single slice MR image in as little as 70 to 100 ms. Multiple adjacent slices (e.g. 30 slices) are acquired covering the complete brain in about 2000 to 3000 ms.

In summary, increase in neuronal activity leads to an increase in oxyHb concentration (i.e. a decrease in local susceptibility) that results mainly in an increase of the MR echo signal of the active brain tissue (see Fig. 1.1).

3. Challenges for clinical use of FMRI

FMRI, even in normal subjects, suffers from a number of physiological, methodological, and technical problems and pitfalls, that become even more important when FMRI is used for diagnosis and treatment in a clinical setting. The physiological BOLD contrast can be altered by the presence of brain pathology. Methodologically, the design of reliable and standardized FMRI paradigms is of utmost importance in clinical FMRI. Also, claustrophobia and patient non-cooperation, especially in more difficult tasks such as cognitive or language task, hinder the use of FMRI in severely ill patients. Finally, technical issues, such as gross head movement and interpretation of the statistical results of the FMRI data are factors to be dealt with. These factors will now be discussed below.

3.1 Physiological challenge: limitations of BOLD FMRI in patients with brain pathology

While the neurovascular (un)coupling is a physiological phenomenon reliably found in normal young volunteers, in a clinical setting, dealing with an altered vascular system in elderly patients and/or pathology of the brain, the BOLD signal can often be disturbed leading to false negative FMRI activations.

Accumulating evidence seems to indicate that the BOLD response in the vicinity of certain tumours does not reflect the electrical neuronal activity as accurately as it does in healthy brain tissue[9–12]. Recent data indicate that cortical BOLD activation can be reduced near glial tumours, both at the edge of the tumour and in normal vascular territories somewhat removed from the tumour[12]. Loss of regional cerebral vasoactivity near these tumours has been suggested to be a contributing factor[9,12]. At the interface of tumours and normal brain, astrocytes and macrophages can release nitric oxide that can regionally increase CBF and decrease the oxygen extraction fraction[13], which may also decrease BOLD signal intensity differences[12]. Tumour-induced changes in regional tissue pH and glucose, lactate, and adenosine triphosphate levels have been documented[14,15], although such effects on BOLD neuronal coupling are not clear. Glial tumours can induce abnormal vessel proliferation in adjacent brain, altering regional CBF, CBV, vasoactivity, and potentially, BOLD contrast.

Other factors, including vasogenic oedema and tumoural haemorrhage, could contribute to the observed decrease in near-lesion BOLD contrast. Despite the theoretical consequences of vasogenic oedema induced dilutional and tissue pressure changes on neurovascular coupling, evidence for a substantial impact on BOLD contrast is lacking in a small number of patients studied. The true impact of vasogenic oedema awaits further investigation in larger patient populations with a range of tumour types. Microhaemorrhages associated with intraparenchymal tumours could hinder the detection of changing susceptibility gradients that provide BOLD contrast, but confirmation of this effect requires verification with histological correlation. Metabolic changes in some brain tumors could induce, for example, tissue pH changes, which may again eliminate the physiological haemodynamic response[16,17]. Finally, also, alterations of microvascular architecture are prone to exist in the neighbourhood of vascular malformations (vascular steal effects).

It is of utmost importance to realize that an absence of FMRI activity in a particular brain region *does NOT mean* that electrical activity within this area is non-existent and, thus, that it is safe to surgically remove this region. We will demonstrate this important point using the following case report, illustrated in Fig. 1.2 — FMRI activity during bilateral finger-tapping versus rest in a patient with a Rolandic tumour (glioma grade 2 within the postcentral gyrus but extending within the 'hand knob' of the pre-central gyrus). In the non-lesioned right hemisphere FMRI activity is observed within the right sensori-motor cortex (SM1; pre- and postcentral gyri), the right premotor cortex (PM), and right parietal cortex (PP). In contrast, in the lesioned left hemisphere, activation is only observed anterior from the tumour in the left premotor cortex (PM). While this FMRI activation map might be interpreted as an absence of electrical neuronal activity within the left SM1 and PP areas (e.g. due to plastic changes and take-over of motor function within the ipsilateral non-lesioned hemisphere), the time traces of the MR signal changes clearly show that this is a false conclusion. Within the left, tumour-invaded hand representation in SM1, the MR signal decreases during performance of the motor task and increases during the rest baseline condition (i.e. the *inverse* BOLD MR signal change than the one expected in normal volunteers). This phenomenon can be explained as a complete lesion-induced neurovascular uncoupling, where oxygen extraction (cause of the initial dip of the BOLD signal) occurs without increase in rCBF and rCBV, resulting in a steady decrease of MR signal during the increased electrical neuronal activity.

To our knowledge, the existence and prevalence of these artifacts is only anecdotal, and still not well studied. As pointed out in an editorial by Bryan and Kraut (1998)[18], these 'negative results' deserve further study.

Finally, it is also important to realize that the BOLD signal can also be influenced by various pharmacological agents. There are indications that antihistaminics reduce the BOLD response; caffeine is a known booster of the BOLD response[19]. It is likely that many more pharmacological agents influence the BOLD response and patients harbouring brain tumours may receive such medication.

3.2 Physiological challenge: brain or vein?

Several authors have raised the concern that FMRI examinations at field strength of 1.5 T images predominately large, draining veins. Although only 3–5% of the water molecules in the gray matter are in the vascular space, the contribution of the intravascular component to the BOLD signal can be substantial, of the order of up to 60% at 1.5 T MRI[20, 21].

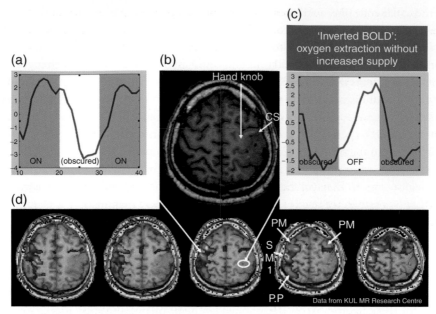

Fig. 1.2 FMRI activity during bilateral finger tapping versus rest in a patient with a Rolandic tumour (glioma gd 2 within the postcentral gyrus but extending within the 'hand knob' of the pre-central gyrus) **(b and d)**. In the non-lesioned right hemisphere, FMRI activity is observed within the right sensorimotor cortex (SM1; pre- and postcentral gyri), the right premotor cortex (PM), and right parietal cortex (PP) **(d)**. In contrast, in the lesioned left hemisphere, activation is only observed anterior from the tumour in the left premotor cortex (PM) **(d)**. While this FMRI activation map might be interpreted as an absence of electrical neuronal activity within the left SM1 and PP areas (e.g. due to plastic changes and take-over of motor function within the ipsilateral non-lesioned hemisphere), the time traces of the MR signal changes clearly show that this is a false conclusion **(a and c)**. Within the left, tumour-invaded hand representation in SM1 **(c)**, the MR signal decreases during performance of the motor task and increases during the rest baseline condition (i.e. the inverse BOLD MR signal change than the one expected in normal volunteers). This phenomenon can be explained as a lesion-induced neurovascular uncoupling, where oxygen extraction occurs without increase in rCBF and rCBV, resulting in a steady decrease of MR signal during the increased electrical neuronal activity.

This can lead to false localization and BOLD signal can be detected in large draining veins, which may be away from the site of neuronal activity. Implementation of imaging parameters confining the FMRI signal toward the site of neuronal activity should be a prerequisite for conducting clinical FMRI examinations. Gao and coworkers[22] have shown that FMR images weighted toward the microcirculation may be obtained at 1.5 T if the pulse sequence is designed for minimizing inflow effects and maximizing BOLD contribution. This can be achieved by acquiring multi-slice, long TR, single-shot, echo-planar images. Use of a higher main magnetic field strength (e.g. 3 T) will also decrease the effect of the draining veins and improve spatial localization, but has the drawback of increased image distortion, a factor decreasing spatial accuracy.

The spatial accuracy of FMRI can be assessed by comparing FMRI activations with gold-standard models, such as intra-cortical stimulation. Such a recent comparison, using the optimal FMRI techniques, revealed that the spatial uncertainty from this drain-ing vein effect was estimated to be no larger than 10 mm[23]. Studies comparing other mapping techniques like magneto-encephalography (MEG) to FMRI have also been performed[24]. Distances between the centres of the MEG and FMRI activation regions were measured and consistent differences (of the order of 10mm) were identified. For example, localization of the primary motor cortex from the FMRI data was consistently more posterior than for the MEG localization. For somatosensory responses, the local-ization of the FMRI activation was inferior and lateral to that of the MEG. Thus, while the MEG dipole and the BOLD FMRI response maximum are in similar regions, the dif-ferent physiological responses are slightly displaced. Consideration of the possible causes for these localization discrepancies is informative. Fundamentally different information is provided by the two techniques, not just with respect to the basis of signal change but also to the time period over which the response is averaged. The MEG 'window' is short (tens of milliseconds). In contrast, the FMRI response is averaged over a much broader time period (seconds). The FMRI response may, therefore, reflect contributions from more than a single electrophysiologically defined dipole in the region of interest.

3.3 Methodological challenge: clinical FMRI acquisition and stimulation paradigms

In order to visualize brain activity reliably in response to sensory, motor, and cognitive tasks, appropriate FMRI paradigms should be developed based on neuropsychological principles.

Obtaining normative FMRI data in healthy subjects is a first step in the development of clinically useful paradigms. However, paradigms need to be adopted for the patient population (e.g. it makes no sense to ask a hemi-paretic patient to perform a motor task with the paretic limbs). Parameters, such as task difficulty and duration of scanning, that are most suitable for clinical populations but without sacrificing image integrity, need to be determined. Certain tasks may require practice outside the scanner to ensure the patient's understanding of what is required of them and the task itself.

Two types of stimulation paradigms are routinely used in research and clinical FRMI: blocked and event-related paradigms (Fig. 1.3). In the historically oldest, blocked FMRI experiment, two or more cognitive or sensorimotor tasks (conditions) are alternated in 'blocks', each block typically lasting 20 to 40 seconds. The advantage of blocked FMRI paradigms is the simplicity of design, relative ease for the subject to comply with the tasks, and straightforwardness of statistical post-processing. These advantages have led to a widespread use of blocked FMRI design in clinical settings. The most commonly mapped functions using blocked designs include sensory functions such as auditory, tac-tile, and visual perception; motor function; and, last but not least, language comprehen-sion and production. Primary motor cortex can easily be identified by alternating blocks of movement with rest[25–33]. However, in patients with mild to severe motor paresis, or in the case of paralysis, indirect localization of the primary motor cortex can be obtained through pure sensory mapping of the adjacent primary sensory cortex by rubbing, stroking, or brushing the body part under investigation (see[28, 34] and Fig. 1.4).

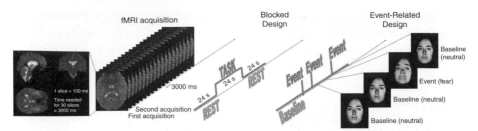

Fig. 1.3 Schematic representation of blocked and event-related FMRI design. In this example, the FMRI acquisition consists of a stack of 30 gradient-echo echo-planar-imaging slices which are acquired every 3000 ms. In a blocked FMRI design, two (or more) tasks are alternated every eight acquisitions (i.e. in blocks of 24 seconds). In an event-related design, events (e.g. faces with fearful expression) are pseudo-randomly presented on a baseline (e.g. faces with neutral expression).

For the mapping of the primary and secondary auditory cortices, different kinds of auditory stimuli can be used, as long as the interference of the MR gradient generated noise is dealt with (for a review on this topic see[35]). Language can be mapped using comprehension and expression tasks (Fig. 1.5). For depicting language expression, word generation tasks involving Broca proper (pars triangularis and opercularis of the inferior frontal gyrus) and other expressive language areas within the middle and superior frontal gyri[28, 36, 37] are used. Most of the time, patients are instructed to perform covert language production tasks, as words spoken aloud would induce artifactual gross head movements. These word generation tasks include picture naming, verbal fluency,

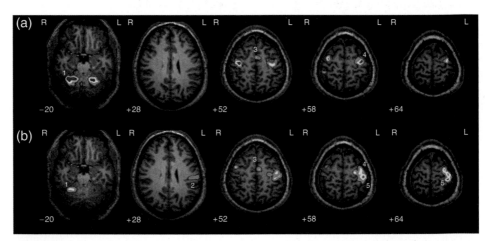

Fig. 1.4 Comparison of bilateral finger tapping (**a**) and left hand brushing (**b**) in a normal volunteer. Bilateral finger tapping activates primary motor cortex (M1, label = 4), supplementary motor area (SMA, label = 3), and cerebellum (label = 1). In comparison, left hand brushing activates mainly the primary sensory cortex (S1, label = 5) but also — due to afferent input — M1 (laber = 4), SMA (label = 3), and cerebellum (label = 1); an additional site of activation corresponds to the secondary sensory cortex (S2, label = 2).

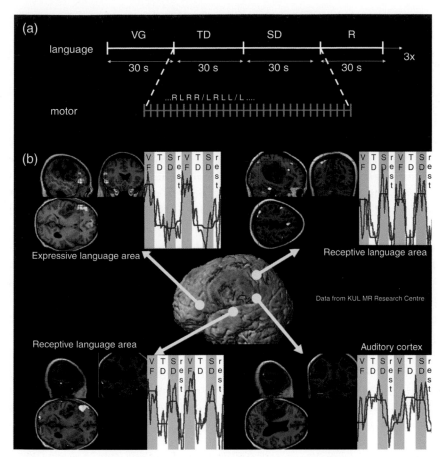

Fig. 1.5 (a) Language paradigm consisting of a covert verb-to-noun generation (VG; e.g. auditorily presented noun 'car' and patient covertly responds 'drive'), tone discrimination (TD; discrimination of tone pitch), semantic discrimination (SD; e.g. patient makes distinction between objects and animals), and rest (R). (b) Right-handed patient with a very large fronto-parieto-temporal tumour in the left hemisphere. The mass effect of the lesion effaces typical anatomical landmarks. The change in MR signal in response to the different tasks compared to rest is used to identify the nodes of the language network: in the auditory cortex the response is the highest during the execution of the TD task; in the receptive language areas, the activity is the highest during the SD task; in the left inferior frontal region, MR signal only increases during the execution of the covert verb-to-noun generation task, thus this area corresponds to the classical Broca's expressive language area. Note the lateralization of Broca's area to the left hemisphere in this right-handed patient.

and verb-to-noun generation. Wernicke's area can be mapped by tasks requiring language comprehension[25, 27]. Most commonly, semantic judgement tasks are used to that purpose. If these tasks are too difficult for the severely ill (cognitively slowed down patients), listening to spoken language or reading written language may be a (less optimal) alternative.

However, in some circumstances the use of blocked designs is less appropriate. If neurophysiological processes suffer from predictability of or habituation to the stimuli, an event-related design is warranted (see Fig. 1.3). Paradigms intended for visualization of emotional processing in the brain are such paradigms. For example, repeated presentations of a set of fearful stimuli during a block of 20 to 40 seconds will not constantly engage the limbic system; there might be a brief response to the first presentation of the fearful stimulus, but subsequent stimuli will induce much less, even no activity, due to the predictability of this design. Conversely, randomized non-predictable single presentations of a fearful stimulus on a baseline of neutral stimuli will reproducibly elicit a brief but strong neuronal response in the limbic system. Thus, in event-related designs, one or more stimuli of interest (e.g. fear-, sad-, and disgust-inducing stimuli) will be (pseudo)randomly presented on a baseline (e.g. neutral stimuli) (see Fig. 1.3). The disadvantages of event-related designs are their relative complexity in set-up and analysis and their slightly decreased statistical power compared to blocked designs.

Nonetheless, event-related designs have entered the clinical setting since disturbance in emotional processing has become of interest recently in diseases such as depression, obsessive compulsive disorder, and phobia. Other examples are the hippocampal function during memory processes in dementia, or even brain processes related to moral aspects (e.g. in kleptomania or pathological lying). An example of an event-related paradigm attempting to study lying can be seen in Fig. 1.6. Subjects had to choose one of five envelopes containing a playing card and to memorize the drawn card. Subsequently, during scanning, they were shown different playing cards and asked question 'do you have this card?'. In order to receive a reward of 15 Euro, they had to answer this question in such a way as to conceal the card they had previously drawn. The activity during (simulated) lying was present in several limbic system structures and frontal cortex. Follow-up experiments are now being undertaken in pathological conditions such as compulsive lying and kleptomania.

Given the vast amount of clinical applications (see below), consensus about the best FMRI paradigms for a given disease do not yet exist. The challenge is to find reliable paradigms both for diagnosis and treatment. One has to keep in mind the (dis)advantages of blocked or event-related designs when designing a clinical experiment. Most importantly, obtaining normative FMRI data in healthy subjects is a first step in the development of clinically useful paradigms.

3.4 Methodological challenge: disentangling expendable versus essential brain regions

Most stimulation paradigms used in clinical FMRI studies elicit activity in a widespread cortical network. For example, a relatively simple motor task such as finger tapping, activates the premotor cortex and the supplementary motor area in addition to the primary sensorimotor cortex. Disentangling primary motor cortex activations from the other activations is highly significant clinically because it has been shown that cortical resection involving the premotor cortex and the supplementary motor area rarely produces major permanent functional deficit, whereas resection of the primary motor cortex does. The challenges for future FMRI studies is to develop stimulation paradigms that differentiate

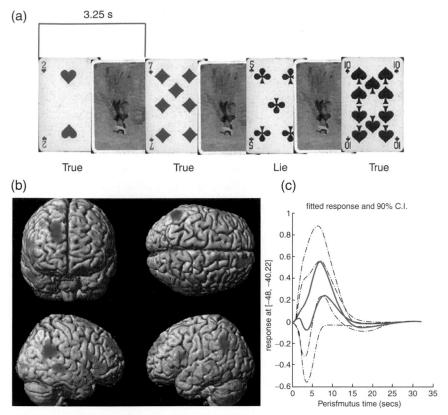

Fig. 1.6 Event-related design of a simulated deception experiment. (**a**) Subject has to conceal the playing card 'five of clubs' which he has previously drawn out of a stack of five playing cards, in order to receive a reward of 15 Euro. During FMRI scanning, different playing cards are visually presented on a screen every 3.5 s and the subject answers truthfully 'no' to the question 'do you have this card?', except for the 'five of clubs', where the subject's 'no' answer now is a lie. (**b**) Areas of increased brain activity during the 'lie' events compared to the 'true' events. (**c**) Time course of the hemodynamic response in such a brain area. Note the increased response when 'lying' as compared to the 'true' event.

between surgically expendable and non-expendable cortical areas. Combinations of FMRI with other techniques such as intra-cortical stimulation and transcranial magnetic stimulation might also help to reach this goal (see below).

3.5 Technical challenge: post-processing of FMRI datasets

The detailed description of post-processing of FMRI falls outside the scope of this chapter and is discussed in detail elsewhere (for one review, see[38]). Briefly, the processing of functional MR brain images involves a number of steps which include correction techniques for bulk head motion, spatial normalization to a standard brain, spatial smoothing, statistical techniques for the reliable separation of the relevant FMRI signal change from the noise, and visualization techniques for localizing activation foci on the anatomy of individual subjects.

However, certain aspects of post-processing are especially important when dealing with patients in a clinical setting, notably artifactual signal induced by head motion, statistical thresholds, and real-time FMRI analysis on the MR scanner console. These will be discussed below.

3.5.1 The effect of bulk head motion

The small intensity changes typically observed in FMRI images (ranging from a fraction of a per cent signal change to a few per cents) can be easily contaminated by a variety of sources. In clinical FMRI, the major contribution to signal artefacts comes from bulk head motion during the functional data series. Another minor contribution comes from physiological brain motion (pulsation of the brain, overlying vessels, and cerebrospinal fluid) driven by the cardiac pulsations[39]. Thus, the primary reason for most failed clinical FMRI examinations is motion. In the study of Krings *et al.* (2001), the most frequent cause for the failure of their clinical exams (15 per cent of their studies) was the presence of head movement artefacts[40].

The motion occurring during an FMRI time series acquisition can be divided into two categories: intra-image motion, which is generally a very fast and sudden motion (i.e. at a time scale smaller than the image acquisition time scale) and inter-image motion, on a time scale between a couple of seconds and minutes, which is a slow movement of the subject (i.e. at a time scale larger than the time necessary to acquire a single image volume). These two subcategories of motion have quite different effects on the acquired image and functional map properties. Intra-image motion, which is typically induced by sudden head movement, results in blurring and ghosting in the older GE-based acquisition sequences, and is less present in the single shot echo-planar imaging in which all data for an image are collected in under 100 ms. But this sudden motion, if very fast, can still result in ghosting artefacts in several slices of the acquired volumes on the resulting EPI images. Slower, longer-lasting motion can also change the contrast in the images. This is especially true if the motion occurs perpendicular to the acquisition plane. Through plane head motion will result in a change of apparent repetition time for the acquisition of the same slice in the different volumes (see Fig. 1.7), which changes the T1 weightings of the tissue for the different slices, thus changing the signal intensity. In other words, the tissue has experienced a different 'spin history'[41].

Motion on a time temporal scale larger than the image acquisition, leads to misregistration of the images within the time series, and makes activation foci undetectable or, even worse, induces artefactual activation, when it is temporally correlated to the stimulus[42]. This will especially have an effect in those regions in the brain that show steep image intensity gradients (e.g. at the edges of the brain or in patients at the border of a T2 hyperintense lesion) which are very prone to these artefacts (Figs. 1.8 and 1.10). The effect of inter-image motion has been shown to be particularly problematic in clinical examinations. Results from Hill *et al.* (2000) indicate that head motion occurred with a greater magnitude in a group of epilepsy patients than in a group of healthy volunteers who underwent the same examination[43].

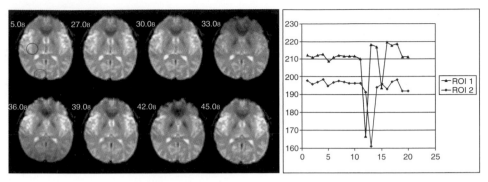

Fig. 1.7 Time series of a volunteer performing a through plane head motion. The time trace shown on the right displays a resulting large signal drop.

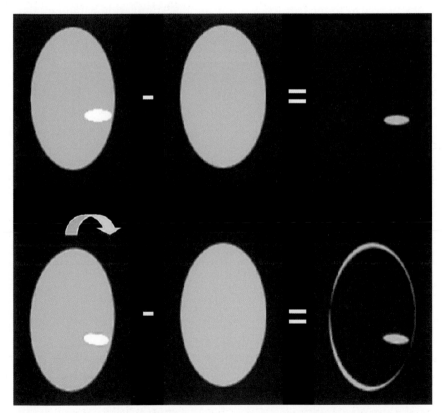

Fig. 1.8 Simulation of the effect of motion between different states of activation on the observed activation. In the situation depicted in the top row, where there is no bulk head motion, the subtraction of the baseline image from the 'activated' image results in the true activation. Conversely, on the bottom row, where the patient slightly rotates the head in the 'activated' image compared to the baseline image, the subtraction of these two images results in the true activated area plus a rim of false activity at the edge of the brain.

3.5.2 Minimizing the effect of bulk head motion in clinical FMRI examinations

Several solutions to correct or minimize this inter-image motion have been proposed by a number of groups. Head movement during the acquisition phase can be restricted by fixation of the head with molds and straps[44, 45] — an intermediate level of head fixation. The use of a 'bite-bar' (a custom molded dental fixation, regularly used in our institution to restrain head motion while imaging volunteers) provides a highly rigid fixation (Fig. 1.9) but can only be used in a limited number of patient studies. The presence of dental prostheses interferes and not all patients can tolerate this kind of fixation. Furthermore, safety precautions preclude its use in those patients who are at risk of having a epileptic seizure during imaging.

Another solution is the use of a posteriori correction of head movement algorithm. Nowadays, integration of such algorithms into the different FMRI analysis packages is standard. The motion correction is achieved by rigid realignment of the consecutively acquired images in the data series with the first image[41, 46–48]. If the patient moved with a frequency unrelated to the frequency of the applied stimulation paradigm, then this realignment post-processing can successfully separate this motion from true activation (Fig. 1.10). As most motion correction algorithms are intensity based, it is also possible that a false motion could be observed in the time series which is actually the result of a large activation at a specific brain region shifting the centre of intensity in a certain direction following the activation paradigm[49].

Most patient motion will be correlated with the applied stimulus[50]. This is certainly true for the different motor paradigms. So, the effect of a patient moving his head at the

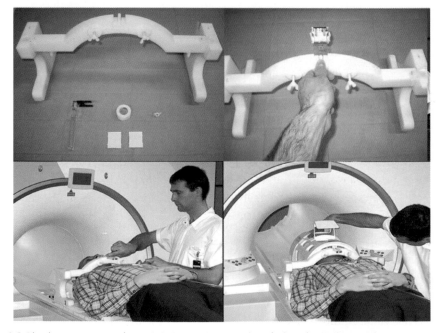

Fig. 1.9 Bite-bar system used to minimize patient motion during the FMRI experiment.

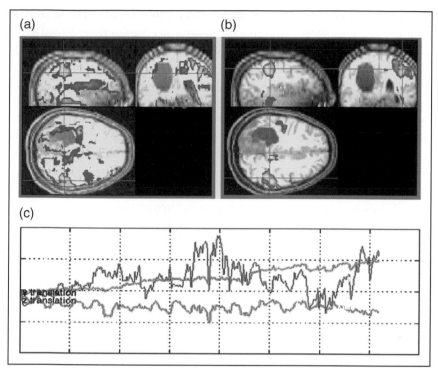

Fig. 1.10 Functional data corrugated with bulk head motion which results in false detection of neuronal activity (**a**). Same data after realignment (**b**). The realignment consisted of an affine coregistration with three rotations (not shown) and three translations (**c**) of the consecutively acquired images in the time series.

start of the task cannot be easily separated from functional effects by their activation period[51]. Several new stimulation paradigms which induce less patient head motion are presently under study. Much attention is given to the differences in anatomico-functional information that can be obtained from active versus passive tasks.

As described earlier, the effect of trough plane motion is a combination of misregistration of the different subsequent BOLD images and the T1-slice effect changing the signal intensity resulting from the change in TR. Therefore, it would be better to adapt the scanning planes in such a way that the maximal observed motion would be in the acquisition plane (e.g. if one expects head nodding from left to right, axial slices should be acquired; if head motion is expected from front to back, acquisition of sagittal slices would minimize the through plane motion). Nowadays, there are also acquisition sequences which adapt to the position of the acquired EPI volume in order to match for the motion of the volunteer. Motion is calculated online and between two consecutive acquired volumes and this information is used to predict the position of the head in the third acquisition. Thus, this technique makes use of a prospective motion correction algorithm, in contrast to the retrospective motion correction techniques used in the analysis tools. As the scan planes are adapted to the motion, the T1 slice effect will also be diminished[52, 53].

If the motion effects still persist in the resulting BOLD activation maps, there is an option in most analysis tools to incorporate the motion parameters calculated in the preprocessing step in the general linear model. By doing so, the signal variability in the voxels, correlating with these motion parameters, will be described in this contrast, decreasing the motion effect in the other contrasts of interest of the stimulation paradigm. Although this will effectively remove motion-induced 'false' activations, it can also remove or decrease the real activation of the motion as correlated with the task. If it was not possible to eliminate the motion during the acquisition phase and the motion correction did not succeed in eliminating all motion (e.g. in the case of paradigm-related motion), there are still motion artefacts present in the results. Some tips to distinguish motion-induced 'false' activations from the real activation induced BOLD activation follow.

Most of the motion-induced false activations are localized at the borders of different structures between which a large signal intensity gradient is shown[54]. The motion-induced signal change typically has a 'ring-like' spatial appearance at these boundaries. In other words, they are observed as a thin rim of hyperactivation in the neighbourhood of large image intensity gradients.

The BOLD haemodynamic response curve typically increases 4 seconds after the onset of stimulation and reaches its maximum 6–8 seconds after stimulation onset. If the movement follows the paradigm, the onset of the movement will be at the same time as the onset of the paradigm. These movement-related signal changes will also follow instantaneously at the start of the movement. Therefore, the temporal profile of the movement-related false activations will be shifted forwards compared to the real activation BOLD temporal profile and coincide with the external profile. The signal intensity change will also be more abrupt compared to the more gradual activation induced BOLD signal intensity change. Movement-related signal changes will also generally display a much higher signal intensity change as compared to the BOLD signal change.

3.5.3 Towards standardized real-time statistical post-processing

Each FMRI experiment generates a huge amount of data, which needs to be analysed rigorously for the best results. Generation of functional activation maps in FMRI experiments requires independent statistical analysis at each of the 100,000 or more voxels of the brain. The basic idea of analysis of functional imaging data is to identify voxels that show signal changes that vary with the changes in the given cognitive or sensorimotor state of interest, across the time course of the experiment. This is quite a challenging problem as the functional MR signal changes are very small (of the order of 0.5 to 5%) and the noise is relatively high (of the same magnitude as the changes of interest), which leads to a high rate of both false negative (Type I) and false positive (Type II) errors. The hypothesis that is tested at each voxel is that there is no effect of the task compared to the baseline condition, and statistical analysis involves making a decision as to whether or not this null hypothesis is true or false. Various statistical tests can then be applied on a voxel by voxel basis, to test the significance of a particular voxel with increased signal associated with a certain brain state. The commonly used one is T statistics. Then, these T statistical maps are superimposed on high-resolution anatomical images to obtain clinically useful FMRI output.

A Type I error constitutes a false positive (i.e. the voxel shows a difference in activation during the task of interest when in reality it does not). A Type II error represents a false negative (i.e. no activation at that voxel when in reality there is). For clinical applications of FMRI, one must consider whether Type I or Type II errors have more deleterious consequences for the patient[55]. For example, in the pre-surgical planning for removing pathologic brain regions, false positives (Type I errors) may bias the surgeon to avoid areas that may not be important to avoid. This could result in incomplete removal of the brain abnormality. In contrast, false negatives (Type II errors) may bias the surgeon to remove too much tissue, possibly leading to an irreversible deficit in function. More research in this field is definitively warranted.

For the most accurate and full analysis, extensive computation may be required, using any of the free or commercial off-line software packages such as SPM (statistical parametric mapping) (*www.fil.ion.ucl.ac.uk/spm*), FSL (fMRI Brain Software Library, http://www.fmrib.ox.ac.uk/fsl/), or brain voyager (*www.brainvoyager.de*) (see Table 1.1). As mentioned earlier, for a quick simple analysis on the MR console, a (near) real-time, 'in-line' BOLD analysis is provided by almost all major MR manufacturers. Although such analysis tools are very comprehensive, they still lack small essential elements, such as co-registration of the functional statistical maps with the anatomy and/or multiplanar reconstruction and/or integration with neuronavigation software (see Table 1.1). An example of a real-time analysis on the scanner console is provided in Fig. 1.11.

Better and better techniques are slowly evolving to solve each of these challenges. For the clinician, the accessibility of MRI promises the freedom to exploit these new methods rapidly. Already, many centres are using FMRI as an adjunct to neurosurgical planning and for the various other applications mentioned below. With the availability of higher tesla magnets, faster sequences, better paradigms, and post-processing tools, the clinical application of this wonderful technique is going to increase in the years to come.

Table 1.1 Possibilities of offline and online (real-time) analysis software packages

Software	MC	SN	SM	Statistics	Cluster	COREG	MPR	Dicom
SPM	Y	Y	Y	GLM	Y	Y	Y	N*
FSL	Y	Y	Y	GLM	Y	Y	Y	N*
Brain voyager	Y	Y	Y	GLM	Y	Y	Y	N*
Online — Philips	Y	N	Y	CC	Y	N	N	N
Online — Siemens	Y	N	Y	GLM	Y	N	Y	N
Online — GE	Y	N	N	CC	N	N	N	N

MC = bulk head motion correction; SN = spatial normalization to standard atlas; SM = spatial smoothing; GLM = statistics using the general linear model; CC = cross-correlation statistics; cluster = threshold on cluster size; COREG = coregistration of anatomical and functional datasets; MPR = multiplanar reformatting; dicom = dicom compatible export of results, for integration with the functional neuronavigation system; N* = dicom conversion of the results is possible using extra software, such as MRICRO, ImageJ or XMedCon; SPM = statistical parametric mapping (http://www.fil.ion.ucl.ac.uk/spm/); FSL = fMRI Brain Software Library (http://www.fmrib.ox.ac.uk/fsl).

(a)   (b)   (c)   (d)

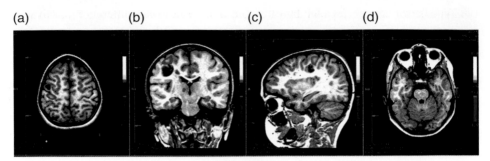

Fig. 1.11 Real-time online analysis on the Siemens Syngo MR console. fMRI activity of left-hand movements versus rest in a patient with a right cystic tumoural lesion superimposed on transversal **(a and d)**, coronal **(b)**, and sagital **(c)** slices. The primary sensorimotor cortex is adjacent, just medially, ventrally, and posteriorly from the tumour.

4. Clinical applications of FMRI

FMRI has been used to study patients with a broad range of neurological disorders, across a wide spectrum of disease severity. The results have provided insights into the mechanism of disease as well as into normal brain function. Many of the important clinical applications of this technique have been described. Some of these are being routinely used in many institutions for patient management.

4.1 Mapping the eloquent cortex

Traditionally, mapping of eloquent areas is achieved by methods such as intraoperative cortical stimulation in the awake patient, implantation of a subdural grid with extraoperative stimulation, or intraoperative recording of sensory-evoked potentials[56, 57]. These methods are accurate but are invasive. FMRI can obtain these data preoperatively and completely non-invasively. Together with its high sensitivity for visualizing brain lesions, FMRI can define the relation between the margin of a lesion and any adjacent functionally significant brain tissue. FMRI has the potential to predict the possible deficits in cognition, in language, or in motor and sensory perceptual functions that would arise from intrinsic lesion expansion, such as bleeding into an arteriovenous malformation, or from therapeutic intervention, such as surgery. This helps the treating physician or the surgeon to explain the relative risk of intervention and non-intervention so that a decision about the treatment option can be made after considering its cost and benefit.

Initially, FMRI studies were primarily concerned with the feasibility and the validity of FMRI compared with corticography[31, 58, 59]. As discussed above, most of the studies revealed good spatial correlation between the two methods. Once a lesion has been localized to the eloquent area, it becomes important to assess the risk that a deficit may follow therapeutic intervention. Yetkin *et al.* showed that when the distance between the representation of brain function (activated area) exceeded 2 cm, the patients showed no post resection deficit and resection was safe. However, as the distance between the lesion and brain function decreased, the rate of postoperative deficit increased[60]. When the lesion margin lay 1 to 2 cm from the zone of activation, 33% of patients showed postoperative deficits.

When the lesion margin lay less than 1 cm from the zone of activation, 50% of patients experienced postoperative deficit. Such information can be helpful when consulting the patient and when deciding on the optimal treatment modality.

FMRI can, therefore, be used to estimate the risk of surgical treatment which, in turn, should improve therapy, offering increased life expectancy and decreased morbidity. However, only very few studies have addressed the effect of FMRI in a neurosurgical context[27,34]. In a retrospective study, Lee *et al.* evaluated the therapeutic efficacy of FMRI and determined how often, and in what ways, FMRI studies influenced the management of individual patients[34]. They evaluated: (a) the use of FMRI to assess the risk associated with and, thus, the feasibility of, proposed surgical resection; (b) the use of FMRI results to guide the placement of the bone flap or of the subdural grids or strips for ictal electroencephalography (EEG) recordings or extraoperative sensorimotor cortical stimulation mapping; and (c) the use of FMRI to help determine whether invasive surgical functional mapping was necessary. In epilepsy patients, FMRI results helped to assess the feasibility of resection in 70% of patients, to plan the surgical procedure in 43%, and to select the patients for invasive mapping in 52%. In tumour patients, FMRI results helped to assess the feasibility in 55%, influenced the planning in 22%, and helped to select patients for invasive surgical functional mapping in 78%.

4.2 Lateralization of language and memory functions in the surgical treatment of epilepsy

Patients with intractable temporal lobe epilepsy (TLE) show improved seizure control or cure following surgery. An understanding of language lateralization is needed for presurgical planning. intracarotid amobarbital testing (IAT) or the Wada test has been the gold standard for identifying lateralization of language and memory functions preoperatively but it is invasive and, therefore, carries risk. FMRI offers a promising non-invasive alternative approach[61]. While there is good agreement between conventional invasive Wada testing and FMRI results, FMRI is more sensitive to involvement of the non-dominant hemisphere. FMRI offers the capability of spatially resolving functional activation within each hemisphere, potentially guiding tailored resections to spare eloquent cortex. The reproducibility of distinct patterns of activation in individual subjects is good, potentially allowing clinical decisions to be made on the basis of results. Binder *et al.*[62] reported a cross validation study comparing language dominance determined by both FMRI and IAT in 22 patients. A semantic decision task was used to activate a distributed network of brain regions in language specialization. Excellent agreement was obtained with both the techniques. There is still some controversy concerning the optimum task for language lateralization. A majority of the studies opine that a covert verbal fluency task yields best correspondence with the Wada test, while others advocate that semantic decision tasks should be used rather than the verbal fluency tasks because the latter may lack the activation of posterior language areas. In our institute, we use a paradigm which includes both verbal fluency and semantic decision (see Fig. 1.5).

FMRI may also be used to assess memory and to identify the epileptogenic focus. In patients who have TLE, the benefit of anterior temporal lobectomy must be weighted against the risks of inducing memory deficits. The development of FMRI paradigms that activate the mesial temporal regions, thought to be critical to forming new explicit memory, has been hampered by the complexity of the memory system. A complex visual scene-encoding task has been used to lateralize mesial temporal lobe memory dysfunction in patients with TLE, and showed good correlation with memory lateralization by IAT[63], while a mental navigation task successfully lateralized temporal lobe seizure foci[64]. Few of the earlier studies of memory function in patients with TLE have suggested that FMRI activation studies might contribute to the localization of the side of ictal activity. Bellgowan *et al.*[65] studied a group of 28 patients who had either left or right TLE and observed that the pattern of activation in the mesial temporal lobe during episodic encoding successfully discriminated those patients who had left ictal activity from those patients who had right ictal activity. However, these studies involved FMRI analysis of a group of patients. It has to be investigated whether these results can be replicated in individual patients.

4.3 Localizing spontaneous ictal activity

With the recent advent of methodologies that allow concurrent EEG and FMRI, it has been possible to localize regional metabolic changes accompanying spike-triggered approaches or using retrospective analysis of continuously acquired data[66, 67]. These techniques capitalize on the temporal resolution of EEG and spatial resolution of FMRI. The approach of concurrent EEG and FMRI recording tends to be more efficient and accurate in comparison with the spike-triggered approach[67]. These techniques may be of particular value in presurgical evaluation of neocortical epilepsy where paroxysmal activity on EEG may remain poorly localized. Also, these techniques may provide new insights into anatomical and pathophysiological correlates of unifocal and multifocal spike discharges.

4.4 FMRI for understanding brain plasticity

Another application of FMRI that has received increasing interest is the study of 'brain plasticity' which includes, for example, the study of recovery of motor function in stroke patients. FMRI could play an important role in determining the prognosis of recovery of function in such patients. Most of the studies on functional recovery after stroke on groups of patients have been performed with positron emission tomography. Because FMRI provides increased spatial resolution and has the ability to study these patients individually and repeatedly from stroke onset to full motor recovery, FMRI has now become the technique of choice.

Cao *et al.* studied the consequences of early ischaemic stroke and demonstrated that there was an increased recruitment of ipsilateral motor cortex during hand movements in children who had hemiparesis from intrauterine stroke[68]. Cramer *et al.* identified increased activation of a motor network in the unaffected hemisphere to a greater extent than found in controls, an increased degree of supplementary motor area activation, and perilesional activation[69]. A study of brain plasticity in patients who have arteriovenous malformations located within the primary motor cortex, revealed three typical patterns of takeover of function: (a) functional displacement within the affected primary motor cortex; (b) activation within the ipsilateral unaffected primary motor cortex; and (c) prominent activation in non-primary motor areas[70]. More recently, Carpentier *et al.*[71] proposed a classification scheme of plasticity with six grades based on inter-hemispheric pixel asymmetry and displacement of activation. Grade 1 represents the normal activation pattern, grade 2 appears to reflect a mass effect, grade 3 reflects the impact of the lesion on the activation (interface disorder) with no clear evidence of plasticity, grade 4 represents possible local plasticity, whereas grade 5 represents definite ipsilateral plasticity, and the grade 6 pattern represents definite contralateral plasticity. As designed, the classification categories, ranging from grades 1 to 6, correspond to levels of reorganization ranging from none to highly reorganized patterns of motor function. A case with grade 6 plasticity is presented in Fig. 1.12.

Another study has described longitudinal cortical reorganization in the auditory brain areas at several intervals (1 week, 5 weeks, and 1 year) after a right cochlear nerve resection for an acoustic neurinoma[72]. Before surgery, the patient had normal bilateral hearing; that is, when auditory stimulation was given to one ear (a) both the ipsilateral and the contralateral auditory cortices were activated but (b) the level of activation in the ipsilateral cortex was approximately one fifth of the level on the contralateral side. After surgery, the patient exhibited sudden and complete hearing loss on the right side. As expected, no cortical activation could be visualized when the resected right ear was stimulated. However, on stimulation of the other ear, an increase in the level of neuronal activity was observed in the ipsilateral auditory cortex at 1 and 5 weeks after surgery, increasing to complete symmetric activation of the left and the right auditory cortices 1 year postoperatively.

Neural correlates of phantom limb symptoms following amputation have been observed, along with an abnormally large region of contralateral motor cortex FMRI activation with stump movement in a patient whose left arm had been amputated at an early age[73]. Differential language lateralization has been observed in deaf patients as compared to hearing subjects[74] and activation of visual cortex has been observed with tactile stimulation in a blind individual[75]. Thulborn *et al.* have applied FMRI to language recovery in stroke patients[76]. Spontaneous redistribution of function to the right hemisphere was observed within days of the stroke and continued for months afterwards.

Clearly, brain plasticity is far from understood. The challenge is to study the physiologic mechanisms behind it. It is unclear why certain stroke patients recover almost completely and why others do not, despite long and intensive rehabilitation. The studies described above demonstrate, however, that longitudinal FMRI studies in individual patients should allow objective measurement of the recovery function and the effects of rehabilitation or other treatment strategies (e.g. neuroprotective drugs) on this recovery.

4.5 **FMRI in guiding therapeutic development**

One of the most exciting prospects of FMRI is to guide therapeutic development, drug development, and response monitoring. The greatest impact may be on areas in which sensitive and objective end points were previously difficult to define (e.g. neurorehabilitation[77]). A similar example is the assessment of outcomes using behavioural therapy, such as for the control of pain. By identifying the biological basis for cognitive and behavioural

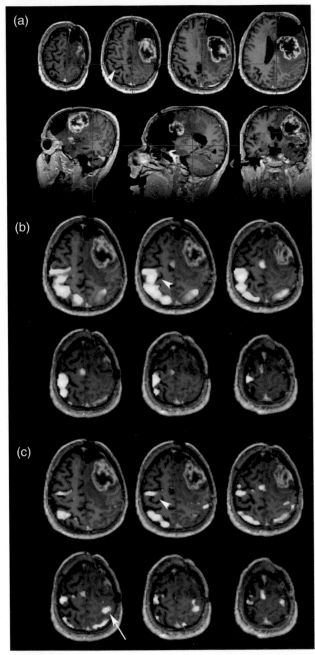

Fig. 1.12 Cortical reorganization of the motor system in a patient with a recurrent glioblastoma multiforma three years after resection of a glioma grade 2 in the right frontal lobe. (**a**) T1w post-contrast anatomical images. (**b**) Activation pattern in response to repetitive left hand clenching versus rest; (**c**) in response to right hand clenching. Arrowheads indicate the position of the right primary motor cortex. The arrow points to the presumed location of the left primary motor cortex. Note the normal pattern of brain activity in B with contralateral activation of the right M1, PM, and bilateral activation pattern of the SMA and parietal proprioceptive regions. The activation pattern in c should be symmetrical to b, but this is not the case. There is some residual activity in the left M1 (arrow) but ipsilateral activation in the right primary motor and premotor cortices is clearly present.

changes, FMRI offers insights into mechanisms of vulnerability and variability of responses to treatments for neurological and psychiatric diseases.

Finally, an emerging application of FMRI is in brain bionics. Implantable stimulators are currently used in the management of a variety of neurological and psychiatric syndromes including Parkinson's disease, epilepsy, chronic pain, non-pulsatile tinnitus (see Fig. 1.13 and[52]), and obsessive compulsive disorder (see Fig. 1.14 and[78]). FMRI can be used to: (a) visualize the hemodynamic effects of neurostimulation ([79]and Fig. 1.14); (b) to guide the placement of electrodes into brain regions under conscious control (Fig. 1.13); and (c) to allow paralysed patients to use motor imagery to control robotic devices[80].

4.6 FMRI helps in identifying preclinical expression of neurodegenerative disease

FMRI can be sensitive to early stages of brain pathology. An illustration of this approach was an FMRI-based memory study of a group of apparently healthy subjects at risk of developing early onset Alzheimer's disease[81]. One year after FMRI scanning, those who were beginning to develop memory problems in early clinical expression of presumed Alzheimer's disease were identified. A significant difference in the pattern and volume of activated cortex with the memory task was found in these subjects relative to those who did not develop memory impairment. The alteration in FMRI activation also correlated with APO-E status and subsequent memory decline.

4.7 Differential diagnosis of neuropsychiatric disorders

Subjects who have recovered from depression have a substantial risk for recurrence of depression, suggesting that there are persistent abnormalities in brain function associated with vulnerability to depression. Smith *et al.* applied a pain-conditioning paradigm to study a group of patients who had recovered from depression and who were not on drug treatment, but were at risk of recurrence of depression[82]. The recovered depressed patients showed an altered FMRI response in the cerebellum relative to healthy controls. This type of study might be used to distinguish between different types of depression or to identify healthy subjects at risk of depression.

Numerous studies have attempted to demonstrate abnormal responses to task activation in a variety of neuropsychiatric syndromes. Alterations in FMRI response to primary sensorimotor or cognitive tasks have been observed in some psychiatric syndromes, but these have been relatively non-specific[83]. For cognitive activation, FMRI studies are further confounded by task performance, since patients typically perform worse than controls. Hence, though limited, the role of FMRI in psychiatry has still to evolve with better techniques and a better understanding of cognitive functions.

4.8 Pharmacological MRI

FMRI techniques are now being increasingly used to investigate regionally specific brain activity associated with the administration of CNS-active drugs. Such techniques offer a relatively non-invasive way to perform pharmacological investigations in experimental animals, healthy human volunteers, and individuals with CNS diseases. However, since

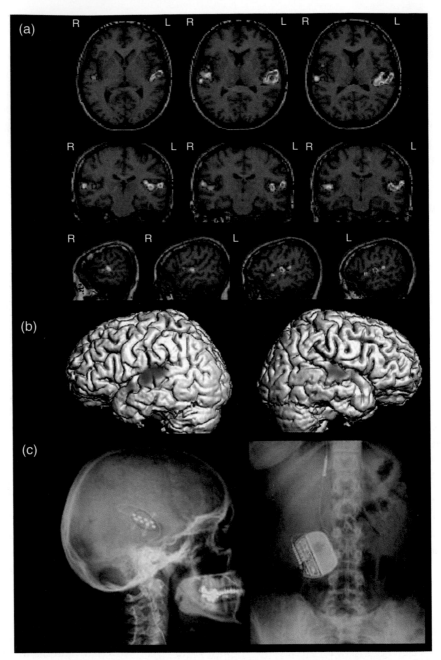

Fig. 1.13 Functional neuronavigation for the guided implantation of an epidural electrode in a patient with left unilateral tinnitus. (**a**) Auditory cortical activation in response to binaural musical stimulation; the right primary auditory cortex has less differential activity due to the spontaneous high level of electrical activity in the right auditory cortex which causes the (phantom) percept of unilateral left tinnitus. (**b**) Same activation represented on 3D surface reconstruction of the brain of the patient. (**c**) Post-operative X-ray showing the location of the epidural electrode projected on the skull (left panel) and of the location of the pacemaker (right panel). Adapted from De Ridder et al[112].

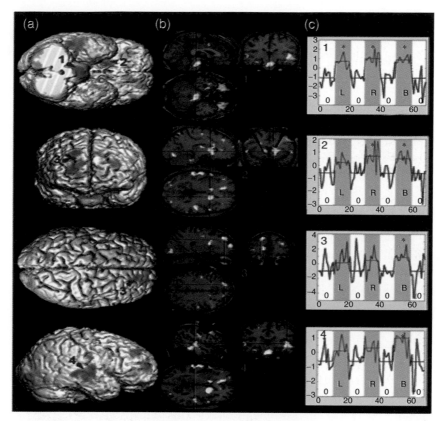

Fig. 1.14 FMRI study showing cortical and subcortical activation in a patient suffering from obsessive compulsive disorder, treated with deep brain stimulation, when brain activity is subtracted during the stimulation-off condition from brain activity shown during the stimulation-on condition, superimposed onto surface reconstructions (**a**) and sections (**b**) of the patient's brain. Regions are labelled as follows: the midline focus in the pons (1), the striatum (2), the focus in the right frontal cortex (3), and the left superior temporal gyrus (4). In the brain sections, the left hemisphere is shown on the right or at the bottom. (**c**) Percentage FMRI signal change (blue line) and statistically modelled signal change (red line) during left (L), right (R), stimulation (B), and no stimulation (0) in the four labelled regions. Conditions for which stimulation versus no stimulation was significant ($P < 0.05$ corrected for multiple comparisons) are indicated by asterisks. Adapted from Nuttin et al[78].

pharmacological agents themselves can interfere with the mechanisms that give rise to the BOLD signal, careful attention to experimental design and data analysis must be exercised[84]. Introduction of a drug into the system could potentially alter the coupling of neural activity along with the rCBF and/or the extraction of oxygen from blood, or may cause local or global cardiovascular changes unrelated to neural activity. Despite all these constraints, FMRI has been successfully used to study acute direct effects of drugs, effects of drugs on task-related activation, chronic effects of drugs, effects of drugs on cerebral metabolism, and variable effects of drugs in different populations[84].

Willson *et al.* have shown recently that dextroamphetamine causes measurable decreases in brain activity in a variety of regions during cognitive tasks. The authors proposed that these changes might be linked to behavioural changes observed after dextroamphetamine administration[85]. Borras and colleagues, using FMRI techniques, have demonstrated that naloxone, even in the absence of psychophysical effects, produces activation in several brain regions that are known to have high levels of mu-opioid receptors and may be involved in endogenous analgesia[86]. This use of FMRI, dubbed 'pharmacological MRI' (phMRI), holds the promise of providing relatively straightforward pharmacodynamic assays and can be used to establish brain penetrability parameters or dose-ranging information for novel therapeutic compounds[87].

5. Future directions of clinical FMRI

Despite its successful application, FMRI has not yet fully reached the status of an established clinical diagnostic procedure. Many of the above mentioned technical, methodological, and physiological limitations contribute to this, justified, lack of acceptance. Combination of FMRI with other (non-invasive) clinical imaging techniques might bring clinical FMRI closer to general acceptance.

5.1 Going to higher field strength: 3T

Recently, 3T whole body MR scanners were introduced into many clinical centres. The doubled field strength (3T compared to 1.5T) has several distinct advantages for FMRI. At 3T, the signal-to-noise ratio (SNR) is roughly twice as large as the SNR at 1.5T[88]. Furthermore, the BOLD effect is roughly doubled in comparison with 1.5T[89, 90], resulting from the increased sensitivity to susceptibility effects. Both advantages of 3T — the increased SNR and increased BOLD sensitivity — work in synergy in FMRI experiments. One example of the increased sensitivity can be seen in Fig. 1.15, a direct comparison of 1.5T and 3T FMRI in the same subject, resulting in increased detectability of subcortical auditory structures at 3T. A drawback of the increased sensitivity at 3T is the increased spatial distortion and signal drop-out artefacts. However, recent promising work has come from another development, notably the use of parallel imaging techniques[91, 92]. Such techniques have the potential to reduce the problems inherent in single-shot EPI imaging sequences, thus reducing the susceptibility related artefacts. Therefore, the combination of 3T and parallel imaging seems to be a very useful one in the clinical setting. The 3T-increased FMRI sensitivity is especially useful in patient examinations, since less time is needed to acquire an FMRI dataset than at 1.5T.

5.2 Disentangling essential versus expendable brain regions

As mentioned above, FMRI lacks the ability to discriminate essential from expendable regions within a network of activations involved in a particular function. This is a particular disadvantage when performing FMRI in the pre-operative work-up of patients with brain tumours, where one would want to identify the relation between essential areas and a brain lesion. Expendable areas could be defined as regions within the network that correlate with the performance of a given neurological function but that are not essential

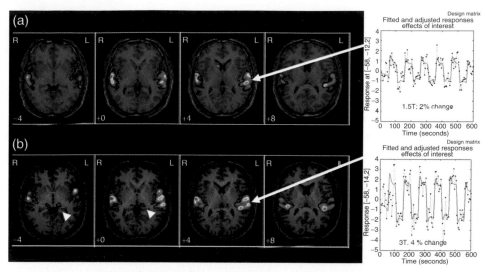

Fig. 1.15 Direct comparison of FMRI at field strengths of 1.5T (**a**) and 3T (**b**) in a single subject, during the presentation of binaural musical stimulation versus rest. Note the differential level of MR signal change that is double (4%) at 3T than at 1.5T (2%). At an identical statistical threshold, this leads to the successful depiction of subcortical activations at 3T only in the medial geniculate body (arrowhead) and inferior colliculus (not shown).

for the correct execution of this function. Intra-operative cortical stimulation — given its ability to reversibly, locally disrupt brain function — can be used to interrogate whether a certain region is critical for the neurological function. Similarly, the intra-arterial amobarbital procedure is commonly employed for assessing hemispheric language and memory dominance. Since this is again a local (one hemisphere) knock-out of function, one can assess whether the activations observed within the language or memory network are crucial or not to the correct execution.

However, both ICS and the Wada test are highly invasive and difficult to perform. Both are very unpleasant to the patient, who experiences unilateral paralysis, the inability to speak, and the inability to understand speech; both are expensive, costing nearly as much as the surgery itself. In addition, the Wada test does not provide information about the localization of language within the hemisphere. Furthermore, ICS requires a surgical procedure itself before any functional information can be obtained.

The combination of FMRI and focal transcranial magnetic stimulation (TMS) might be an interesting alternative to ICS and/or Wada testing. TMS is a non-invasive technique able to produce focal, transient, and fully reversible disruption of cortical network function during the performance of cognitive, sensory, or motor tasks[93]. Effectively, TMS utilizes an electromagnet to cause a very temporary disruption in the firing of neurons at the site of stimulation. TMS has a relative high spatial resolution and recent advances in image processing[94] have allowed for the refinement of TMS by combining MRI modalities with TMS using a neuronavigation system to measure the position of the stimulating coil and map this position onto a MRI dataset. In this way it is possible to pinpoint very specific areas of cortex for transcranial magnetic stimulation. Where FMRI cannot tell us whether an area is necessary for the task we are investigating, stimulating the same area with TMS and observing the effects of the stimulation on behaviour can tell us if that area is required for the task. The combination of FMRI and TMS might also be used to study cortical plasticity in response to the presence of tumours and other lesions (cortical dysplasia, stroke, etc.)[95].The only limitation of TMS is its limited efficacy in disrupting deeper brain structures or cortical areas that are difficult to reach due to the skull shape (e.g. posterior fossa due to the neck, temporal lobe due to interposition of the ears). Nonetheless, the combination of FMRI and TMS deserves more research attention.

5.3 The brain is composed of gray AND white matter

A major criticism of FMRI is that it is sensitive to cortical changes but provides no or only limited information about white matter fibre tracts and connections. For a comprehensive understanding of normal and pathological brain function, information about the neuronal networks consisting of cortical activations and anatomical connections is warranted. Combining FMRI with techniques which provide information about white matter connectivity might bring us closer to this understanding.

Diffusion tensor imaging (DTI) is a modification of the MRI technique and is sensitive to Brownian motion of water molecules in biological tissues[96, 97]. This new clinical method can demonstrate the orientation and integrity of white matter fibres in vivo[98]. Within cerebral white matter, water molecules diffuse more freely along the direction of axonal fascicles than across them, arising from the restriction of free water diffusion by the axonal membrane, axonal microtubuli, and the axonal myelin sheath[99–101]. Such directional dependence of diffusivity is termed 'anisotropy'. An integrated MR measure of water diffusion in at least six non-collinear directions is used to calculate the diffusion tensor (D), from which fractional anisotropy (FA — the amount of anisotropy) and the directionally averaged mean diffusivity (Dav) can be derived[102]. By combining anisotropy data with the directionality, it is possible to obtain estimates of fibre orientation. This has led to fibre tractography (FT) in which three-dimensional pathways of white matter tracts are reconstructed by sequentially piecing together discrete and shortly spaced estimates of fibre orientation to form continuous trajectories[103–105].

The power of the combined use of FMRI and DTI lies in the fact that both techniques can be performed using the same MR machine, in a single imaging session. Valuable information about the major white matter connections can be obtained through FT, using the FMRI-activated regions as starting points for the FT algorithm. Doing so, corticospinal and corticobulbar tracts, arcuate, uncinate, inferior, and superior longitudinal fasciculi, corpus callosum, and cerebellar peduncles are some of the major fibre bundles that can be readily depicted[98,106]. An example of the tracking of the arcuate fasciculus (the classical direct pathway between Broca's and Wernicke's language regions[107]), in a normal subject, can be seen in Fig. 1.16.

DTI has been proposed as a technique suitable for presurgical planning in brain tumour patients[108–110]. It has the potential to establish spatial relationships between eloquent white matter and tumour borders, provide information essential to preoperative planning,

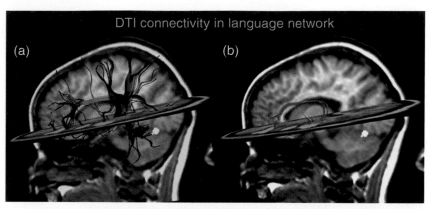

Fig. 1.16 Combined FMRI and DTI in a normal subject. (**a**) Fibre bundles originating from a ROI corresponding to the activation site of Wernicke's area: Wernicke is anatomically interconnected with the temporal pole, cerebellum, parietal lobe, peri-rolandic region, and frontal areas. (**b**) DTI fibre tracking between Wernicke's and Broca's regions: depiction of the classical direct arcuate fasciculus.

and improve the accuracy of surgical risk assessments preoperatively. Several recent studies[108, 109, 111] showed that the combined use of FMRI and DTI can provide a better estimation of the proximity of tumour borders to eloquent brain systems subserving language, speech, vision, motor, and premotor functions. In the study of Ulmer and coworkers[108], twice as many eloquent structures were localized to within 5 mm of tumour borders when DTI and FMRI were utilized for preoperative planning, compared to that afforded by FMRI alone. Additionally, a low regional complication rate of surgery (4%) observed in this series suggests that preoperative planning with these combined techniques may improve surgical outcomes compared to that previously reported in the literature.

We would like to emphasize this point by the illustrative case shown in Fig. 1.17. This 31-year-old right-handed patient with a low grade glioma in the left supramarginal and angular gyri underwent FMRI with verbal fluency tasks in order to assess the language network. The FMRI activity in Broca's and Wernicke's areas is more than 20 mm distance from the radiological tumour border and applying the 'golden rule' here would lead to the (false) conclusion that it is safe to remove the tumour. DTI with fibre tracking depicting the arcuate bundle between Wernicke's and Broca's areas shows that the bundle seems to be displaced medially by the mass effect of the lesion and its middle part is adjacent to the tumour border. It is likely that a resection of the tumour would lead to an injury of the arcuate fasciculus which, functionally, would result in a severe conduction aphasia.

Larger studies specifically designed to establish the accuracy and predictive value of combined FMRI and DTI in brain tumour patients are warranted to substantiate our preliminary observations, but it is our conviction that the single use of FMRI without knowledge of the white matter connections will prove to be unethical in the near future.

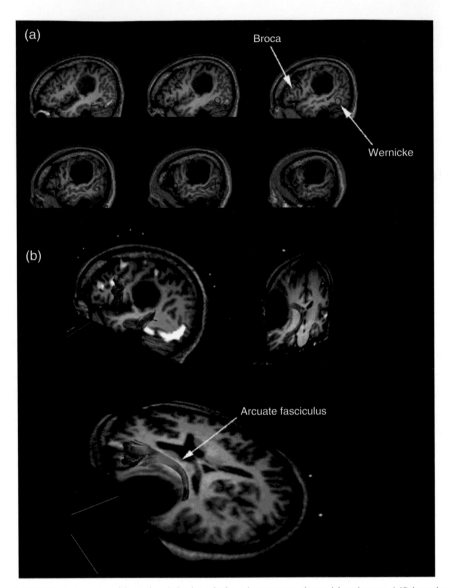

Fig. 1.17 Thirty-one-year-old, male, right-handed patient presenting with seizures. MR imaging revealed a low-grade tumoral mass in the left supramarginal and angular gyri. (**a**) FMRI during a verbal fluency task depicts a left lateralized language, with Wernicke's area in the middle temporal gyrus and Broca in the inferior frontal gyrus. Both eloquent areas are at distance from the lesion. (**b**) DTI with fibre tracking depicting the arcuate bundle between Wernicke's and Broca's. The bundle seems to be displaced medially by the mass effect of the lesion and its middle part is adjacent to the tumour border.

6. **Conclusions**

The development of applications of FMRI for diagnostic and therapeutic purposes in patients with neurological, neurosurgical, or psychiatric diseases is a fast developing field. Physiological, methodological, and technical problems have to be taken into account when performing clinical FMRI. Nonetheless, solutions for these problems are currently under development and results are very promising. Together with other techniques, such as TMS and DTI, clinical FMRI seems to have a bright future.

References

1. Villringer A. Understanding functional neuroimaging methods based on neurovascular coupling. *Adv Exp Med Biol* 1997;**413**:177–93.

2. Duong TQ, Kim DS, Ugurbil K, Kim SG. Spatiotemporal dynamics of the BOLD FMRI signals: toward mapping submillimeter cortical columns using the early negative response. *Magn Reson Med* 2000;**44**(2):231–42.

3. Ogawa S, Lee TM, Kay AR, Tank DW. Brain magnetic resonance imaging with contrast dependent on blood oxygenation. *Procs Natl Acad Sci USA* 1990;**87**(24):9868–72.

4. Bandettini PA, Wong EC, Hinks RS, Tikofsky RS, Hyde JS. Time course EPI of human brain function during task activation. *Magn Reson Med* 1992;**25**(2):390–7.

5. Frahm J, Bruhn H, Merboldt KD, Hanicke W. Dynamic MR imaging of human brain oxygenation during rest and photic stimulation. *J Magn Reson Imaging* 1992;**2**(5):501–5.

6. Kwong KK, Belliveau JW, Chesler DA, Goldberg IE, Weisskoff RM, Poncelet BP, *et al*. Dynamic magnetic resonance imaging of human brain activity during primary sensory stimulation. *Proc Natl Acad Sci USA* 1992;**89**(12):5675–9.

7. Thulborn KR, Waterton JC, Matthews PM, Radda GK. Oxygenation dependence of the transverse relaxation time of water protons in whole blood at high field. *Biochem Biophys Acta* 1982;**714**(2):265–70.

8. Mansfield P, Maudsley AA. Medical imaging by NMR. *Br J Radiol* 1977;**50**(591):188–94.

9. Holodny AI, Schulder M, Liu WC, Wolko J, Maldjian JA, Kalnin AJ. The effect of brain tumors on BOLD functional MR imaging activation in the adjacent motor cortex: implications for image-guided neurosurgery. *American Journal of Neuroradiology* 2000;**21**(8):1415–22.

10. Ulmer JL, Krouwer HG, Mueller WM, Ugurel MS, Kocak M, Mark LP. Pseudo-reorganization of language cortical function at fMR imaging: a consequence of tumor-induced neurovascular uncoupling. *American Journal of Neuroradiology* 2003;**24**(2):213–7.

11. Ulmer JL, Hacein–Bey L, Mathews VP, Mueller WM, Deyoe EA, Prost RW, *et al*. Lesion-induced pseudo-dominance at functional magnetic resonance imaging: implications for preoperative assessments. *Neurosurgery* 2004;**55**(3):569–79.

12. Schreiber A, Hubbe U, Ziyeh S, Hennig J. The influence of gliomas and nonglial space-occupying lesions on blood-oxygen-level-dependent contrast enhancement. *American Journal of Neuroradiology* 2000;**21**(6):1055–63.

13. Whittle IR, Collins F, Kelly PAT, Ritchie I, Ironside JW. Nitric oxide synthase is expressed in experimental malignant glioma and influences tumour blood flow. *Acta Neurochirurgica* 1996;**138**(7):870–5.

14. Hossmann KA, Linn F, Okada Y. Bioluminescence and fluoroscopic imaging of tissue Ph and metabolites in experimental brain tumors of cat. *Nmr in Biomedicine* 1992;**5**(5):259–64.

15. Linn F, Seo K, Hossmann KA. Experimental transplantation gliomas in the adult cat brain. 3: regional biochemistry. *Acta Neurochirurgica* 1989;**99**(1–2):85–93.

16. Hund–Georgiadis M, Mildner T, Georgiadis D, Weih K, von Cramon DY. Impaired hemodynamics and neural activation? A FMRI study of major cerebral artery stenosis. *Neurology* 2003;**61**(9):1276–9.

17. Fujiwara N, Sakatani K, Katayama Y, Murata Y, Hoshino T, Fukaya C, *et al*. Evoked-cerebral blood oxygenation changes in false-negative activations in BOLD contrast functional MRI of patients with brain tumors. *Neuroimage* 2004;**21**(4):1464–71.

18. Bryan RN, Kraut M. Functional magnetic resonance imaging: you get what you (barely) see. *American Journal of Neuroradiology* 1998;**19**:991–2.

19. Laurienti PJ, Field AS, Burdette JH, Maldjian JA, Yen YF, Moody DM. Dietary caffeine consumption modulates FMRI measures. *Neuroimage* 2002;**17**(2):751–7.

20. Kennan RP, Zhong J, Gore JC. Intravascular susceptibility contrast mechanisms in tissues. *Magn Reson Med* 1994;**331**(1):9–21.

21. Boxerman JL, Bandettini PA, Kwong KK, Baker JR, Davis TL, Rosen BR, *et al*. The intravascular contribution to FMRI signal change: Monte Carlo modeling and diffusion-weighted studies in vivo. *Magn Reson Med* 1995;**34**(1):4–10.

22. Gao JH, Miller I, Lai S, Xiong TJ, Fox PT. Quantitative assessment of blood inflow effects in functional MRI signals. *Magn Reson Med* 1996;**36**(2):314–9.

23. Turner R. How much cortex can a vein drain? Downstream dilution of activation-related cerebral blood oxygenation changes. *Neuroimage* 2002;**16**(4):1062–7.

24. Stippich C, Freitag P, Kassubek J, Soros P, Kamada K, Kober H, *et al*. Motor, somatosensory and auditory cortex localization by FMRI and MEG. *Neuroreport* 1998;**9**(9):1953–7.

25. Maldjian J, Atlas SW, Howard RS, Greenstein E, Alsop D, Detre JA, *et al*. Functional magnetic resonance imaging of regional brain activity in patients with intracerebral arteriovenous malformations before surgical or endovascular therapy. *Journal of Neurosurgery* 1996;**84**(3):477–83.

26. Latchaw RE, Hu XP, Ugurbil K, Hall WA, Madison MT, Heros RC. Functional magnetic resonance imaging as a management tool for cerebral arteriovenous malformations. *Neurosurgery* 1995;**37**(4):619–25.

27. Atlas SW, Howard RS, Maldjian J, Alsop D, Detre JA, Listerud J, *et al*. Functional magnetic resonance imaging of regional brain activity in patients with intracerebral gliomas: findings and implications for clinical management. *Neurosurgery* 1996;**38**(2):329–37.

28. Dymarkowski S, Sunaert S, Van Oostende S, Van Hecke P, Wilms G, Demaerel P, *et al*. Functional MRI of the brain: localisation of eloquent cortex in focal brain lesion therapy. *European Radiology* 1998;**8**(9):1573–80.

29. Hirsch J, Ruge MI, Kim KHS, Correa DD, Victor JD, Relkin NR, *et al*. An integrated functional magnetic resonance imaging procedure for preoperative mapping of cortical areas associated with tactile, motor, language, and visual functions. *Neurosurgery* 2000;**47**(3):711–21.

30. Yetkin FZ, Mueller WM, Morris GL, McAuliffe TL, Ulmer JL, Cox RW, *et al*. Functional MR activation correlated with intraoperative cortical mapping. *American Journal of Neuroradiology* 1997;**18**(7):1311–5.

31. Lehericy S, Duffau H, Cornu P, Capelle L, Pidoux B, Carpentier A, *et al*. Correspondence between functional magnetic resonance imaging somatotopy and individual brain anatomy of the central region: comparison with intraoperative stimulation in patients with brain tumors. *Journal of Neurosurgery* 2000;**92**(4):589–98.

32. Sabbah P, Foehrenbach H, Dutertre G, Nioche C, DeDreuille O, Bellegou N, *et al*. Multimodal anatomic, functional, and metabolic brain imaging for tumor resection. *Clinical Imaging* 2002;**26**(1):6–12.

33. Roux FE, Ibarrola D, Tremoulet M, Lazorthes Y, Henry P, Sol JC, *et al*. Methodological and technical issues for integrating functional magnetic resonance imaging data in a neuronavigational system. *Neurosurgery* 2001;**49**(5):1145–56.

34. Lee CC, Ward HA, Sharbrough FW, Meyer FB, Marsh WR, Raffel C, *et al*. Assessment of functional MR imaging in neurosurgical planning. *American Journal of Neuroradiology* 1999;**20**(8):1511–9.

35. Sunaert S. Functional MR imaging of hearing. In: Lemmerling M, Kollias SS (ed.) *Radiology of the Petrous Bone*, 1st edn, Springer–Verlag, Berlin/Heidelberg/New York; 2003, p. 223–35.

36. Rutten GJM, van Rijen PC, van Veelen CWM, Ramsey NF. Language area localization with three-dimensional functional magnetic resonance imaging matches intrasulcal electrostimulation in Broca's area. *Annals of Neurology* 1999;**46**(3):405–8.

37. Roux FE, Boulanouar K, Lotterie JA, Mejdoubi M, Lesage JP, Berry I. Language functional magnetic resonance imaging in preoperative assessment of language areas: correlation with direct cortical stimulation. *Neurosurgery* 2003;**52**(6):1335–45.

38. Turner R, Howseman A, Rees GE, Josephs O, Friston K. Functional magnetic resonance imaging of the human brain: data acquisition and analysis. *Exp Brain Res* 1998;**123**(1–2):5–12.

39. Dagli MS, Ingeholm JE, Haxby JV. Localization of cardiac-induced signal change in FMRI. *Neuroimage* 1999;**9**(4):407–15.

40. Krings T, Reinges MHT, Erberich S, Kemeny S, Rohde V, Spetzger U, *et al*. Functional MRI for presurgical planning: problems, artefacts, and solution strategies. *Journal of Neurology, Neurosurgery, and Psychiatry* 2001;**70**(6):749–60.

41. Friston KJ, Williams S, Howard R, Frackowiak RSJ, Turner R. Movement-related effects in FMRI time-series. *Magn Reson Med* 1996;**35**(3):346–55.

42. Hajnal JV, Myers R, Oatridge A, Schwieso JE, Young IR, Bydder GM. Artifacts due to stimulus correlated motion in functional imaging of the brain. *Magn Reson Med* 1994;**31**(3):283–91.

43. Hill DL, Smith AD, Simmons A, Maurer CR, Cox TC, Elwes R, Brammer M, Hawkes DJ, Polkey CE. Sources of error in comparing functional magnetic resonance imaging and invasive electrophysiological recordings. *J Neurosurg* 2000;**93**(2):214–23.

44. Debus J, Essig M, Schad LR, Wenz F, Baudendistel K, Knopp MV, *et al*. Functional magnetic resonance imaging in a stereotactic setup. *Magn Reson Imaging* 1996;**14**(9):1007–12.

45. Fitzsimmons JR, Scott JD, Peterson DM, Wolverton BL, Webster CS, Lang PJ. Integrated RF coil with stabilization for FMRI human cortex. *Magn Reson Med* 1997;**38**(1):15–8.

46. Friston KJ, Holmes AP, Poline JB, Grasby PJ, Williams SC, Frackowiak RS, *et al*. Analysis of FMRI time-series revisited. *Neuroimage* 1995;**2**(1):45–53.

47. Bellon E, Feron M, Maes F, Hoe LV, Delaere D, Haven F, *et al*. Evaluation of manual vs semi-automated delineation of liver lesions on CT images. *Eur Radiol* 1997;**7**(3):432–8.

48. Maes F, Collignon A, Vandermeulen D, Marchal G, Suetens P. Multimodality image registration by maximization of mutual information. *IEEE Trans Med Imaging* 1997;**16**(2):187–98.

49. Biswal BB, Hyde JS. Contour-based registration technique to differentiate between task- activated and head motion-induced signal variations in FMRI. *Magn Reson Med* 1997;**38**(3):470–6.

50. Hill DL, Smith AD, Simmons A, Maurer CR, Cox TC, Elwes R, *et al*. Sources of error in comparing functional magnetic resonance imaging and invasive electrophysiological recordings. *J Neurosurg* 2000;**93**(2):214–23.

51. Hajnal JV, Myers R, Oatridge A, Schwieso JE, Young IR, Bydder GM. Artifacts due to stimulus correlated motion in functional imaging of the brain. *Magn Reson Med* 1994;**31**(3):283–91.

52. Ward HA, Riederer SJ, Grimm RC, Ehman RL, Felmlee JP, Jack CR. Prospective multiaxial motion correction for FMRI. *Magn Reson Med* 2000;**43**(3):459–69.

53. Thesen S, Heid O, Mueller E, Schad LR. Prospective acquisition correction for head motion with image-based tracking for real-time FMRI. *Magn Reson Med* 2000;**44**(3):457–65.

54. Weisskoff RM. Functional MRI: are we all moving towards artifactual conclusions? Or FMRI fact or fancy? *NMR Biomed* 1995;**8**(3):101–3.

55. Desmond JE, Chen SHA. Ethical issues in the clinical application of FMRI: factors affecting the validity and interpretation of activations. *Brain and Cognition* 2002;**50**(3):482–97.

56. Berger MS, Cohen WA, Ojemann GA. Correlation of motor cortex brain mapping data with magnetic resonance imaging. *J Neurosurg* 1990;**72**(3):383–7.

57. Gregorie EM, Goldring S. Localization of function in the excision of lesions from the sensorimotor region. *J Neurosurg* 1984;**61**(6):1047–54.

58. Jack CR, Thompson RM, Butts RK, Sharbrough FW, Kelly PJ, Hanson DP, *et al*. Sensory-motor cortex — correlation of presurgical mapping with functional MR imaging and invasive cortical mapping. *Radiology* 1994;**190**(1):85–92.

59. Puce A. Comparative assessment of sensorimotor function using functional magnetic resonance imaging and electrophysiological methods. *J Clin Neurophysiol* 1995;**12**(5):450–9.

60. Yetkin FZ, Ulmer JL, Mueller W, Cox RW, Klosek MM, Haughton VM. Functional magnetic resonance imaging assessment of the risk of postoperative hemiparesis after excision of cerebral tumors. *International Journal of Neuroradiology* 1998;**4**(4):253–7.

61. Adcock JE, Wise RG, Oxbury JM, Oxbury SM, Matthews PM. Quantitative FMRI assessment of the differences in lateralization of language-related brain activation in patients with temporal lobe epilepsy. *Neuroimage* 2003;**18**(2):423–38.

62. Binder JR, Swanson SJ, Hammeke TA, Morris GL, Mueller WM, Fischer M, *et al*. Determination of language dominance using functional MRI: a comparison with the Wada test. *Neurology* 1996;**46**(4):978–84.

63. Detre JA, Maccotta L, King D, Alsop DC, Glosser G, D'Esposito M, *et al*. Functional MRI lateralization of memory in temporal lobe epilepsy. *Neurology* 1998;**50**(4):926–32.

64. Jokeit H, Okujava M, Woermann FG. Memory FMRI lateralizes temporal lobe epilepsy. *Neurology* 2001;**57**(10):1786–93.

65. Bellgowan PS, Binder JR, Swanson SJ, Hammeke TA, Springer JA, Frost JA, *et al*. Side of seizure focus predicts left medial temporal lobe activation during verbal encoding. *Neurology* 1998;**51**(2):479–84.

66. Krakow K, Woermann FG, Symms MR, Allen PJ, Lemieux L, Barker GJ, *et al*. EEG-triggered functional MRI of interictal epileptiform activity in patients with partial seizures. *Brain* 1999;**122**(Pt 9):1679–88.

67. Lemieux L, Krakow K, Fish DR. Comparison of spike-triggered functional MRI BOLD activation and EEG dipole model localization. *Neuroimage* 2001;**14**(5):1097–104.

68. Cao Y, Vikingstad EM, Huttenlocher PR, Towle VL, Levin DN. Functional magnetic resonance studies of the reorganization of the human hand sensorimotor area after unilateral brain injury in the perinatal period. *Proc Natl Acad Sci USA* 1994;**91**(20):9612–6.

69. Cramer SC, Nelles G, Benson RR, Kaplan JD, Parker RA, Kwong KK, *et al*. A functional MRI study of subjects recovered from hemiparetic stroke. *Stroke* 1997;**28**(12):2518–27.

70. Alkadhi H, Kollias SS, Crelier GR, Golay X, Hepp–Reymond MC, Valavanis A. Plasticity of the human motor cortex in patients with arteriovenous malformations: a functional MR imaging study. *American Journal of Neuroradiology* 2000;**21**(8):1423–33.

71. Carpentier AC, Constable RT, Schlosser MJ, de Lotbiniere A, Piepmeier JM, Spencer DD, Awad IA. Patterns of functional magnetic resonance imaging activation in association with structural lesions in the rolandic region: a classification system. *Journal of Neurosurgery* 2001;**94**(6):946–54.

72. Bilecen D, Seifritz E, Radu EW, Schmid N, Wetzel S, Probst R, *et al*. Cortical reorganization after acute unilateral hearing loss traced by FMRI. *Neurology* 2000;**54**(3):765–7.

73. Dettmers C, Liepert J, Adler T, Rzanny R, Rijntjes M, van SR, *et al*. Abnormal motor cortex organization contralateral to early upper limb amputation in humans. *Neurosci Lett* 1999;19;**263**(1):41–4.

74. Neville HJ, Bavelier D, Corina D, Rauschecker J, Karni A, Lalwani A, *et al.* Cerebral organization for language in deaf and hearing subjects: biological constraints and effects of experience. *Proc Natl Acad Sci USA* 1998;**95**(3):922–9.

75. Sadato N, Hallett M. FMRI occipital activation by tactile stimulation in a blind man. *Neurology* 1999;**52**(2):423.

76. Thulborn KR, Carpenter PA, Just MA. Plasticity of language-related brain function during recovery from stroke. *Stroke* 1999;**30**(4):749–54.

77. Johansen–Berg H, Dawes H, Guy C, Smith SM, Wade DT, Matthews PM. Correlation between motor improvements and altered FMRI activity after rehabilitative therapy. *Brain* 2002;**125**(Pt 12):2731–42.

78. Nuttin BJ, Gabriels LA, Cosyns PR, Meyerson BA, Andreewitch S, Sunaert SG, *et al.* Long-term electrical capsular stimulation in patients with obsessive-compulsive disorder. *Neurosurgery* 2003;**52**(6):1263–72.

79. Rezai AR, Lozano AM, Crawley AP, Joy ML, Davis KD, Kwan CL, *et al.* Thalamic stimulation and functional magnetic resonance imaging: localization of cortical and subcortical activation with implanted electrodes. Technical note. *J Neurosurg* 1999;**90**(3):583–90.

80. Kennedy PR, Bakay RA. Restoration of neural output from a paralyzed patient by a direct brain connection. *Neuroreport* 1998;**9**(8):1707–11.

81. Bookheimer SY, Strojwas MH, Cohen MS, Saunders AM, Pericak–Vance MA, Mazziotta JC, *et al.* Patterns of brain activation in people at risk for Alzheimer's disease. *N Engl J Med* 2000;**343**(7):450–6.

82. Smith KA, Ploghaus A, Cowen PJ, McCleery JM, Goodwin GM, Smith S, *et al.* Cerebellar responses during anticipation of noxious stimuli in subjects recovered from depression. Functional magnetic resonance imaging study. *Br J Psychiatry* 2002;**181**:411–5.

83. Callicott JH, Weinberger DR. Neuropsychiatric dynamics: the study of mental illness using functional magnetic resonance imaging. *Eur J Radiol* 1999;**30**(2):95–104.

84. Salmeron BJ, Stein EA. Pharmacological applications of magnetic resonance imaging. *Psychopharmacol Bull* 2002;**36**(1):102–29.

85. Willson MC, Wilman AH, Bell EC, Asghar SJ, Silverstone PH. Dextroamphetamine causes a change in regional brain activity in vivo during cognitive tasks: a functional magnetic resonance imaging study of blood oxygen level-dependent response. *Biological Psychiatry* 2004;**56**(4):284–91.

86. Borras MC, Becerra L, Ploghaus A, Gostic JM, DaSilva A, Gonzalez RG, *et al.* FMRI measurement of CNS responses to naloxone infusion and subsequent mild noxious thermal stimuli in healthy volunteers. *Journal of Neurophysiology* 2004;**91**(6):2723–33.

87. Leslie RA, James MF. Pharmacological magnetic resonance imaging: a new application for functional MRI. *Trends in Pharmacological Sciences* 2000;**21**(8):314–8.

88. Edelstein WA, Glover GH, Hardy CJ, Redington RW. The intrinsic signal-to-noise ratio in NMR imaging. *Magn Reson Med* 1986;**3**(4):604–18.

89. Jezzard P, Turner R. Magnetic resonance imaging methods for study of human brain function and their application at high magnetic field. *Comput Med Imaging Graph* 1996;**20**(6):467–81.

90. Turner R, Jezzard P, Wen H, Kwong KK, Le BD, Zeffiro T, *et al.* Functional mapping of the human visual cortex at 4 and 1.5 tesla using deoxygenation contrast EPI. *Magn Reson Med* 1993;**29**(2):277–9.

91. Sodickson DK, Manning WJ. Simultaneous acquisition of spatial harmonics (SMASH): fast imaging with radiofrequency coil arrays. *Magn Reson Med* 1997;**38**(4):591–603.

92. Pruessmann KP, Weiger M, Scheidegger MB, Boesiger P. SENSE: sensitivity encoding for fast MRI. *Magn Reson Med* 1999;**42**(5):952–62.

93. Epstein CM, Figiel GS, McDonald WM, Mazon–Leece J, Figiel L. Rapid rate transcranial magnetic stimulation in young and middle-aged refractory depressed patients. *Psychiatric Annals* 1998;**28**(1):36–9.

94. Krings T, Chiappa KH, Foltys H, Reinges MHT, Cosgrove GR, Thron A. Introducing navigated transcranial magnetic stimulation as a refined brain mapping methodology. *Neurosurgical Review* 2001;**24**(4):171–9.

95. Rutten GJM, Ramsey NF, van Rijen PC, Franssen H, van Veelen CWM. Interhemispheric reorganization of motor hand function to the primary motor cortex predicted with functional magnetic resonance imaging and transcranial magnetic stimulation. *Journal of Child Neurology* 2002;**17**(4):292–7.

96. Lebihan D. Diffusion, perfusion and functional magnetic resonance imaging. *Journal des Maladies Vasculaires* 1995;**20**(3):209–14.

97. Basser PJ, Pierpaoli C. Microstructural and physiological features of tissues elucidated by quantitative-diffusion-tensor MRI. *Journal of Magnetic Resonance Series B* 1996;**111**(3): 209–19.

98. Wakana S, Jiang HY, Nagae–Poetscher LM, van Zijl PCM, Mori S. Fiber tract-based atlas of human white matter anatomy. *Radiology* 2004;**230**(1):77–87.

99. Lebihan D, Breton E, Lallemand D, Grenier P, Cabanis E, Lavaljeantet M. MR imaging of intravoxel incoherent motions — application to diffusion and perfusion in neurologic disorders. *Radiology* 1986;**161**(2):401–7.

100. Moseley ME, Cohen Y, Kucharczyk J, Mintorovitch J, Asgari HS, Wendland MF, *et al.* Diffusion-weighted MR imaging of anisotropic water diffusion in cat central nervous system. *Radiology* 1990;**176**(2):439–45.

101. Pierpaoli C, Jezzard P, Basser PJ, Barnett A, DiChiro G. Diffusion tensor MR imaging of the human brain. *Radiology* 1996;**201**(3):637–48.

102. Basser PJ, Pierpaoli C. A simplified method to measure the diffusion tensor from seven MR images. *Magnetic Resonance in Medicine* 1998;**39**(6):928–34.

103. Mori S, Crain BJ, Chacko VP, van Zijl PCM. Three-dimensional tracking of axonal projections in the brain by magnetic resonance imaging. *Annals of Neurology* 1999;**45**(2):265–9.

104. Basser PJ, Pajevic S, Pierpaoli C, Duda J, Aldroubi A. In vivo fiber tractography using DT-MRI data. *Magnetic Resonance in Medicine* 2000;**44**(4):625–32.

105. Mori S, Kaufmann WE, Davatzikos C, Stieltjes B, Amodei L, Fredericksen K, *et al.* Imaging cortical association using diffusion-tensor-based tracts in the human brain axonal tracking. *Magnetic Resonance in Medicine* 2002;**47**(2):215–23.

106. Thomas B, Eyssen M, Peeters RR, Molenaers G, Van Hecke P, De Cock P, *et al.* Quantitative diffusion tensor imaging in cerebral palsy due to periventricular white matter injury. *Brain* 2005; in press.

107. Catani M, Jones DK, Ffytche DH. Perisylvian language networks of the human brain. *Annals of Neurology* 2005;**57**(1):8–16.

108. Ulmer JL, Salvan CV, Mueller WM, Krouwer HG, Stroe GO, Aralasmak A, *et al.* The role of diffusion tensor imaging in establishing the proximity of tumor borders to functional brain systems: implications for preoperative risk assessments and postoperative outcomes. *Technology in Cancer Research & Treatment* 2004;**3**(6):567–76.

109. Hendler T, Pianka P, Sigal M, Kafri M, Ben–Bashat D, Constantini S, *et al.* Delineating gray and white matter involvement in brain lesions: three-dimensional alignment of functional magnetic resonance and diffusion-tensor imaging. *Journal of Neurosurgery* 2003;**99**(6): 1018–27.

110. Wilms G, Demaerel P, Sunaert S. Intra-axial brain tumours. *European Radiology* 2005;**15**(3):468–84.

111. Parmar H, Sitoh YY, Yeo TT. Combined magnetic resonance tractography and functional magnetic resonance imaging in evaluation of brain tumors involving the motor system. *Journal of Computer Assisted Tomography* 2004;**28**(4):551–6.

112. De Ridder D, De Mulder G, Walsh V, Muggleton N, Sunaert S, Moller A. Magnetic and electrical stimulation of the auditory cortex for intractable tinnitus – case report. *Journal of Neurosurgery* 2004;**100**(3):560–4.

2

Preoperative assessment: motor function

Gunther Fesl and Tarek A. Yousry

1. Introduction

With the advent of FMRI, it was quickly recognized that a new tool might be available for the preoperative mapping of motor function. The motor system was extensively studied in both healthy volunteers and also in patients. The clear relationship between the activation of the primary motor cortex and the corresponding electrophysiological response even led to the use of intraoperative mapping as a method to validate motor FMRI. Today, preoperative motor FMRI seems to be the major clinical application of a method that has become an indispensable tool of research.

2. The motor system

2.1 Components and their anatomic location

Motor control is a complex organized process that involves several motor, sensory, and associative areas. Anatomically, the motor cortex, neocortical association areas, the basal ganglia, the cerebellum, the brainstem, and the spinal cord are involved.

The main cortical motor areas include the primary motor cortex (M1), the supplementary motor area (SMA), the presupplementary motor area (pre-SMA), the cingulate motor area (CMA), the premotor area (pre-MA) and the prefrontal cortex (PFC)[1]. The location of these areas is usually described using the Brodmann classification which subdivides the cortex into more than 40 areas using cytoarchitectonic criteria (Fig. 2.1).

2.1.1 The primary motor cortex (M1)

Part of the precentral gyrus (BA 4). M1 extends from the anterior part of the paracentral lobule on the medial surface, over the cerebral margin, and down the convexity along the crown and posterior face of the precentral gyrus. Its antero-posterior extent is broader superiorly and on the medial surface. From there, BA 4 tapers progressively downward toward the sylvian fissure. Just above the sylvian fissure and behind the inferior frontal gyrus, BA 4 becomes restricted to a narrow strip along the posterior face of the precentral gyrus, within the central sulcus[1] (Figs. 2.1 and 2.2).

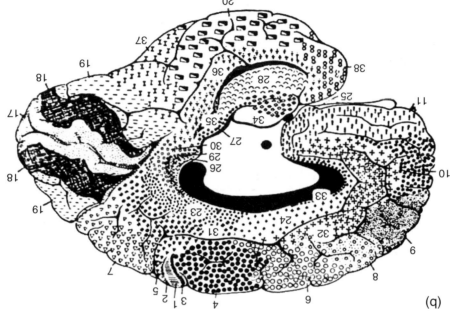

(b)

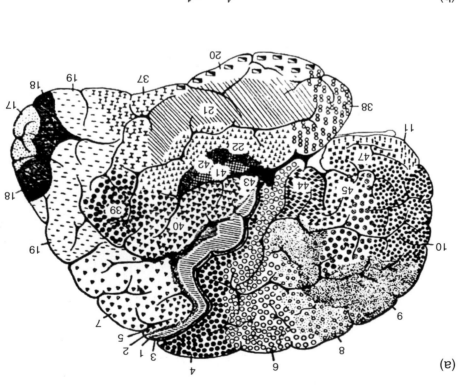

(a)

Fig. 2.1 Cytoarchitecture of the human cortex. Convexity (**a**) and medial (**b**) surface views of Brodmann's areas. Symbols indicate Brodmann's parcellation of the cortex into the cytoarchitectonic areas that are denoted by Brodmann's areas (BA) numbers[1].

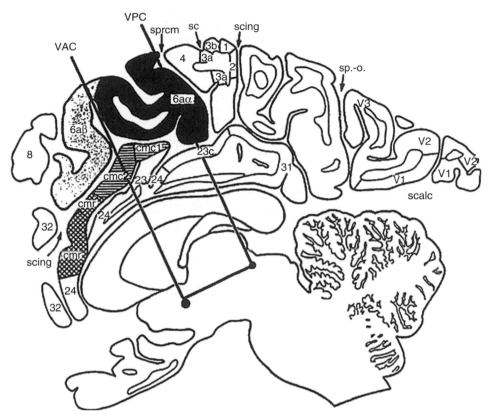

Fig. 2.2 Mesial motor areas (SMA, pre-SMA, and CMA) on the medial parasagittal plane, orientated with anterior to the reader's left (AC = anterior commissure; PC = posterior commissure). The VAC and VPC are the vertical lines erected to the AC–PC line at AC (VAC) and PC (VPC)[1,2]. The cytoarchitectonic areas are numbered after Brodmann and Vogt[1,3,4]. Black areas show the position of the SMA on the medial surface of the hemisphere; grey shows the position of the pre-SMA; cross-hatching indicates the rostral portion of the cingulate motor area (cmr); whereas the horizontal lines show the caudal portion of the cingulate motor area (cmc), itself divided into parts one and two (scing = cingulate sulcus; sc = central sulcus; sprcm = medial precentral sulcus; sp-o = parietal occipital sulcus; scalc = calcarine sulcus; V1–V3 are the visual cortical areas).

2.1.2 The supplementary motor area (SMA)

(Synonyms: SMA proper, caudal SMA, posterior SMA, M2, F3.) Is situated on the medial surface of the hemisphere in the paracentral lobule and posterior portion of the superior (medial) frontal gyrus (BA 6a alpha, medial). Its specific site varies among individuals but it is typically found in relation to the medial precentral sulcus. Zilles *et al.* reports that the SMA is located between two vertical planes perpendicular to the anterior commissure-posterior commissure (AC-PC) line, one vertical at the anterior commissure (VAC) and the other vertical at the posterior commissure (VPC)[2] (Figs. 2.1 and 2.2). Anatomically, the SMA is bordered anteriorly by the pre-SMA, posteriorly by the primary motor cortex, laterally by the premotor cortex on the convexity, and ventrally (inferiorly) by the posterior CMA[1].

2.1.3 The pre-supplementary motor area (pre-SMA)

(Synonyms: rostral SMA, anterior SMA, F3, supplementary negative area). Lies along the medial face of the superior (medial) frontal gyrus just anterior to the SMA (BA 6a beta, medial). It shows individual variability. According to Zilles *et al.*, it lies predominantly anterior to VAC. The pre-SMA borders posteriorly on the SMA, laterally on the anterior portion of the premotor cortex on the convexity, and ventrally (inferiorly) on the anterior cingulate motor area[1] (Figs. 2.1 and 2.2).

2.1.4 The cingulate motor area (CMA)

Composed of two portions: a rostral CMA (cmr) and a caudal CMA (cmc). These appear to correspond to the functionally defined anterior cingulate motor area (cmr) and posterior cingulate area (cmc). The CMA corresponds to BA 24c and BA 24d (and perhaps to the posterior portion of BA 32, BA 32 of Vogt[3,4]. The CMA lies in the superior (dorsal) and inferior (ventral) banks of the cingulate sulcus. The cmr lies entirely rostral to VAC. The cmc flanks VAC but lies entirely anterior to the VPC[1] (Figs. 2.1 and 2.2).

2.1.5 The premotor area (pre-MA)

(Synonym M2). Extends along the frontal convexity to occupy contiguous portions of the superior frontal gyrus, the middle frontal gyrus, and the precentral gyrus (BA 6a alpha (convexity), BA 6a beta (convexity) and BA 6b). The dorsal pre-MA lies within the posterior portions of the superior and middle frontal gyri. The ventral pre-MA occupies the anterior face and part of the crown of the precentral gyrus anterior to the primary motor area (M1). Like M1, the ventral portion of pre-MA progressively tapers inferiorly. An additional small area, BA6b, lies further inferiorly, superior to the sylvian fissure and anterior to the motor face area[1] (Figs. 2.1 and 2.2).

2.1.6 The prefrontal cortex (PFC)

Is situated anterior to the pre-MA (BA 9, 10, and 46). The PFC lies along the frontal convexity in the superior and middle frontal gyri and extends onto the medial surface of the frontal lobe along the superior (medial) frontal gyrus[1] (Fig. 2.1).

2.2 Function

2.2.1 Hierarchy and parallelism

The motor cortices exhibit dual features, some hierarchical and some parallel.

Hierarchical model The right dorsolateral PFC (BA 9, 46) is involved in the decision of what to do and when to do it. The pre-SMA is concerned with selection of and preparation for the specific movements required. The SMA proper plays a role in the initiation of and the correct performance of the movements, especially internally generated, self-initiated movements without external cues, and M1 signals the correct sets of motor neurons in the cord. In such hierarchy, the PFC projects to all premotor areas. The SMA and CMA project to the pre-MA and M1[1].

Distributed multiparallel model Here, the ventral pre-MA, SMA, and CMA may all project directly to M1, as well as to each other. The pre-SMA, however, is not regarded as projecting directly to M1. Instead it projects to M1 only, indirectly through the SMA or the CMA.

Dum and Strick studied the multiparallel aspect of motor processing for the cervical cord in monkeys by injecting retrograde tracers into the cord[5]. They found that direct corticospinal neurons passed to the cervical cord from M1, the pre-MA, the SMA, and the anterior and posterior CMA (cmr and cmc). These are the same areas that also send projection fibres to M1. The total number of direct corticospinal neurons to the arm from all non-M1 areas equalled or exceeded the number from M1 itself[1].

2.2.2 Cortical somatotopy

Besides the fine somatotopy in the primary motor cortex (BA4) (see next chapter), a cruder somatotopy is found in the SMA, the pre-SMA, and in the cingulate motor cortex[1,6]. Cortical zones seem to correspond to broad regions, such as head, trunk, upper and lower extremities, rather than to individual motion units.

2.2.3 Assessment with FMRI

As mentioned earlier, the motor system was one of the first systems to be studied by FMRI[7–10]. Several studies investigated the influence of different modulators like task complexity, frequency, force, handedness, habituation, and learning on the magnitude of signal change, activation size, or activation pattern[11–19]. This understanding is important when designing a paradigm, especially in the context of clinical use. However, even with well-controlled, simple movements, the whole network of cortical motor areas can be displayed[20]. The contribution of the different areas may, therefore, be more quantitative in nature rather than exclusively specific to a certain aspect of motor behaviour.

Although the whole motor system must be considered as one functional unit, lesions in the primary motor cortex lead to serious and long-lasting paresis, whereas lesions in other cortical motor areas often cause weak and transient symptoms[21,22]. For these reasons, the primary objective of preoperative FMRI is the identification of M1.

3. The primary motor cortex

3.1 The central region (M1)

The central region is composed of the precentral gyrus (PreCG) anteriorly, postcentral gyrus (PostCG) posteriorly, subcentral gyrus (SubCG) inferiorly, and the paracentral lobule superiorly, all arrayed around the central sulcus (Rolandic sulcus)[23]. Classically, the central sulcus (CS) is divided into three genua (knees)[23–25]. The superior genu lies along the medial segment of the central sulcus and has its convexity directed anteriorly. The middle genu lies lateral to the superior genu, has its convexity directed posteriorly, and corresponds to the motor hand knob[26]. The inferior genu of the CS is the next curve found along the lateral surface and has its convexity directed anteriorly. The segment of the CS situated inferolateral to the inferior genu has been described as being nearly straight[27].

However, in a recent study, the CS of only 3% hemispheres showed the 'classic' straight course. In the great majority of hemispheres (97%), the CS had between two and four additional curves, with two additional curves being the most frequent pattern (69%)[28].

3.2 Localization of M1

As detailed above (2.1), M1 extends from the anterior part of the paracentral lobule on the medial surface, down the convexity, along the crown and posterior face of the precentral gyrus[1]. BA 4 is known to cover the surface of the anterior bank of the central sulcus medially with a gradient decreasing from medial to lateral[29]. However, the exact borders of the primary motor cortex cannot be determined macroanatomically because the borders of BA 4 show considerable variation[30]. This might explain the occurrence of motor activation in the posterior bank of the central sulcus. Furthermore, BA 4 is not homogeneous but can be subdivided into an area BA 4 a (anterior) and BA 4 p (posterior). This subdivision is based on differences in the cytoarchitecture, quantitative distributions of transmitter binding sites, and function[31].

3.3 Anatomical landmarks for identification

Various anatomical and functional methods have been developed to assist with the identification of the central sulcus. The anatomical methods can be subdivided into those relying on deep and those relying on superficial landmarks[32–38]. Deep landmarks such as the anterior and posterior commissure (AC-PC) were used to construct a coordinate system, which permits the assignment of anatomical structures like the central sulcus to specific coordinates, allowing its identification in all three planes[38]. This method was initially developed for stereotactic purposes and is especially useful for targeting deep structures such as the thalamic nuclei. Its reliability, however, decreases with increasing distance from the centre towards the periphery. Its reliability in identifying the central sulcus is, therefore, limited[39]. Superficial landmarks can be divided into direct landmarks located in the central region, or indirect landmarks, which have a specific relationship with components of the central region (Fig. 2.3).

Several methods have been described in the axial plane; the following are the most useful (see also Fig. 2.3):

a) **The knob**: the motor hand area is located on a specific protrusion of the precentral gyrus (knob, inverted omega, or horizontal epsilon), which is found at the middle genu of the central sulcus opposite to the intersection of the superior frontal sulcus and the precentral sulcus. The characteristic shape of this protrusion is the single most useful sign to directly identify the central sulcus. Although of less typical shape on the surface, the middle genu has been shown to be also a useful landmark in neurosurgery.

b) **The lateral axial method**: the superior frontal sulcus meets the precentral sulcus in a near right angle. The sulcus behind is the central sulcus[37].

c) **The medial axial method**: the ramus marginalis of the sulcus cinguli forms a 'bracket' with the ramus of the opposite hemisphere ('bracket sign'). The central sulcus is the sulcus which enters the bracket anteriorly[40].

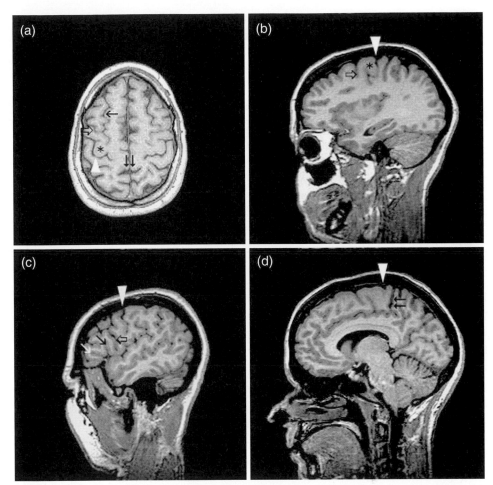

Fig. 2.3 Anatomical landmarks for the identification of the central sulcus demonstrated on axial (**a**) and sagittal (**b**, **c**, and **d**) MPRAGE reconstructions. The central sulcus is indicated by the white arrowhead in images a, b, c, and d. The asterisk marks the motor hand area, a typical omega shaped protrusion (knob) in the upper precentral gyrus (a) appearing as a posteriorly directed hook in the sagittal plane (b). The lateral and medial axial method can be reproduced on image a, the lateral and medial sagittal methods are demonstrated with image c and d. (Transparent arrow = precentral sulcus; horizontal black arrow = superior frontal sulcus; parallel black arrows = marginal ramus of the cingulate sulcus; oblique white arrow = anterior horizontal ramus of the sylvian fissure; oblique black arrow = anterior ascending ramus of the sylvian fissure).

d) **The white matter pattern**: the white matter can be divided into six sections at the level of the centrum semiovale (superior frontal gyrus, medial frontal gyrus, precentral gyrus, postcentral gyrus, inferior parietal lobule, and precuneus), in order to locate the accompanied cortical structures [32].

In the sagittal plane, three methods have been described (see Fig. 2.3):

a) **The medial sagittal method**: the ramus marginalis of the sulcus cinguli can be easily identified as postero-superior continuation of the cingulate sulcus. The central sulcus forms a small indentation into the paracentral lobule anterior to the ramus[36].

b) **The hook**: the motor hand area (knob in the axial plane) has the appearance of a posteriorly directed hook. This hook is found on the section that displays the insula.

c) **Lateral sagittal method**: the anterior horizontal ramus and the anterior ascending ramus of the sylvian fissure are identified. The precentral sulcus lies behind, followed by the central sulcus[33].

3.4. M1 somatotopy

Functionally, the primary motor and primary somatosensory areas are organized somatotopically. The term 'somatotopy' refers to the topographic organization of function along the cortex. It is a map of the sites at which smaller or larger regions of cortex form functional units that correspond to body parts or to motions across a joint [1]. Classically, the somatotopy of M1 is given by the motor homunculus[41,42]. The homunculus was verified with various brain mapping techniques including cortical stimulation, evoked potentials, PET, MEG, TMS, and also FMRI[42–53].

In several studies, functional MRI showed its potential to accurately map primary motor function and to verify the homunculus along the precentral gyrus (e.g. [54–56]) (Fig. 2.4). Even small-scale somatotopical organization of finger-specific activation was described[57,58].

The locations of the somatotopical regions have been well demonstrated with respect to each other (relative position), but poorly defined in absolute position. Thus far, only the hand motor area has been shown to map to a characteristic protuberance of the posterior face of the precentral gyrus (the motor hand knob)[26]. The primary motor tongue area is known to lie close to the sylvian fissure, but no specific cortical anatomical configuration defines the site of the primary motor tongue area (MTA). However, its position can be approximated by the intersection between the central sulcus and the cella media of the lateral ventricles[28]. The primary motor foot area is known to lie close to the 'mantelkante' in the paracentral lobule.

4. Preoperative FMRI in Rolandic tumours

4.1 Preoperative identification of the motor cortex

4.1.1 Indication and limitation of anatomical landmarks

The management of tumours located in the central region is dependant on their exact relationship with the functional anatomy of the motor system. A location of the primary motor function adjacent to or even within the tumour would lead to conservative management.

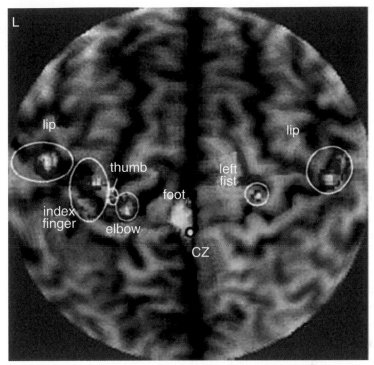

Fig. 2.4 FMRI evaluation of somatotopic representation in human primary motor cortex examining foot, elbow, fist, thumb, index, finger, and lip movements. Combination of group analyses with SPM96 and ISOVIEW 2D evaluation of distances from CZ (coordinate of the intersection of the interhemispheric fissure and the central sulcus) to the activation maxima in the contralateral precentral sulcus[55].

A separation of tumour and functional cortex, on the other hand, opens the window to more active intervention which aims at combining radical treatment with preservation of function. It is, therefore, important to determine, preoperatively, the relationship between tumour and motor function. This relationship can be assessed directly by localizing the functional areas themselves or, indirectly, by identifying those anatomical structures that have a stable and constant relationship with these functional areas, the precentral gyrus and the postcentral gyrus.

The identification of these anatomical structures was for decades at the centre of preoperative planning. All neuroradiological methods available at the time (such as radiography, ventriculography, and angiography) were used to that purpose. The advent of cross-sectional imaging (CT, MR) changed the situation by allowing, for the first time, the non-invasive direct evaluation of cerebral structures. Methods were therefore developed to enable a reliable identification of the central region, first in the axial plane and, later, with the advent of MR, in the sagittal plane (see Section 3.3). The successful use of these methods is based on the stability of the anatomical relationships of the structures of the central region.

However, these anatomical methods have their limitations. The anatomical relationships can be distorted by a tumour, making the use of any anatomical landmark impossible.

Furthermore, as the anatomical structures are surrogate markers for the functional areas, anatomical methods cannot assess the change of the relationship between anatomical structure and the function usually residing in it. Such a change can, for instance, be induced by a slow-growing tumour. To address the limitations of the anatomical methods, it was important to introduce functional methods into the preoperative planning procedures, namely PET and FMRI.

4.1.2 FMRI and other functional methods

Functional methods such as SPECT, PET, TMS, MEG, and FMRI have all been used to identify the central region. The main advantages of FMRI in comparison to the other methods are its non-invasiveness, its capability of providing anatomical and functional information, and its ubiquity. In addition, MRI provides exquisite information on the morphology and location of lesions.

FMRI based on the BOLD effect does not require contrast, can be repeated immediately, and for several times. The functional information obtained through FMRI covers the whole brain and all cortical regions including the depth of the sulci. FMRI is also characterized by high spatial resolution and a reasonable temporal resolution that currently meets the needs of preoperative localization of function. Although mainly performed at a field strength of 1.5T, it can also be performed at 1.0T[59–61]. The new generation of MR scanners offers specific analysis programs that allow a fast display of FMRI results and could make user-dependent off-line processing unnecessary. Although some of these programs await validation, their development clearly indicates the progress towards the technical feasibility of performing FMRI in a clinical context.

The various functional methods, however, reflect different physiological mechanisms. A direct comparison between these methods is, therefore, difficult. A validation of one functional method by another one is only meaningful in a specifically defined context.

In the context of preoperative assessment of the motor cortex, intraoperative electrical corticography (ECC) was seen as the gold standard. The fundamental difference between FMRI and ECC is that the first detects areas activated by a specific function, whereas the latter detects the areas which, when externally activated, affect a specific function. From a neurosurgical point of view, however, the question that needs to be answered is the location of the primary motor sensory cortex and, in that respect, both methods can be compared with each other.

Many studies have compared the results obtained through the two methods, FMRI and ECC. All described a good agreement between these techniques[62–69] (Fig. 2.5), though it should be taken into account that the accuracy of ECC is reported to be around 10mm[70]. This agreement between FMRI and ECC was defined either with respect to the location of the activated area or the location of the central sulcus. When comparing the location of the activated area, a good agreement was defined to be present when the activation was located on the same gyrus[63], within the same gyrus[65], or when measurements showed that the difference between the two methods was not significant[71]. An overlap of up to 2cm between the two methods was found in between 63% and 100%[72–76]. The areas activated by FMRI, however, were found to be larger than those identified by ECC[73,77] (Fig. 2.6).

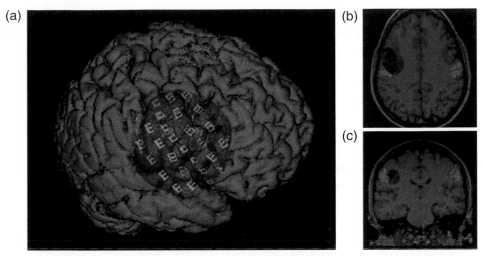

Fig. 2.5 Thirty-year-old female patient suffering from an astrocytoma grade III in the right frontal lobe. (**a**) Overlay of the intraoperative photograph onto the 3D surface reconstruction of the patient's brain. (**b, c**) The ipsilateral primary motor tongue area assessed by FMRI is adjacent to the posterior border of the tumor. (**a**) DCC led to a speech arrest at stimulation point 22, 23, and 26, demonstrating a good agreement between FMRI and DCC results.

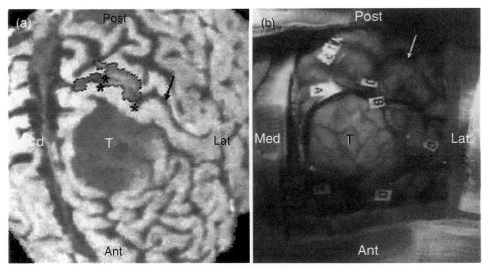

Fig. 2.6 Correspondence between FMR images and cortical stimulation using intraoperative photographs. (**a**) Surface rendering of the cortex obtained in a patient with a left premotor low-grade glioma who was performing hand movement. The activated area is projected on the surface of the cortex in red around the central sulcus *(arrow,* both panels). (**b**) Intraoperative view of the same patient obtained in the same orientation as that shown in a. Letters outline the tumour margins. Numerals correspond to the sites of stimulation that elicited hand movements. The positive sites are labelled in a by asterisks. (Ant = anterior; Lat = lateral; Med = medial; Post = posterior; T = tumour)[73].

Interestingly, no false positive or false negative FMRI activations were reported[77]. Both FMRI and ECC were equally successful in identifying the central sulcus[78,79].

A methodological problem in these direct comparisons is the transfer of data obtained through ECC onto an MR image with the FMRI data. This problem has now been addressed through the use of navigation systems. ECC coordinates can be co-registered into the virtual space of the navigation system, thereby allowing direct quantitative comparisons with FMRI data[70] with an application of 2–3mm 'under good conditions' and up to 7mm 'following a bad registration'[80]. More relevant, from a neurosurgical point of view however, is the ability to co-register FMRI data into the virtual space, which is the precondition to the use of FMRI data not only for preoperative management but also intraoperatively.

4.1.3 PET

PET examination for assessing function of the somatosensory system is performed either using 15-O H_2O PET to assess the perfusion or using FDG PET to assess the metabolism. The advantage of the former is its superior temporal resolution, whereas the advantages of the latter are the superior signal-to-noise ratio, the independence from a cyclotrone, and the option of co-investigating the tumour's metabolism[81,82]. The studies which compared PET data with invasive mapping showed a good agreement between both methods[83–86]. The few studies that have compared data from PET data with those from FMRI also revealed a good agreement[87–91].

4.1.4 SPECT

SPECT assesses blood flow and has been used to identify functional areas, despite its comparatively poor temporal and spatial resolution[92]. The main advantage of SPECT seems to lie in its comparatively lower costs[93].

4.1.5 MEG and EEG

EEG can directly measure the cortical electrical activity, whereas MEG assesses this activity indirectly by measuring the induced magnetic field. The major advantage of both methods is their excellent temporal resolution[94]. Using complex 'dipole source' algorithms, the origin of the activation is projected onto point source, which does not allow the assessment of the volume of the activated cortex. Comparative studies of motor function between FMRI and MEG showed a difference of up to 10mm. This discrepancy was explained by the different physiological mechanisms assessed by each of these methods[95,96].

It was shown, however, that both FMRI and EEG can reliably identify the central sulcus preoperatively[97] and that MEG and SSEP completely concur on the identification of the central sulcus[98]. MEG can, therefore, be used as a tool to assist in the preoperative decision making process[99,100].

4.1.6 TMS

Transcranial magnetic stimulation (TMS) is a direct, simple, non-invasive, cost-effective tool which can reliably assess motor function[53,101–106]. The best mapping accuracy which may be obtained with TMS is about 0.5cm[75].

4.1.7 Multimodal comparisons

Assessing the motor hand and motor foot areas, Krings *et al.* compared the value of FMRI, FDG PET, TMS, and ECC. An excellent overlap was found between FMRI and the other methods. Only in one patient did FMRI and PET yield different results, but ECC confirmed the FMRI results[75] (Fig. 2.7). Similar results were obtained by other studies comparing FMRI with FDG PET or H_2O PET and ECC[81,107].

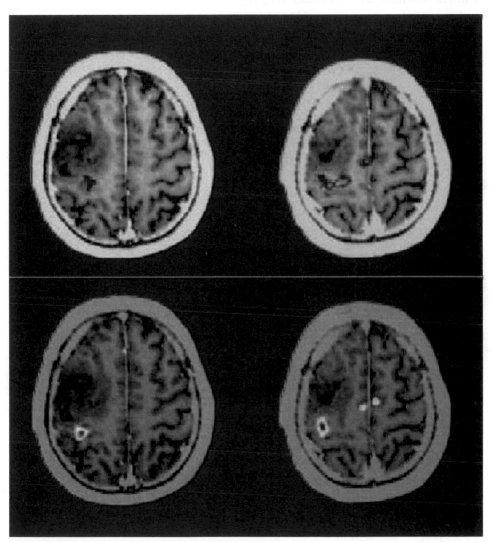

Fig. 2.7 Comparison of FMRI and PET finger tapping results of the left hand (upper row: FMRI; lower row: PET). In this patient with a mild paresis of his left upper limb, activation is seen in the primary motor cortex and the supplementary motor area in both modalities in exactly matching cortical regions[75].

4.1.8 Clinical use

The main use of FMRI in the context of surgery in the central and peri-central region is the identification of the primary motor cortex. There is general agreement that FMRI is a reliable tool in identifying the central sulcus and the primary motor sensory cortex in healthy volunteers, as well as in patients with distorted anatomy caused by various pathologies such as arachnoid cysts or intra- or extra-axial tumours (e.g. [62–66, 68–70,72,73,78,79,108–126]).

In an attempt to assess the clinical impact of FMRI on the management of patients with tumours, Lee *at al.* found that FMRI had an influence on the decision of the feasibility of surgery in 55%, on the decision of selecting patients for non-invasive mapping in 78%, and on the planning of the procedure in 22% of patients with tumours. From this, they determined the therapeutic efficacy to be 89%[112].

Not surprisingly, the chances of a postoperative deficit were found to increase with the decreased distance between tumour margin and the area of activation. A distance of more than 2cm was considered to be safe (0% deficit); a distance of 1–2cm was associated with a deficit in 33%; and a distance of 1cm or less was associated with a deficit of 50%[127]. A different study found a distance of 5mm between tumour margin and activation to be a 'significant predictor' of a postoperative deficit and recommended an ECC if the distance was below 10 mm and to 'completely' resect the tumour if the distance was more than 10mm[119].

It should be noted that motor cortical activation was found adjacent to the tumours[65,109,115,117] as well as within the tumour[73,128], which underlines the role of FMRI in determining the feasibility of surgery.

The successful identification of the central sulcus and precentral gyrus is reported to range from 89% to 100% in technically successful studies[64,129] using FMRI. It should be noted, however, that a motor paradigm can lead to an activation in the precentral gyrus, pre- and postcentral gyrus, or only the postcentral gyrus. The postcentral activation is to be expected as any motor paradigm also activates the sensory system. It has also been shown that sulcal 'activation' can be found in a vein in the central sulcus[130]. Such 'activation' is very useful for the purpose of identification of the CS.

In a different approach, FMRI was used to assess the relationship between anatomical structures and their functional role. This led to the identification of a functional anatomical landmark — the motor hand area (hand knob) in the precentral gyrus. The stability of the functional anatomical relationship of this structure was the basis for the description of a new landmark. Although this landmark was identified through FMRI, it is now used without it as it has become the most important landmark in identifying the central region.

The question whether FMRI can replace ECC is not resolved yet. FMRI can provide reliable information for the location of the motor sensory cortex and of the central region. ECC has, however, the advantage of providing functional information intraoperatively. Advances in neuronavigation and the possibility of performing intraoperative FMRI could address this issue.

In addition to the information mentioned above on the anatomical location of function, FMRI can provide information on the changes associated with the presence of a space-occupying lesion. Depending on the lesion size and location, different patterns of activation

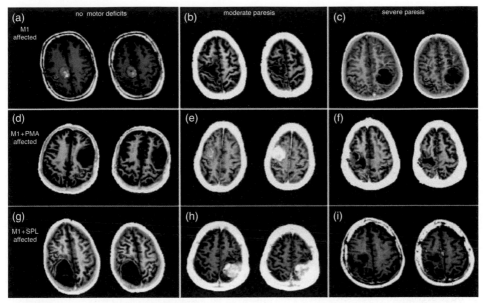

Fig. 2.8 Examples for nine different subgroups of patients (lesions affecting M1, M1 and PMA, M1 and SPL, with three different degrees of paresis each). Patients without motor deficits present with a strong activation within the primary motor cortex, whereas secondary motor areas do not show activity (**a**), (**d**), and (**g**). Both patients with moderate (**b**), (**e**), and (**h**) and severe (**c**), (**f**), and (**i**) paresis have additional activity in SMA and, depending on the lesion location, also in PMA and SPL. Activation in primary motor cortex decreases with increasing degree of paresis[133].

were observed. These can encompass a decrease in perlesional activation[74,115,131], a shift from primary to secondary motor areas[74,128,132,133], or a shift to homologous areas of the unaffected hemisphere[114].

It was also shown that an increase in the grade of paresis was associated with a decrease in the perilesional activation and an increase in the activation of secondary motor areas[133] (Fig. 2.8).

It should be noted that the absence of activation does not signify the absence of functional cortex. It was shown using FMRI and ECC that preoperatively absent activation in the primary motor cortex can return, described as a 'sudden unmasking', after tumour resection[134,135].

4.2 Methodology

4.2.1 Prerequisites for the clinical use of FMRI

Preoperative FMRI should enable a quick and reliable localization of function. The clinical use of FMRI has to be simple in its set-up and paradigms and has to be fast in its analysis. The combination of user friendly automatization of the various procedural steps and the adequate training of staff will help the performance of FMRI studies as a routine procedure. Furthermore, integration of the FMRI data into a neuronavigation system will allow the intraoperative use of data[118,136,137].

4.2.2 MR scanner, FMRI signal and sequence

High-field MR scanners with powerful gradient systems are prerequisites for the application of FMRI. However, with 1.0T and conventional gradient systems, good results were also obtained.[59–61] Scanners at 1.5T are nevertheless the standard at which most of the clinical FMRI studies are currently performed and the added value of 3T scanners in the clinical set-up is still to be shown.

Three different factors affect the FMRI signal —the change of the local cerebral blood flow, the local cerebral blood volume, and the relative share of oxyhaemoglobin and deoxyhaemoglobin in the capillary and venous blood[138].

Different FMRI techniques either measure different factors or different proportions of the previously mentioned factors. The BOLD technique enables the detection of local alterations of the oxyhaemoglobin:deoxyhaemoglobin ratio which is affected by the local cerebral blood flow and blood volume[10, 139–141].The arterial spin labelling (ASL) technique measures alterations of the cerebral blood flow[142, 143], and MR perfusion assesses both cerebral blood flow and cerebral blood volume[144–146].

Among the various functional MR techniques, the BOLD technique emerged as the main FMRI technique. It is a non-invasive technique which, in contrast to MR perfusion, does not require the administration of a contrast agent[147]. Furthermore, the signal-to-noise ratio of the BOLD technique is higher than that of the ASL technique, thereby offsetting the capability of ASL to detect a 35–38% difference in signal intensity between rest and activity[147] (compared to only 1–5% for BOLD)[147, 148]. Moreover, the temporal resolution of the ASL is limited by the time the tagged blood needs to enter the imaging slices and is, therefore, inferior to the temporal resolution of the BOLD technique[138].

The BOLD effect itself can be assessed with spin echo (SE) or with gradient echo (GE) sequences[149]. Initially, FLASH (fast low angle shot) GE sequences were used, which allowed only a limited coverage of the head and a limited temporal resolution. Echo planar imaging (EPI), however, allowed a higher temporal resolution combined with complete coverage of the head, albeit with reduced spatial resolution. FLASH GE sequences were, therefore, replaced by EPI GE sequences[59]. While voxel sizes of about 4*4*4 mm were sufficient for some time, a higher spatial resolution has been increasingly demanded for clinical applications[150]. The limiting factor of increasing spatial resolution is the deterioration of the signal-to-noise ratio.

Although GE EPI sequences are clearly more sensitive than the SE EPI sequences in the detection of the BOLD effect[151], they are more sensitive to susceptibility effects, thereby leading to stronger distortions and more border artefacts.

The selection of the sequence (independent of local hardware and software prerequisites) is, therefore, a compromise between BOLD signal harvest, spatial resolution, temporal resolution, examination time, signal-to-noise ratio, and acceptable artefacts.

4.2.3 Task design

FMRI using the BOLD technique is currently based on assessing local signal intensity changes. At least two different conditions which can be compared are therefore required. To perform this comparison, two different experimental designs are available for the examination of simple motor tasks. These are the block design and the event-related design.

Block design During continuous image acquisition, different conditions are repeated in predefined time blocks. For the examination of primary motor function, this usually means the performance of a certain movement during active blocks vs. absolute rest during the control blocks. These blocks can either alternate (ABABAB) or be performed consecutively (AAABBB). Better results are gained with the alternating design[152]. Times of 14 to 60 seconds have been reported to be the optimum for one block length[70,109,114,153]. This enables the assessment of multiple scans during the plateau phase of a condition.

Block design results reflect a sum activation of all active phases vs. rest with high statistical power.

Event-related design Event-related designs allow the examination of activation caused by single events but the statistical power is inferior and the experimental set-up is more demanding (compared to block designs)[154–156].

Marquart *et al.* compared single-event designs and block trials for simple motor tasks. They found that for the tongue and the toe movement tasks, which may produce some head motion artefacts, the single-event paradigm provides a useful alternative to the block-design method for identifying the sensorimotor cortex or SMA. However, it does not achieve a greater percentage of activation within primary motor areas. For the finger movement task, which does not usually produce head motion artefacts, the block-design method generally produced a greater percentage of activated pixels in the sensorimotor cortex or SMA than did the single-event method[157].

Reviewing the literature, we found that most of the research groups performing preoperative FMRI apply block designs (e.g. [62,64–66,69,73,77–79,93,109,112–115,117,123,150,158,159]). Standard paradigms for detecting the precentral gyrus are the examination of a finger or hand movement, often in combination with an examination of a foot, mouth, or tongue movement (e.g. [128]). Movements may be self paced or externally triggered by visual or acoustic stimuli. Self-paced movements result in higher activations compared with externally triggered movements[7]. Higher task complexity, frequency, and force also affects the pattern of activation[11,12,160]. Whereas simple fist clenching activates mainly the primary motor hand area of the contralateral hemisphere, finger tapping in a fixed sequence activates additional motor areas like the SMA, the ipsilateral M1 area, the premotor areas, the primary somatosensory areas, and the superior parietal areas. Increasing the task complexity also increases the activation of the contralateral superior parietal areas, the contralateral inferior parietal areas (to a lesser extent), and the ipsilateral superior parietal areas[7,11,161].

However, paradigms considered for clinical use should be as simple as possible. Complicated tasks may lead to poor compliance and useless results[162]. It is important to check the patient's ability to perform the task and to monitor the patient's performance of that task (visually or with response buttons)[111]. If no activation is detected, a repetition of the measurement may help to confirm absent activation. Additional examination of the non-affected side helps in assessing the difference in the level of activation between the affected and the non-affected hemisphere[111]. In the case of patients with severe paresis who are unable to perform a motor task or in the case of children, passive sensory stimuli can be used to detect the postcentral gyrus[163]. Alternatively, motor imagery can be used in adults to activate the central region[164,165].

In summary, reliable localization of motor function in rolandic tumours may be achieved with simple hand, foot, mouth, or tongue movements using the block-design approach. Different groups introduced time-optimized protocols[113,118]. These protocols may be used as models which can be adjusted according to the local hard and software environment.

4.2.4 Postprocessing

The acquired EPI scans may be converted first or may be exported directly to an external postprocessing computer. Several commercial or free postprocessing software packages are available (e.g. SPM: *http://www.fil.ion.ucl.ac.uk/spm/*; FSL: *http://www.FMRIb. ox.ac.uk/fsl/*; AFNI: *http://afni.nimh.nih.gov/afni/*; Brain Voyager: *www.brainvoyager.com*; MEDx: *medx.sensor.com*; Stimulate: *www.cmrr.umn.edu/stimulate/*; VoxBo: *www. voxbo.org*)[166–168] Some centres use their own 'homemade' software.

In this section, the most important postprocessing steps are presented:

Image registration and transformation Movement artefacts are caused by unintentional head movements, the physiological cyclic heart function, and respiration. Head movements cannot be avoided completely, even with foam pads or strips. They can cause false negative and false positive activations[169]. Motion correction which co-registers and reslices successive image volumes to a single reference volume is, therefore, the first step that has to precede any other postprocessing steps.

Smoothing The relative signal change detected with BOLD FMRI ranges between 1% and 5 % depending on the anatomical location and the technical equipment (hardware and software)[147,148]. Processes that improve the signal-to-noise ratio or the signal-to-artefact ratio such as smoothing (convolving the data with a Gaussian (smoothing) kernel) are, therefore, used. Temporal and spatial smoothing have the advantage of improving signal-to-noise ratios. However, spatial smoothing leads to a deterioration of image resolution[150,170,171]. The compromise between improving the SNR and loss of spatial information has to be made carefully.

Statistics As mentioned previously, several commercial and free postprocessing software programs exist[167,168,172,173]. Different statistical methods are implemented in these programs such as parametric tests (e.g. t-test, general linear model), nonparametric tests (e.g. Kolmogorov–Smirnov procedure, permutation, jack-knife and bootstrap techniques), and multivariate tests.

A complementary approach to hypothesis-driven analyses is data-driven analyses like the independent component analysis (ICA). It assumes that FMRI data can be modelled by identifying sets of voxels whose activity varies together over time and is maximally different from the activity in other sets[174].

A general recommendation cannot be made as there is no 'best statistic'. While it is indeed true that in a particular context some statistical procedures are better than others, it is nearly always the case that many different procedures apply equally well[175]. Besides the implemented statistics, other arguments like handling, automatization, postprocessing time, and data import and export features need also to be considered.

Data presentation The final postprocessing step is the presentation of the FMRI results. The degree of complexity of this step should be related to the aim of the study. If the aim is to identify the central sulcus preoperatively and take a decision on the indication for surgery or the need for intraoperative ECC, then a simple superimposition of the FMRI data on the anatomical image is sufficient. However, inaccurate superimpositions can result from differences in the geometric distortion between the various sequences used such as EPI (FMRI) and SE/FSE (anatomical images) and from signal losses due to small- and large-scale static field inhomogeneities in the EPI images. The degree of mislocalization can be estimated by presenting the FMRI results on the EPI source images. The obtained anatomical information is of course inferior, but matching mistakes can be avoided. The problem of distortion can also be addressed by using a specific sequence design such as a multi-echo reference scan which allows simultaneous correction of ghost and geometric distortion artefacts in EPI[176].

If the aim is to use the data for planning of the procedure, then a more elaborate presentation is required. Such a presentation could be a 3D reconstruction with the FMRI data and the tumour presented in different colours. Ideally, however, the data should be directly transferred into a neuronavigation system, thereby making the previously acquired data available intraoperatively[70,80,89,93,114,137,177–181] (Fig. 2.9).

4.3 Limitations

The previously described advantages of FMRI led to its widespread use especially in the context of the preoperative assessment of motor function. There are, however, some methodological problems, which restrict the power and the applicability of FMRI. These problems can lead to an inaccurate display of activation or to the detection of false negative or false positive activations and can, thereby, have serious clinical implications. If a real activation is not displayed (false negative), a resection of that area can cause a severe paresis. If false activation is displayed (false positive), the resection will be less radical than anticipated, which may have an effect on the tumour regrowth, although a substantial controversy surrounds this issue.

4.3.1 Movement artefacts and clinical status

Stimulus correlated movements can lead to false negative as well as to false positive activations[169,182]. The main reasons for failing to detect activation are unintentional head movement or a bad clinical status[65,70,79,112,115,129]. Krings *et al.* showed that both factors were related to each other, suggesting that a severe paresis makes movement artefacts more likely[183]. Movement artefacts are more frequently observed with tasks that activate proximal muscles than with tasks that activate distal muscles. But it should be noted that movement artefacts are not only the result of unintentional head movement but can also result from cyclic heart function and respiration[184]. While some FMRI groups inspect the serial EPI scans or plots of registration results for suspicious drifts before deciding whether a movement correction is necessary or not, other groups perform an automated

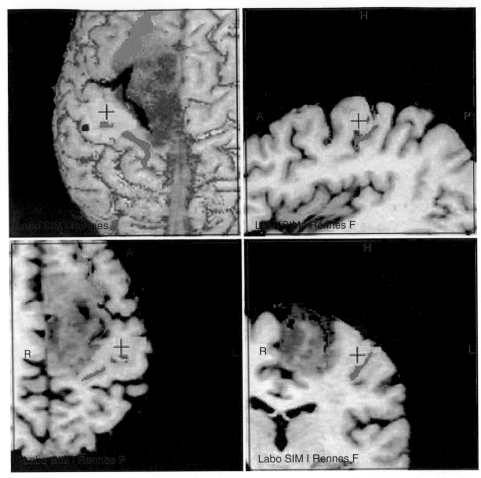

Fig. 2.9 View produced by SIM 3D software for planning stages, showing MR imaging. Overlay: sulcal and functional information for neuronavigation: (**a**) volume-rendered view and (**c**) axial, (**d**) coronal, and (**b**) sagittal sections intersecting at cursor location (red cross). Sulci: PFS (light blue), PrCS (dark blue), and CS (green). Functional imaging: motor FMR imaging (yellow), motor MEG (magenta), and somesthetic MEG (orange)[178].

movement correction in every case. However, it should be noted that 3D correction algorithms can result in signal decrease due to data interpolation.

4.3.2 Tumour and oedema

Although it has been shown that FMRI can detect activation in the vicinity of a tumour or within the tumour itself, the presence of a tumour as such can change or even suppress the FMRI activation. The degree to which the tumour can influence the FMRI signal depends on its histology, the presence of oedema, and the distance between the tumour and the area of activation[185].

Tumour histology has an important effect on the peri- and intra-tumoural activation pattern[128]. Gliomas and glioblastomas, in particular, lead to a clearer reduction of the FMRI activation[131,186]. It is suggested that reduced BOLD response near gliomas is related to the actual cortical invasion which affects neurovascular coupling before influencing the neuronal activation. The neurovascular coupling seems to break down before the cortical function is severely affected. A second, long-distance mechanism relates to the metabolism derangement and neurotransmitter distribution. The release of nitric oxide by reactive astrocytes and macrophages at the brain–glioma interface, for instance, results in luxury perfusion and a reduced oxygen extraction fraction leading to reduced BOLD contrast enhancement[186]. It has also been proposed that a reduction of BOLD contrast near a glioma is due to a loss of autoregulation of the tumour vasculature and a changed venous response resulting from compression of neighbouring vasculature[131]. This reduced activation is, however, not caused by a local destruction of neurons. Duffau et al. found more positive cortical stimulation points, in the form of a sudden unmasking, shortly after tumour resection[135]. Similarly, Roux et al. found postoperative function in the precentral gyrus in contrast to the preoperative FMRI findings and to the negative preoperative cortical stimulation results. They concluded from this that healthy peritumoural cortex may be preserved, even if it could not be detected preoperatively with either method[134]. Furthermore, Fujiwara et al. found that the use of near infrared spectroscopy (NIRS) led to an increase of deoxyhaemoglobin in the vicinity of tumours during task performance in 7 of 12 patients. This increase of deoxyhaemoglobin was responsible for an inferior BOLD signal and smaller FMRI activation, despite the presence of cortical function as shown by ECC[187]. Using NIRS, another group also found a local decrease of the BOLD signal after glioma resection, despite clinical improvement[188].

All these studies show that reduced FMRI activation close to cerebral tumours is not necessarily the result of a neuronal loss. There is enough evidence suggesting that a reduced BOLD answer may be a consequence of neovascularization and a disturbed autoregulation with changes in metabolism and blood flow which has to be expected in high-grade tumours or tumours with oedema.

4.3.3 Venous signal

Another factor that can lead to inaccuracies in the localization of function relates to the mainly intravascular origin of the BOLD signal at 1.5T scans[138,189]. This intravascular signal, however, can be of microvascular as well as of macrovascular origin. The latter originates from large draining veins, which can be located at a mean distance of 1cm and up to 2.8 cm from the maximum parenchymal activation[70,110,183,190,191]. It is suggested that activated areas almost always include a venous vessel and consist of surrounding gray matter and CSF. The FMRI signal changes can be described by extravascular dephasing effects in both gray matter and CSF around a venous vessel in combination with intravascular effects. In that hypothesis, it is assumed that almost all BOLD effects stem from the same source — a single vein[192]. Compared to the activation in the parenchyma, the 'activated' veins can be recognized by their tubular structure and their superficial course in the central sulcus. They can, therefore, be used to identify the central sulcus[130].

Furthermore, the signal change detected in big draining veins is about twice as high as that found in activated parenchyma. This problem could be addressed by using higher magnetic fields, in which the component of the parenchymal activation increases[66].

4.3.4 Compliance

An obvious prerequisite for a successful FMRI examination is a compliant patient. The patient needs to be adequately informed about the examination and its relevance to his management. The paradigms should be rehearsed sufficiently, so that a flawless examination is possible. This can be further supported by easily recognizable visual or auditory queues to trigger the active epochs. Auditory queues in motor FMRI examinations have the advantage that the patients can keep their eyes closed, thereby avoiding visual input, whereas auditory input in the form of scanner noise is unavoidable anyway. False negative activations based on lacking compliance are avoidable with trained personnel and adequate patient preparation.

4.3.5 FMRI experiment and its postprocessing

The magnitude of signal change and the number and size of the presented activations are influenced by a number of factors which can be divided into extrinsic and intrinsic factors. Extrinsic factors include the selection of the sequence, the study design (run length, block length, number of the active and passive scans, etc.), the motor task (complexity, frequency, amplitude), and the various postprocessing steps[11,128,136,150,181]. The intrinsic (physiological and pathological) factors that influence the FMRI activations include, among others, age[193–195], gender[196], attention and stress[197], individual skills, arterial disease[198], and physiological and pharmacological modulation[199–201]. All these can influence the BOLD signal or the height and size of the activations. Furthermore, the display of this activation depends on the threshold used, thereby underlining the statistical character of these results. In the absence of absolute quantitative methods, it is therefore currently not possible to assess the relationship between the limits of the 'real' area of activation and the planned resection borders.

4.3.6 Reliability

To assess and to compare the location of activated areas, centres of the masses (COMs) or (geometric) centres of gravity (COGs) were described. They indicate a geometric centre of an activated cluster composed of a defined number of voxels. These COMs of motor cortex activation were found to be highly reproducible (within 3 mm)[202,203]. The amplitude and size of activation, however, was found to be highly variable between repetitions[88,202–205] and is, therefore, not a reliable correlate for activation[204].

4.3.7 Neuronavigation

Various factors influence the accuracy of neuronavigational systems which is assessed by the application accuracy. Application accuracy describes the difference between imaging, registration and technical deviation and can range from 2 mm to 7 mm[80]. Main factors are the geometrical distortion of the functional scans and the steps of the registration process itself[110,136]. After the beginning of the surgery, two additional factors — the positional shift and the brainshift — can cause inaccuracies of up to 2.5cm, making neuronavigational guidance useless[80,137,206–211]. Intra-operative update of image data could overcome this problem.

5. Conclusion

Functional MRI is an important tool in the preoperative assessment of patients with tumours affecting the central region. FMRI can reliably both identify the central region and display motor function. It can assess the changes of cortical activation induced by a tumour — changes that correlate with the clinical signs of these patients. The FMRI results can be comprehensively displayed and the information seems to be easy to access. Probably for these reasons, neurosurgeons started regarding this tool as a prerequisite for evaluating patients with tumours affecting the central region. The possibility of integrating this functional information with the anatomical data into a navigation system underlines this development. It has to be mentioned, however, that important issues have not been addressed yet. The lack of activation, for example, does not indicate the absence of functional tissue. The correlation between the size of the activated area and the size of the activated tissue is not clear; and the ideal threshold that would display this activation as close as possible to reality has also yet to be defined. It is, therefore, important to use the FMRI results in the corresponding clinical context and to avoid relying on them alone when making decisions on patient's management.

References

1. Naidich, T.P. *et al.* The motor cortex: anatomic substrates of function. *Neuroimaging Clin N Am*, 2001. **11**(2):171–93, vii–viii.
2. Zilles, K. *et al.* Anatomy and transmitter receptors of the supplementary motor areas in the human and nonhuman primate brain. *Adv Neurol*, 1996. **70**:29–43.
3. Vogt, C. and Vogt, O. Allgemeine Ergebnisse unserer Hirnforschung. *J Psychol Neurol*, 1919. **25**:279–461.
4. Vogt, C. and Vogt, O. Die vergleichend-architektonische und vergleichend-reizphysiologische Felderung der Grosshirnrinde unter besonderer Beruecksichtigung der menschlichen Naturwissenschaften. *Naturwissenschaften*, 1926. **14**:1190–4.
5. Dum, R.P. and Strick, P.L. The origin of corticospinal projections from the premotor areas in the frontal lobe. *J Neurosci*, 1991. **11**(3):667–89.
6. Fontaine, D., Capelle, L., and Duffau, H. Somatotopy of the supplementary motor area: evidence from correlation of the extent of surgical resection with the clinical patterns of deficit. *Neurosurgery*, 2002. **50**(2):297–303; discussion 303–5.
7. Rao, S.M. *et al.* Functional magnetic resonance imaging of complex human movements. *Neurology*, 1993. **43**(11):2311–8.
8. Connelly, A. *et al.* Functional mapping of activated human primary cortex with a clinical MR imaging system. *Radiology*, 1993. **188**(1):125–30.
9. Constable, R.T. *et al.* Functional brain imaging at 1.5 T using conventional gradient echo MR imaging techniques. *Magn Reson Imaging*, 1993. **11**(4):451–9.
10. Kwong, K.K. *et al.* Dynamic magnetic resonance imaging of human brain activity during primary sensory stimulation. *Proc Natl Acad Sci USA*, 1992. **89**(12):5675–9.

11. Yousry, I., Naidich, T.P., and Yousry, T.A. Functional magnetic resonance imaging: factors modulating the cortical activation pattern of the motor system. *Neuroimaging Clin N Am*, 2001. **11**(2):195–202, viii.

12. Kastrup, A. *et al.* Changes of cerebral blood flow, oxygenation, and oxidative metabolism during graded motor activation. *Neuroimage*, 2002. **15**(1):74–82.

13. Wiese, H. *et al.* Movement preparation in self-initiated versus externally triggered movements: an event-related FMRI-study. *Neurosci Lett*, 2004. **371**(2–3):220–5.

14. Verstynen, T.D. *et al.* Ipsilateral motor cortex activity during unimanual hand movements relates to task complexity. *J Neurophysiol*, 2005 Mar; **93**(3): 1209–22. Epub 2004 Nov 3.

15. Krings, T. *et al.* Cortical activation patterns during complex motor tasks in piano players and control subjects. A functional magnetic resonance imaging study. *Neurosci Lett*, 2000. **278**(3):189–93.

16. Tanji, J. Sequential organization of multiple movements: involvement of cortical motor areas. *Annu Rev Neurosci*, 2001. **24**:631–51.

17. Tanji, J. and Mushiake, H. Comparison of neuronal activity in the supplementary motor area and primary motor cortex. *Brain Res Cogn Brain Res*, 1996. **3**(2):143–50.

18. Stephan, K.M. *et al.* The role of ventral medial wall motor areas in bimanual co-ordination. A combined lesion and activation study. *Brain*, 1999. **122** (Pt 2):351–68.

19. Van Oostende, S. *et al.* FMRI studies of the supplementary motor area and the premotor cortex. *Neuroimage*, 1997. **6**(3):181–90.

20. Kollias, S.S. *et al.* Identification of multiple nonprimary motor cortical areas with simple movements. *Brain Res Rev*, 2001. **36**(2–3):185–95.

21. Olivier, A. Surgical strategies for patients with supplementary sensorimotor area epilepsy. the Montreal experience. *Adv Neurol*, 1996. **70**:429–43.

22. Zentner, J. *et al.* Functional results after resective procedures involving the supplementary motor area. *J Neurosurg*, 1996. **85**(4):542–9.

23. Yousry, T.A. Naming the central sulcus and its components. *International Journal of Neuroradiology*, 1998. Vol. **4**(No. 3):178–82.

24. Broca, P. Nomenclature cérébrale. *Revue d' Antropologie*, 1878. **1**:193–236.

25. Déjérine, J. *Anatomie des centres nerveux.* 1895, Paris: Rueff et Cie.

26. Yousry, T.A. *et al.* Localization of the motor hand area to a knob on the precentral gyrus. A new landmark. *Brain*, 1997. **120** (Pt 1):141–57.

27. Sastre Janer, F.A. *et al.* Three-dimensional reconstruction of the human central sulcus reveals a morphological correlate of the hand area. *Cereb Cortex*, 1998. **8**(7):641–7.

28. Fesl, G. *et al.* Inferior central sulcus: variations of anatomy and function on the example of the motor tongue area. *Neuroimage*, 2003. **20**(1):601–10.

29. Rademacher, J. *et al.* Variability and asymmetry in the human precentral motor system. A cytoarchitectonic and myeloarchitectonic brain mapping study. *Brain*, 2001. **124**(Pt 11): 2232–58.

30. Amunts, K. and Zilles, K. Advances in cytoarchitectonic mapping of the human cerebral cortex. *Neuroimaging Clin N Am*, 2001. **11**(2):151–69, vii.

31. Geyer, S. *et al.* Two different areas within the primary motor cortex of man. *Nature*, 1996. 382(6594):805–7.

32. Iwasaki, S. *et al.* Identification of pre- and postcentral gyri on CT and MR images on the basis of the medullary pattern of cerebral white matter. *Radiology*, 1991. 179(1):207–13.

33. Naidich, T.P., Valavanis, A.G., and Kubik, S. Anatomic relationships along the low-middle convexity: Part I–Normal specimens and magnetic resonance imaging. *Neurosurgery*, 1995. **36**(3):517–32.

34. Talairach, J. and Tournoux, P. *Co-planar Stereotactic Atlas of the Human Brain.* 1988, New York: Thieme.

35. Steinmetz, H., Furst, G., and Freund, H.J. Variation of perisylvian and calcarine anatomic landmarks within stereotaxic proportional coordinates. *AJNR Am J Neuroradiol*, 1990. **11**(6):1123–30.

36. Sobel, D.F. *et al.* Locating the central sulcus: comparison of MR anatomic and magnetoencephalographic functional methods (see comments). *AJNR Am J Neuroradiol*, 1993. **14**(4):915–25.

37. Kido, D.K. *et al.* Computed tomographic localization of the precentral gyrus. *Radiology*, 1980. **135**(2):373–7.

38. Talairach, J. and Tournoux, P. *Referentially oriented cerebral MRI anatomy.* 1993, Stuttgart, New York: Thieme

39. Steinmetz, H., Furst, G., and Freund, H.J. Cerebral cortical localization: application and validation of the proportional grid system in MR imaging. *J Comput Assist Tomogr*, 1989. **13**(1):10–19.

40. Naidich, T.P. and Brightbill, T.C. Systems for localizing fronto-parietal gyri and sulci on axial CT and MRI. *International Journal of Neuroradiology*, 1996. **2**(4):313–338.

41. Foerster, O. Motorische felder und bahnen, in *Handbuch der Neurologie* (ed. O. Bumke and O. Foerster). 1936, Springer–Verlag: Berlin, p. 1–357.

42. Penfield, W. and Rasmussen, T. *The cerebral cortex in man. A clinical study of localisation of function.* 1950, New York: Macmillan.

43. Penfield, W. and Boldrey, E. Somatic motor and sensory representation in the cerebral cortex of man as studied by electrical stimulation. *Brain*, 1937. **60**:389–443.

44. Foerster, O., The motor cortex in man in the light of Hughlings Jackson's doctrines. *Brain*, 1936. **59**:135–59.

45. Urasaki, E. *et al.* Cortical tongue area studied by chronically implanted subdural electrodes – with special reference to parietal motor and frontal sensory responses. *Brain*, 1994. **117**(Pt 1)117–32.

46. Uematsu, S. *et al.* Motor and sensory cortex in humans: topography studied with chronic subdural stimulation. *Neurosurgery*, 1992. **31**(1):59–71; discussion 71–2.

47. Libet, B. Electrical stimulation of cortex in human subjects, and conscious sensory aspects., in somatosensory system. Handbook of sensory physiology (ed. A. Iggo). 1973, Springer–Verlag: Berlin, p. 743–90.

48. Woolsey, C.N., Erickson, T.C., and Gilson, W.E. Localization in somatic sensory and motor areas of human cerebral cortex as determined by direct recording of evoked potentials and electrical stimulation. *J Neurosurg*, 1979. **51**(4):476–506.

49. Grafton, S.T. *et al.* Somatotopic mapping of the primary motor cortex in humans: activation studies with cerebral blood flow and positron emission tomography. *J Neurophysiol*, 1991. **66**(3):735–43.

50. Fox, P.T., Burton, H., and Raichle, M.E. Mapping human somatosensory cortex with positron emission tomography. *J Neurosurg*, 1987. **67**(1):34–43.

51. Cheyne, D., Kristeva, R., and Deecke, L. Homuncular organization of human motor cortex as indicated by neuromagnetic recordings. *Neurosci Lett*, 1991. **122**(1):17–20.

52. Nakamura, A. *et al.* Somatosensory homunculus as drawn by MEG. *Neuroimage*, 1998. **7**(4 Pt 1):377–86.

53. Krings, T. *et al.* Functional magnetic resonance imaging and transcranial magnetic stimulation: complementary approaches in the evaluation of cortical motor function. *Neurology*, 1997. **48**(5):1406–16.

54. Rao, S.M. *et al.* Somatotopic mapping of the human primary motor cortex with functional magnetic resonance imaging. *Neurology*, 1995. **45**(5):919–24.

55. Lotze, M. *et al.* FMRI evaluation of somatotopic representation in human primary motor cortex. *Neuroimage*, 2000. **11**(5 Pt 1):473–81.

56. Rotte, M., Kanowski, M., and Heinze, H.J. Functional magnetic resonance imaging for the evaluation of the motor system: primary and secondary brain areas in different motor tasks. *Stereotact Funct Neurosurg*, 2002. **78**(1):3–16.

57. Beisteiner, R. *et al*. Finger somatotopy in human motor cortex. *Neuroimage*, 2001. **13**(6 Pt 1):1016–26.

58. Hlustik, P. *et al*. Somatotopy in human primary motor and somatosensory hand representations revisited. *Cereb Cortex*, 2001. **11**(4):312–21.

59. Fellner, C. *et al*. Functional MRI of the motor cortex using a conventional gradient system: comparison of FLASH and EPI techniques. *Magn Reson Imaging*, 1998. **16**(10):1171–80.

60. van der Kallen, B.F. *et al*. Activation of the sensorimotor cortex at 1.0 T: comparison of echo-planar and gradient-echo imaging. *AJNR Am J Neuroradiol*, 1998. **19**(6):1099–104.

61. Papke, K. *et al*. Clinical applications of functional MRI at 1.0 T: motor and language studies in healthy subjects and patients. *Eur Radiol*, 1999. **9**(2):211–20.

62. Chapman, P.H. *et al*. Functional magnetic resonance imaging for cortical mapping in pediatric neurosurgery. *Pediatr Neurosurg*, 1995. **23**(3):122–6.

63. Conesa, G. *et al*. EPI functional MRI: a useful tool for preoperative rolandic fissure localization. *Front Radiat Ther Oncol*, 1999. **33**:23–7.

64. Dymarkowski, S. *et al*. Functional MRI of the brain: localisation of eloquent cortex in focal brain lesion therapy. *Eur Radiol*, 1998. **8**(9):1573–80.

65. Mueller, W.M. *et al*. Functional magnetic resonance imaging mapping of the motor cortex in patients with cerebral tumors. *Neurosurgery*, 1996. **39**(3):515–20; discussion 520–1.

66. Jack, C.R. Jr. *et al*. Sensory motor cortex: correlation of presurgical mapping with functional MR imaging and invasive cortical mapping. *Radiology*, 1994. **190**(1):85–92.

67. Puce, A. *et al*. Functional magnetic resonance imaging of sensory and motor cortex: comparison with electrophysiological localization. *J Neurosurg*, 1995. **83**(2):262–70.

68. Cosgrove, G.R., Buchbinder, B.R., and Jiang, H. Functional magnetic resonance imaging for intracranial navigation. *Neurosurg Clin N Am*, 1996. **7**(2):313–22.

69. Pujol, J. *et al*. Presurgical identification of the primary sensorimotor cortex by functional magnetic resonance imaging. *J Neurosurg*, 1996. **84**(1):7–13.

70. Kim, P.E. and Singh, M. Functional magnetic resonance imaging for brain mapping in neurosurgery. *Neurosurg Focus*, 2003. **15**(1):E1.

71. Yousry, T.A. *et al*. Topography of the cortical motor hand area: prospective study with functional MR imaging and direct motor mapping at surgery. *Radiology*, 1995. **195**(1):23–9.

72. Yetkin, F.Z. *et al*. Functional MR activation correlated with intraoperative cortical mapping. *AJNR Am J Neuroradiol*, 1997. **18**(7):1311–5.

73. Lehericy, S. *et al*. Correspondence between functional magnetic resonance imaging somatotopy and individual brain anatomy of the central region: comparison with intraoperative stimulation in patients with brain tumors. *J Neurosurg*, 2000. **92**(4):589–98.

74. Fandino, J. *et al*. Intraoperative validation of functional magnetic resonance imaging and cortical reorganization patterns in patients with brain tumors involving the primary motor cortex. *J Neurosurg*, 1999. **91**(2):238–50.

75. Krings, T. *et al*. Metabolic and electrophysiological validation of functional MRI. *J Neurol Neurosurg Psychiatry*, 2001. **71**(6):762–71.

76. Roux, F.E. *et al*. Usefulness of motor functional MRI correlated to cortical mapping in Rolandic low-grade astrocytomas. *Acta Neurochir (Wien)*, 1999. **141**(1):71–9.

77. Roux, F.E. *et al*. Cortical intraoperative stimulation in brain tumors as a tool to evaluate spatial data from motor functional MRI. *Invest Radiol*, 1999. **34**(3):225–9.

78. Hirsch, J. *et al*. An integrated functional magnetic resonance imaging procedure for preoperative mapping of cortical areas associated with tactile, motor, language, and visual functions. *Neurosurgery*, 2000. **47**(3):711–21; discussion 721–2.

79. Tomczak, R.J. *et al*. FMRI for preoperative neurosurgical mapping of motor cortex and language in a clinical setting. *J Comput Assist Tomogr*, 2000. **24**(6):927–34.

80. Steinmeier, R. *et al.* Surgery of low-grade gliomas near speech-eloquent regions: brainmapping versus preoperative functional imaging. *Onkologie*, 2002. **25**(6):552–7.

81. Krings, T. *et al.* Functional MRI and 18F FDG-positron emission tomography for presurgical planning: comparison with electrical cortical stimulation. *Acta Neurochir (Wien)*, 2002. **144**(9):889–99; discussion 899.

82. Gupta, N.C., Nicholson, P., and Bloomfield, S.M. FDG-PET in the staging work-up of patients with suspected intracranial metastatic tumors. *Ann Surg*, 1999. **230**(2):202–6.

83. Bittar, R.G. *et al.* Localization of somatosensory function by using positron emission tomography scanning: a comparison with intraoperative cortical stimulation. *J Neurosurg*, 1999. **90**(3):478–83.

84. Kaplan, A.M. *et al.* Functional brain mapping using positron emission tomography scanning in preoperative neurosurgical planning for pediatric brain tumors. *J Neurosurg*, 1999. **91**(5):797–803.

85. Vinas, F.C. *et al.* [15O]-water PET and intraoperative brain mapping: a comparison in the localization of eloquent cortex. *Neurol Res*, 1997. **19**(6):601–8.

86. Schreckenberger, M. *et al.* Localisation of motor areas in brain tumour patients: a comparison of preoperative [18F]FDG-PET and intraoperative cortical electrostimulation. *Eur J Nucl Med*, 2001. **28**(9):1394–403.

87. Bittar, R.G. *et al.* Presurgical motor and somatosensory cortex mapping with functional magnetic resonance imaging and positron emission tomography. *J Neurosurg*, 1999. **91**(6):915–21.

88. Ramsey, N.F. *et al.* Functional mapping of human sensorimotor cortex with 3D BOLD FMRI correlates highly with H2(15)O PET rCBF. *J Cereb Blood Flow Metab*, 1996. **16**(5):755–64.

89. Braun, V. *et al.* Multimodal cranial neuronavigation: direct integration of functional magnetic resonance imaging and positron emission tomography data: technical note. *Neurosurgery*, 2001. **48**(5):1178–81; discussion 1181–2.

90. Kinahan, P.E. and Noll, D.C. A direct comparison between whole-brain PET and BOLD FMRI measurements of single-subject activation response. *Neuroimage*, 1999. **9**(4):430–8.

91. Joliot, M. *et al.* FMRI and PET of self-paced finger movement: comparison of intersubject stereotaxic averaged data. *Neuroimage*, 1999. **10**(4):430–47.

92. Nishiyama, Y. *et al.* Visualization of the motor activation area using SPECT in neurosurgical patients with lesions near the central sulcus. *J Nucl Med*, 2000. **41**(3):411–5.

93. Sabbah, P. *et al.* Multimodal anatomic, functional, and metabolic brain imaging for tumor resection. *Clin Imaging*, 2002. **26**(1):6–12.

94. Krings, T. *et al.* Accuracy of electroencephalographic dipole localization of epileptiform activities associated with focal brain lesions. *Ann Neurol*, 1998. **44**(1):76–86.

95. Kober, H. *et al.* Correlation of sensorimotor activation with functional magnetic resonance imaging and magnetoencephalography in presurgical functional imaging: a spatial analysis. *Neuroimage*, 2001. **14**(5):1214–28.

96. Stippich, C. *et al.* Motor, somatosensory and auditory cortex localization by FMRI and MEG. *Neuroreport*, 1998. **9**(9):1953–7.

97. Nimsky, C. *et al.* Integration of functional magnetic resonance imaging supported by magnetoencephalography in functional neuronavigation. *Neurosurgery*, 1999. **44**(6):1249–55; discussion 1255–6.

98. Ganslandt, O. *et al.* Functional neuronavigation with magnetoencephalography: outcome in 50 patients with lesions around the motor cortex. *J Neurosurg*, 1999. **91**(1):73–9.

99. Ganslandt, O. *et al.* Magnetic source imaging supports clinical decision making in glioma patients. *Clin Neurol Neurosurg*, 2004. **107**(1):20–6.

100. Ossenblok, P. *et al.* Magnetic source imaging contributes to the presurgical identification of sensorimotor cortex in patients with frontal lobe epilepsy. *Clin Neurophysiol*, 2003. **114**(2):221–32.

101. Krings, T. *et al.* Stereotactic transcranial magnetic stimulation: correlation with direct electrical cortical stimulation. *Neurosurgery*, 1997. **41**(6):1319–25; discussion 1325–6.

102. Asakura, T. *et al*. Identification of the cerebral motor cortex by focal magnetic stimulation: clinical application to neurosurgical patients. *Stereotact Funct Neurosurg*, 1994. **63**(1–4):177–81.

103. Boroojerdi, B. *et al*. Localization of the motor hand area using transcranial magnetic stimulation and functional magnetic resonance imaging. *Clin Neurophysiol*, 1999. **110**(4):699–704.

104. Krings, T. *et al*. Multimodality neuroimaging: research and clinical applications. *Neurol Clin Neurophysiol*, 2001. **2001**(1):2–11.

105. Krings, T. *et al*. Introducing navigated transcranial magnetic stimulation as a refined brain mapping methodology. *Neurosurg Rev*, 2001. **24**(4):171–9.

106. Krings, T. *et al*. Navigated transcranial magnetic stimulation for presurgical planning–correlation with functional MRI. *Minim Invasive Neurosurg*, 2001. **44**(4):234–9.

107. Reinges, M.H. *et al*. Preoperative mapping of cortical motor function: prospective comparison of functional magnetic resonance imaging and [15O]-H2O-positron emission tomography in the same co-ordinate system. *Nucl Med Commun*, 2004. **25**(10):987–97.

108. Sunaert, S. and Yousry, T.A. Clinical applications of functional magnetic resonance imaging. *Neuroimaging Clin N Am*, 2001. **11**(2):221–36, viii.

109. Sunaert, S. *et al*. Functional magnetic resonance imaging (FMRI) visualises the brain at work. *Acta Neurol Belg*, 1998. **98**(1):8–16.

110. Golder, W. Functional magnetic resonance imaging – basics and applications in oncology. *Onkologie*, 2002. **25**(1):28–31.

111. Moritz, C. and Haughton, V. Functional MR imaging: paradigms for clinical preoperative mapping. *Magn Reson Imaging Clin N Am*, 2003. **11**(4):529–42, v.

112. Lee, C.C. *et al*. Assessment of functional MR imaging in neurosurgical planning. *AJNR Am J Neuroradiol*, 1999. **20**(8):1511–9.

113. Stippich, C. *et al*. Preoperative functional magnetic resonance tomography (FMRI) in patients with rolandic brain tumors: indication, investigation strategy, possibilities and limitations of clinical application. *Rofo*, 2003. **175**(8):1042–50.

114. Wilkinson, I.D. *et al*. Motor functional MRI for pre-operative and intraoperative neurosurgical guidance. *Br J Radiol*, 2003. **76**(902):98–103.

115. Atlas, S.W. *et al*. Functional magnetic resonance imaging of regional brain activity in patients with intracerebral gliomas: findings and implications for clinical management. *Neurosurgery*, 1996. **38**(2):329–38.

116. Hammeke, T.A. *et al*. Functional magnetic resonance imaging of somatosensory stimulation. *Neurosurgery*, 1994. **35**(4):677–81.

117. Krings, T. *et al*. Functional magnetic resonance mapping of sensory motor cortex for image-guided neurosurgical intervention. *Acta Neurochir (Wien)*, 1998. **140**(3):215–22.

118. Heilbrun, M.P., Lee, J.N., and Alvord, L. Practical application of FMRI for surgical planning. *Stereotact Funct Neurosurg*, 2001. **76**(3–4):168–74.

119. Krishnan, R. *et al*. Functional magnetic resonance imaging-integrated neuronavigation: correlation between lesion-to-motor cortex distance and outcome. *Neurosurgery*, 2004. **55**(4):904–15.

120. Latchaw, R.E. and Hu, X. Functional MR imaging in the evaluation of the patient with epilepsy. Functional localization. *Neuroimaging Clin N Am*, 1995. **5**(4):683–93.

121. Nitschke, M.F. *et al*. Preoperative functional magnetic resonance imaging (FMRI) of the motor system in patients with tumours in the parietal lobe. *Acta Neurochir (Wien)*, 1998. **140**(12):1223–9.

122. Pardo, F.S. *et al*. Functional cerebral imaging in the evaluation and radiotherapeutic treatment planning of patients with malignant glioma. *Int J Radiat Oncol Biol Phys*, 1994. **30**(3):663–9.

123. Ternovoi, S.K. *et al*. Localization of the motor and speech zones of the cerebral cortex by functional magnetic resonance tomography. *Neurosci Behav Physiol*, 2004. **34**(5):431–7.

124. Righini, A. *et al*. Functional MRI: primary motor cortex localization in patients with brain tumors. *J Comput Assist Tomogr*, 1996. **20**(5):702–8.

125. Witt, T.C. *et al.* Preoperative cortical localization with functional MRI for use in stereotactic radiosurgery. *Stereotact Funct Neurosurg*, 1996. **66**(1–3):24–9.

126. Vlieger, E.J. *et al.* Functional magnetic resonance imaging for neurosurgical planning in neurooncology. *Eur Radiol*, 2004. **14**(7):1143–53.

127. Yetkin, F.Z. *et al.* Functional magnetic resonance imaging assessment of the risk of postoperative hemiparesis after excision of cerebral tumours. *Int J Neuroradiol*, 1998. **4**: 253–7.

128. Roux, F.E. *et al.* Motor functional MRI for presurgical evaluation of cerebral tumors. *Stereotact Funct Neurosurg*, 1997. **68**(1–4 Pt 1):106–11.

129. Pujol, J. *et al.* Clinical application of functional magnetic resonance imaging in presurgical identification of the central sulcus. *J Neurosurg*, 1998. **88**(5):863–9.

130. Yousry, T.A. *et al.* The central sulcal vein: a landmark for identification of the central sulcus using functional magnetic resonance imaging. *J Neurosurg*, 1996. **85**(4):608–17.

131. Holodny, A.I. *et al.* The effect of brain tumors on BOLD functional MR imaging activation in the adjacent motor cortex: implications for image-guided neurosurgery. *AJNR Am J Neuroradiol*, 2000. **21**(8):1415–22.

132. Carpentier, A.C. *et al.* Patterns of functional magnetic resonance imaging activation in association with structural lesions in the rolandic region: a classification system. *J Neurosurg*, 2001. **94**(6):946–54.

133. Krings, T. *et al.* Activation in primary and secondary motor areas in patients with CNS neoplasms and weakness. *Neurology*, 2002. **58**(3):381–90.

134. Roux, F.E. *et al.* Functional MRI and intraoperative brain mapping to evaluate brain plasticity in patients with brain tumours and hemiparesis. *J Neurol Neurosurg Psychiatry*, 2000. **69**(4):453–63.

135. Duffau, H. Acute functional reorganisation of the human motor cortex during resection of central lesions: a study using intraoperative brain mapping. *J Neurol Neurosurg Psychiatry*, 2001. **70**(4):506–13.

136. Stippich, C. *et al.* Functional magnetic resonance imaging: physiological background, technical aspects and prerequisites for clinical use. *Rofo*, 2002. **174**(1):43–9.

137. Rutten, G.J. *et al.* Toward functional neuronavigation: implementation of functional magnetic resonance imaging data in a surgical guidance system for intraoperative identification of motor and language cortices. Technical note and illustrative case. *Neurosurg Focus*, 2003. **15**(1):E6.

138. Chen, W. and Ogawa, S. Principles of BOLD functional MRI, in *Functional MRI* (ed. C.T.W. Moonen and P.A. Bandettini). 2000, Springer: Berlin, Heidelberg, New York. p. 103–113.

139. Bandettini, P.A. and Ungerleider, L.G. From neuron to BOLD: new connections. *Nat Neurosci*, 2001. **4**(9):864–6.

140. Ogawa, S. *et al.* Intrinsic signal changes accompanying sensory stimulation: functional brain mapping with magnetic resonance imaging. *Proc Natl Acad Sci USA*, 1992. **89**(13):5951–5.

141. Ogawa, S. *et al.* Brain magnetic resonance imaging with contrast dependent on blood oxygenation. *Proc Natl Acad Sci USA*, 1990. **87**(24):9868–72.

142. Detre, J.A. *et al.* Perfusion imaging. *Magn Reson Med*, 1992. **23**(1):37–45.

143. Kim, S.G. Quantification of relative cerebral blood flow change by flow-sensitive alternating inversion recovery (FAIR) technique: application to functional mapping. *Magn Reson Med*, 1995. **34**(3):293–301.

144. Belliveau, J.W. *et al.* Functional mapping of the human visual cortex by magnetic resonance imaging. *Science*, 1991. **254**(5032):716–9.

145. Zigun, J.R. *et al.* Measurement of brain activity with bolus administration of contrast agent and gradient-echo MR imaging. *Radiology*, 1993. **186**(2):353–6.

146. Frank, J.A. *et al.* Measurement of relative cerebral blood volume changes with visual stimulation by 'double-dose' gadopentetate-dimeglumine-enhanced dynamic magnetic resonance imaging. *Invest Radiol*, 1994. **29** Suppl 2:S157–60.

147. Li, T.Q. *et al.* Assessment of hemodynamic response during focal neural activity in human using bolus tracking, arterial spin labeling and BOLD techniques. *Neuroimage*, 2000. **12**(4):442–51.

148. Bandettini, P.A. *et al.* Time course EPI of human brain function during task activation. *Magn Reson Med*, 1992. **25**(2):390–7.

149. Kennan, R.P. Gradient echo and spin echo methods for functional MRI, in *Functional MRI* (ed. C.T.W. Moonen and P.A. Bandettini). 2000, Springer: Berlin, Heidelberg, New York, p. 127–136.

150. Yoo, S.S. *et al.* Evaluating requirements for spatial resolution of FMRI for neurosurgical planning. *Hum Brain Mapp*, 2004. **21**(1):34–43.

151. Bandettini, P.A. *et al.* Spin-echo and gradient-echo EPI of human brain activation using BOLD contrast: a comparative study at 1.5 T. *NMR Biomed*, 1994. **7**(1–2):12–20.

152. Mohamed, F.B. *et al.* Investigation of alternating and continuous experimental task designs during single finger opposition FMRI: a comparative study. *J Comput Assist Tomogr*, 2000. **24**(6):935–41.

153. Zarahn, E., Aguirre, G., and D'Esposito, M. A trial-based experimental design for FMRI. *Neuroimage*, 1997. **6**(2):122–38.

154. Aguirre, G.K. and D'Esposito, M. Experimental design for brain FMRI, in *Functional MRI*, (ed. C.T.W. Moonen and P.A. Bandettini). 2000, Springer: Berlin, Heidelberg, New York, p. 369–80.

155. Birn, R.M., Cox, R.W., and Bandettini, P.A. Detection versus estimation in event-related FMRI: choosing the optimal stimulus timing. *Neuroimage*, 2002. **15**(1):252–64.

156. Liu, T.T. *et al.* Detection power, estimation efficiency, and predictability in event-related FMRI. *Neuroimage*, 2001. **13**(4):759–73.

157. Marquart, M., Birn, R., and Haughton, V. Single- and multiple-event paradigms for identification of motor cortex activation. *AJNR Am J Neuroradiol*, 2000. **21**(1):94–8.

158. Bittar, R.G., Ptito, A., and Reutens, D.C. Somatosensory representation in patients who have undergone hemispherectomy: a functional magnetic resonance imaging study. *J Neurosurg*, 2000. **92**(1):45–51.

159. Nimsky, C., Ganslandt, O., and Fahlbusch, R. Functional neuronavigation and intraoperative MRI. *Adv Tech Stand Neurosurg*, 2004. **29**:229–63.

160. Rao, S.M. *et al.* Relationship between finger movement rate and functional magnetic resonance signal change in human primary motor cortex. *J Cereb Blood Flow Metab*, 1996. **16**(6):1250–4.

161. Wexler, B.E. *et al.* An FMRI study of the human cortical motor system response to increasing functional demands. *Magn Reson Imaging*, 1997. **15**(4):385–96.

162. Price, C.J. and Friston, K.J. Scanning patients with tasks they can perform. *Hum Brain Mapp*, 1999. **8**(2–3):102–8.

163. Lee, C.C., Jack, Jr. C.R., and Riederer, S.J. Mapping of the central sulcus with functional MR: active versus passive activation tasks. *AJNR Am J Neuroradiol*, 1998. **19**(5):847–52.

164. Rodriguez, M. *et al.* Hand movement distribution in the motor cortex: the influence of a concurrent task and motor imagery. *Neuroimage*, 2004. **22**(4):1480–91.

165. Stippich, C., Ochmann, H., and Sartor, K. Somatotopic mapping of the human primary sensorimotor cortex during motor imagery and motor execution by functional magnetic resonance imaging. *Neurosci Lett*, 2002. **331**(1):50–4.

166. Friston, K.J. *et al.* Statistical parametric maps in functional imaging: a general linear approach. *Hum Brain Mapp*, 1995. **2**:189–210.

167. Cox, R.W. AFNI: software for analysis and visualization of functional magnetic resonance neuroimages. *Comput Biomed Res*, 1996. **29**(3):162–73.

168. Gold, S. *et al.* Functional MRI statistical software packages: a comparative analysis. *Hum Brain Mapp*, 1998. **6**(2):73–84.

169. Hajnal, J.V. *et al.* Artifacts due to stimulus correlated motion in functional imaging of the brain. *Magn Reson Med*, 1994. **31**(3):283–91.

170. Yoo, S.S., Guttmann, C.R., and Panych, L.P. Multiresolution data acquisition and detection in functional MRI. *Neuroimage*, 2001. **14**(6):1476–85.

171. Chen, N.K. *et al.* Selection of voxel size and slice orientation for FMRI in the presence of susceptibility field gradients: application to imaging of the amygdala. *Neuroimage*, 2003. **19**(3):817–25.

172. Friston, K.J., Jezzard, P., and Turner, R. Analysis of functional MRI time series. *Hum Brain Mapp*, 1994. **1**:153–171.

173. Bandettini, P.A. *et al.* Processing strategies for time-course data sets in functional MRI of the human brain. *Magn Reson Med*, 1993. **30**(2):161–73.

174. McKeown, M.J. *et al.* Analysis of FMRI data by blind separation into independent spatial components. *Hum Brain Mapp*, 1998. **6**(3):160–88.

175. Lange, N. Statistical procedures for functional MRI, in *Functional MRI* (ed. C.T.W. Moonen and P.A. Bandettini). 2000, Springer: Berlin, Heidelberg, New York, p. 301–36.

176. Schmithorst, V.J., Dardzinski, B.J., and Holland, S.K. Simultaneous correction of ghost and geometric distortion artifacts in EPI using a multiecho reference scan. *IEEE Trans Med Imaging*, 2001. **20**(6):535–9.

177. Kamada, K. *et al.* Visualization of the eloquent motor system by integration of MEG, functional, and anisotropic diffusion-weighted MRI in functional neuronavigation. *Surg Neurol*, 2003. **59**(5):352–61; discussion 361–2.

178. Jannin, P. *et al.* Integration of sulcal and functional information for multimodal neuronavigation. *J Neurosurg*, 2002. **96**(4):713–23.

179. Schulder, M. *et al.* Functional image-guided surgery of intracranial tumors located in or near the sensorimotor cortex. *J Neurosurg*, 1998. **89**(3):412–8.

180. McDonald, J.D. *et al.* Integration of preoperative and intraoperative functional brain mapping in a frameless stereotactic environment for lesions near eloquent cortex. Technical note. *J Neurosurg*, 1999. **90**(3):591–8.

181. Roux, F.E. *et al.* Methodological and technical issues for integrating functional magnetic resonance imaging data in a neuronavigational system. *Neurosurgery*, 2001. **49**(5):1145–56; discussion 1156–7.

182. Seto, E. *et al.* Quantifying head motion associated with motor tasks used in FMRI. *Neuroimage*, 2001. **14**(2):284–97.

183. Krings, T. *et al.* Functional MRI for presurgical planning: problems, artefacts, and solution strategies. *J Neurol Neurosurg Psychiatry*, 2001. **70**(6):749–60.

184. Jack, C.R.J. *et al.* The role of functional MRI in planning perirolandic surgery, in *Functional MRI* (ed. C.T.W. Moonen and P.A. Bandettini). 2000, Springer: Berlin, Heidelberg, New York, p. 539–550.

185. Krings, T. *et al.* Factors related to the magnitude of T2* MR signal changes during functional imaging. *Neuroradiology*, 2002. **44**(6):459–66.

186. Schreiber, A. *et al.* The influence of gliomas and nonglial space-occupying lesions on blood-oxygen-level-dependent contrast enhancement. *AJNR Am J Neuroradiol*, 2000. **21**(6):1055–63.

187. Fujiwara, N. *et al.* Evoked-cerebral blood oxygenation changes in false-negative activations in BOLD contrast functional MRI of patients with brain tumors. *Neuroimage*, 2004. **21**(4):1464–71.

188. Murata, Y. *et al.* Decreases of blood oxygenation level–dependent signal in the activated motor cortex during functional recovery after resection of a glioma. *AJNR Am J Neuroradiol*, 2004. **25**(7):1242–6.

189. Boxerman, J.L. *et al.* The intravascular contribution to FMRI signal change: Monte Carlo modeling and diffusion-weighted studies in vivo. *Magn Reson Med*, 1995. **34**(1):4–10.

190. Segebarth, C. *et al.* Functional MRI of the human brain: predominance of signals from extracerebral veins. *Neuroreport*, 1994. **5**(7):813–6.

191. Krings, T. *et al.* MR blood oxygenation level-dependent signal differences in parenchymal and large draining vessels: implications for functional MR imaging. *AJNR Am J Neuroradiol*, 1999. **20**(10):1907–14.

192. Hoogenraad, F.G. *et al.* Quantitative differentiation between BOLD models in FMRI. *Magn Reson Med*, 2001. **45**(2):233–46.

193. Hesselmann, V. *et al.* Age related signal decrease in functional magnetic resonance imaging during motor stimulation in humans. *Neurosci Lett*, 2001. **308**(3):141–4.

194. Nielson, K.A. *et al.* Comparability of functional MRI response in young and old during inhibition. *Neuroreport*, 2004. **15**(1):129–33.

195. Riecker, A. *et al.* Relation between regional functional MRI activation and vascular reactivity to carbon dioxide during normal aging. *J Cereb Blood Flow Metab*, 2003. **23**(5):565–73.

196. Kastrup, A. *et al.* Gender differences in cerebral blood flow and oxygenation response during focal physiologic neural activity. *J Cereb Blood Flow Metab*, 1999. **19**(10):1066–71.

197. Loubinoux, I. *et al.* Within-session and between-session reproducibility of cerebral sensorimotor activation: a test–retest effect evidenced with functional magnetic resonance imaging. *J Cereb Blood Flow Metab*, 2001. **21**(5):592–607.

198. Hamzei, F. *et al.* The influence of extra- and intracranial artery disease on the BOLD signal in FMRI. *Neuroimage*, 2003. **20**(2):1393–9.

199. Chollet, F. Pharmacologic modulation of human cerebral activity: contribution of functional neuroimaging. *Neuroimaging Clin N Am*, 2001. **11**(2):375–80, x.

200. Laurienti, P.J. *et al.* Dietary caffeine consumption modulates FMRI measures. *Neuroimage*, 2002. **17**(2):751–7.

201. Dietrich, T. *et al.* Effects of blood estrogen level on cortical activation patterns during cognitive activation as measured by functional MRI. *Neuroimage*, 2001. **13**(3):425–32.

202. Marshall, I. *et al.* Repeatability of motor and working-memory tasks in healthy older volunteers: assessment at functional MR imaging. *Radiology*, 2004. **233**(3):868–77.

203. Alkadhi, H. *et al.* Reproducibility of primary motor cortex somatotopy under controlled conditions. *AJNR Am J Neuroradiol*, 2002. **23**(9):1524–32.

204. McGonigle, D.J. *et al.* Variability in FMRI: an examination of intersession differences. *Neuroimage*, 2000. **11**(6 Pt 1):708–34.

205. Miki, A. *et al.* Reproducibility of visual activation in functional MR imaging and effects of postprocessing. *AJNR Am J Neuroradiol*, 2000. **21**(5):910–5.

206. Hartkens, T. *et al.* Measurement and analysis of brain deformation during neurosurgery. *IEEE Trans Med Imaging*, 2003. **22**(1):82–92.

207. Spetzger, U. *et al.* Error analysis in cranial neuronavigation. *Minim Invasive Neurosurg*, 2002. **45**(1):6–10.

208. Nabavi, A. *et al.* Serial intraoperative magnetic resonance imaging of brain shift. *Neurosurgery*, 2001. **48**(4):787–97; discussion 797–8.

209. Reinges, M.H. *et al.* Course of brain shift during microsurgical resection of supratentorial cerebral lesions: limits of conventional neuronavigation. *Acta Neurochir (Wien)*, 2004. **146**(4):369–77; discussion 377.

210. Trantakis, C. *et al.* Investigation of time-dependency of intracranial brain shift and its relation to the extent of tumor removal using intra-operative MRI. *Neurol Res*, 2003. **25**(1):9–12.

211. Reinges, M.H. *et al.* Virtual pointer projection of the central sulcus to the outside of the skull using frameless neuronavigation — accuracy and applications. *Acta Neurochir (Wien)*, 2000. **142**(12):1385–9; discussion 1389–90.

3

Preoperative assessment: language

Geert–Jan Rutten and Franck–Emmanuel Roux

1. Introduction

Brain surgery aims at optimal treatment of a lesion with minimal damage to healthy brain tissue, in order to spare the patient from any (new) neurological deficit. This not only requires a priori knowledge about the nature, location, and extent of the lesion and neighbouring anatomical structures (e.g. the vascular architecture) but also about the location of functionally important brain structures (i.e. the (sub)cortical areas that are indispensable or 'critical' for normal sensorimotor or cognitive function). Despite the importance of both these structural and functional aspects in resective brain surgery, routine and easily applicable clinical techniques only exist for identification and localization of the structural lesion. Nowadays, information from structural neuroimaging techniques such as CT or MRI is a prerequisite for any brain surgical intervention. In clear contrast, in the majority of these procedures, localization of function still relies on models that were developed over a century ago.

These models are predominantly based on the results of post-mortem studies of brain-lesioned patients with neurological deficits, and strongly link specific functions to specific anatomical landmarks and cortical topography. For language, this resulted in the formulation of the classical model that describes the language system as composed primarily of two cortical regions in the left hemisphere: the areas of Broca and Wernicke. Although no clear anatomical definition of these areas exists, they are usually defined, as respectively, the posterior part of the left inferior frontal gyrus and the posterior part of the left perisylvian region. However, over the years, it has been recognized that potential language cortex is much larger than previously thought, whereas language areas themselves can be much smaller and highly variable in both extent and location[1]. Clinicians and researchers have gradually come to realize that, for individual patients, the classical language model has little predictive value. Contrary to the general clinical assumption that is formulated in the Broca–Wernicke model, there seems no simple one-to-one relationship between structure and function. This holds true, in particular, for neurosurgical patients, where brain lesions may have changed structural or functional brain topography. A better understanding of the cerebral representation of language function is clearly needed in order to predict and explain the effects of brain surgery more accurately.

Recent alternative language models (largely based on the results of neurolinguistic and functional imaging studies) propose a more dynamic network view, where multiple regions are interconnected that each serve specific language functions. A particular language function is likely to be represented by a network of several brain areas and, vice versa, brain areas can be involved in different kinds of functions. There seems a considerable variability in the topography of these more distributed language systems, even in normal subjects. These findings explain why 'fixed' language models are not sufficient for presurgical planning and that techniques are required that are able to identify each individual's network of critical functional areas to optimize surgical treatment.

This was already recognized in the 1930s, when clinical techniques were introduced to predict whether or not the planned surgical intervention might compromise critical language areas (i.e. to estimate the risk of postoperative language deficits). These techniques (electrocortical stimulation mapping (ESM) and, later, the amobarbital (or Wada) test) are still considered the gold standards for the localization and lateralization of critical language functions respectively[2]. Although, in particular, ESM has offered a substantially new and different clinical view on language functions, these techniques are not often used in general brain surgery. Although undoubtedly related to the fact that these techniques are elaborate and invasive, and have several methodological limitations, presumably the most important reason for their lack of use is the fact that, in the surgeon's experience, indirect localization of function via cortical topography often proves to be a reasonable concept in terms of postoperative functional outcome. It should be realized, however, that any language-model based planning strategy may result in suboptimal surgical treatment.

Would there be a method that could quickly and reliably localize critical language functions without harming the patient, it would surely become part of the standard presurgical workup for many brain surgical procedures. FMRI can potentially fulfil these demands. Despite promising initial results, however, it is not yet used as a clinical tool for language mapping, as it has proven to be difficult to develop standardized FMRI protocols that can live up to the results of the current clinical methods. In this chapter, we will discuss prerequisites that have to be met for neurosurgical use of language FMRI and review current problems and solutions.

2. Language

2.1 The significance of language for cognition

Language is a form of communication that is unique to humans. It is the outward expression of our thoughts and experiences and, as such, plays a critical role in almost all aspects of our life. 'Aphasia' denotes a disturbance of language processing caused by a dysfunction in specific brain regions[3]. As a result of this disturbance, the two-way communication process between inner thoughts and the symbols and grammar that constitute language is disrupted, which in turn compromises the formulation and/or comprehension of language[4]. Language processes operate in different modalities: in addition to verbal output, reading, or writing, it can, for instance, also involve visuomotor forms of communication (e.g. sign language in deaf people). Language is considered to be relatively independent from sensorimotor and other cognitive functions, and is also not a disorder of thought[5]. Patients who have suffered brain damage can have severe language deficits while maintaining otherwise normal cognitive functions and, alternatively, in patients with disorders of thought (e.g. schizophrenia) language function is usually normal. Furthermore, brain lesions can selectively affect a particular aspect of language processing, so language functions can operate, in part, via spatially distinct subsystems. For instance, some patients have a rather selective impairment for naming of living things as compared to the naming of non-living things, or have a selective deficit for the processing of nouns or verbs[6–9].

There is no unequivocal definition of 'language', nor is there a definite neurobiological substrate for the various language functions. Language features can be subdivided into the following broad categories: phonology (the sound of words), orthography (the spelling of words), semantics (knowledge of the world), and syntax (knowledge of grammatical relationships between words). The definition of language as 'a form of communication' seems too inclusive, as it covers the many processes that are supportive to language processing but are not necessarily involved in the processing of linguistic content. Examples are physiological, attentional, or arousal processes. Whether there are specialized subsystems that sustain these processes during language function remains to be established.

It is important to realize that language (or any other function) is represented on many different functional and anatomical levels, from spatiotemporal firing patterns of groups of neurons to the interaction between entire cortical regions. As such, the 'definition' of language in terms of a neural substrate is rather dependent on the questions asked. Neurosurgeons are interested in the cortical and subcortical representation of function (on a relative coarse scale of mm), as they need to know whether damage to a particular area will affect language function. Considering the importance of surgical intervention in patients with intractable epilepsy or brain lesions, subtle or transient aphasic deficits that follow surgery may sometimes be regarded as acceptable. A non-invasive, routine, and easily applicable tool for identification of areas that, when damaged, result in permanent and significant language deficits (i.e. identification of 'critical' language areas) is currently not available. Development of FMRI for this purpose would aid more effective and safer surgery.

2.2 Clinical models and theories

2.2.1 Lesion studies

At the end of the nineteenth century, Wernicke and Lichtheim provided the first systematic analyses of the relationship between brain damage and aphasia. They stated that the anterior half of the brain was concerned with motor movements and the posterior part (including the temporal lobe) with the processing of sensory information[10]. They also set up language models that consisted of several brain areas that were interconnected and correctly predicted a number of language disorders that would result from damage to some of the presumed connections[11]. This clinical concept has changed little over time and remains the basis of current language models and aphasia research. In its most general form (and as often found in contemporary clinical textbooks), the model consists of two cortical areas in the left hemisphere: an inferior frontal 'expressive' language area (Broca's area, for planning and execution of speech) and a temporoparietal 'receptive' language area (Wernicke's area, for analysis and identification of linguistic stimuli) that are connected via a large white matter tract (the articulate fasciculus). The classical language model includes the angular gyrus, that represents the perception of written language. As there is no unequivocal definition of Wernicke's area, this area is not always included in the various definitions in the literature[12–14]. For historical reviews of these language models, see Penfield and Roberts[2], Young[15], and Doody[16].

With the development of structural imaging techniques (starting with CT at the end of the 1980s), lesions could be delineated in vivo and with more precision. These studies largely confirmed the former results of post-mortem studies but also added 'new' language areas to the list. For instance, there is now widespread evidence for the involvement of several subcortical structures (e.g. basal ganglia) in language function, as initially suggested by Marie and Dejerine in the beginning of the twentieth century[2,17–20]. A different source of information came from the studies of patients who had undergone surgical resection of brain areas[2]. These studies were particularly relevant as they were able to demonstrate that resection of large parts of the brain did *not* result in postoperative language deficits and, therefore, were not critical for language function.

2.2.2 Neuropsychological studies

It is important to note that the classical language model is based on deficits in the processing of words. It was not until the 1970s that studies began analysing deficits in sentence processing and recognized that, for instance, Broca's aphasics can have problems with comprehension of syntax[21,22]. When studies began focussing more on the cognitive deficits of brain-lesioned patients, it was realized that the classical language model, with its two separated areas for production and comprehension, is only a crude approximation to the variety of aphasic disturbances that can be found in patients. Furthermore, the classical language model also does not account for prosody (i.e. the modulation of speech via intonation, tempo, loudness, and timing) and the bodily movements that normally accompany verbal communication. These are language features that convey information beyond that transmitted by the factual words and sentences, and are thought to be mediated by the right hemisphere[23]. It has been demonstrated that focal damage to the right hemisphere can affect prosody (with significant psychosocial disability) without disturbance of the propositional element of language[24].

Linguistic studies demonstrated that different language functions can function as relatively independent subsystems as, for instance, the processing of word meaning can be impaired while phonological, orthographical, and syntactical processing is spared after brain injury. Even specific semantic knowledge in itself can be fractionated, as category-specific deficits have been found with selective naming of persons, animals, and tools, supporting the hypothesis that retrieval of knowledge from concrete entities in different conceptual domains depends on partially segregated neural systems[25,26]. Several other observations contrast with the classical language model[27–29] and this led to a change in the conceptualization of the neural architecture presumed to underlie language functions. It is no longer thought to be comprised of a few brain centres but instead viewed as the result of synchronized activity in parallel organized neural networks made up of many cerebral regions[6,30,31]. As these models are bound by few, if any, anatomical constraints, they are not very useful for clinical practice.

2.2.3 Electrocortical stimulation mapping

Intraoperative electrocortical stimulation mapping (ESM) was the first technique that allowed examination of a part of the brain in action[32,33]. ESM works on the observation that electrical stimulation of certain parts of the cortex can arrest or disturb ongoing speech and language functions in the awake patient, and it assumes that these areas, when resected, would produce postoperative aphasia (ESM studies have in fact coined the term 'critical language area'). In the 1930s, ESM had become a standard part of the surgical treatment of medically intractable epilepsy and was routinely used for language mapping to tailor the extent of frontal or temporal lobe removals[2,34].

From ESM studies, several observations were made that contrasted with the classical lesion-derived language model. It was found that ESM-derived language areas are usually small ($1–2cm^2$) and distributed (i.e. in between these areas, no stimulation-induced language errors are found), in contrast with the relatively large areas of Broca and Wernicke that were deduced from lesion studies. Language areas detected with ESM are also found in a much wider area than described in the classical language models and the location is highly variable between patients[2,35–37]. There is no single frontal or temporoparietal area where stimulation-induced language errors are found in all patients. ESM provided evidence for a number of 'new' language areas in the supplementary motor cortex (SMA)[2], basal-temporal cortex[38–40], thalamus[41–43], and, more recently, premotor cortex and insula[44–46]. From ESM results, it can be argued that language cortex shows a modular design and functions via parallel processes and that different cortical sites are frequently involved in different language functions. (See Ojemann[34] for an extensive discussion on this subject.)

2.2.4 Functional neuroimaging

Functional neuroimaging techniques are a valuable adjunct to the lesion-deficit approach. Their principles rest on the assumption that there is a relationship between brain function and cerebral blood dynamics. In other words, when two experimental conditions give rise to two different patterns of neural activity (as measured via neurophysiological correlates), one may assume that they are engaged in functionally distinct cognitive operations. Foremost advantage of functional neuroimaging techniques is that any sensorimotor or cognitive function of interest can, in principle, be studied once appropriate experimental conditions are devised, so it is not limited to the region of the brain that has been damaged, nor to the function that is disturbed. FMRI and PET can, therefore, study brain areas that are involved in functional reorganization following brain injury and rehabilitation of function[47–56]. Another advantage is that subjects without neurological impairments can be studied, and this allows modelling of language in a population that is free from the effects of pathology and potential reorganization of function, and also permits study of individual differences in brain organization. Functional neuroimaging techniques additionally provide information about the dynamics of neural activity. By studying the interactions between different brain regions, one can explore the role of functional networks that sustain particular functions.

Investigations of the functional neuroanatomy of language have witnessed a remarkable progress over the last few years thanks to functional neuroimaging techniques. See, for reviews, Price *et al.*[57,58], Mesulam[59], and Binder[60]. To some extent, results are consistent with the features of the classical language model[57]. However, in general, a wider and more variable network of language-related areas is found, presumably because these techniques not only yield areas that are *critical* for function (as in the lesion-deficit approach) but also areas that *participate* in function[61]. For instance, functional neuroimaging studies consequently show involvement of areas surrounding the (left) inferior frontal sulcus in various language tasks. Topographically, these dorsolateral prefrontal areas are distinct from the classical Broca's language area. Activation in these areas need not necessarily reflect language processing per se but might, for instance, be related to working memory[62–64]. In fact, FMRI studies find an increasing number of 'new' areas that seem to be related to language processing. This is presumably explained by the fact that more and more tasks are constructed that target a particular aspect of language function that have not yet been consequently tested in brain-lesioned patients (at least not in such detail).

There are certainly also apparent inconsistencies when functional imaging studies are compared to findings from neuropsychological and clinical–anatomical studies[58]. For example, many PET and FMRI studies have suggested a role for the inferior frontal cortex in semantic processing while there are, in general, no major language comprehension deficits in patients with left frontal lesions and 'Broca's aphasia'[3,62,65–67]. Another apparent contradiction exists between the clinical evidence for hemispheric language dominance (which in the greater majority of healthy subjects and patients is unilateral and left-sided) and functional imaging techniques that consequently indicate language-related areas in both hemispheres (albeit often with an asymmetrical distribution)[12,68–70]. To what extent this relates to the inability of functional neuroimaging to selectively identify only critical language areas or to the inability of current clinical techniques to identify the more subtle aspects of language processing remains to be established. These questions will be addressed in more detail in the rest of this chapter.

2.3 The need for brain mapping techniques

Current clinical language models and surgical planning strategies are predominantly based on the results of lesion studies for a reason that seems, at least at first glance, very intuitive and valid — when a particular part of the brain is destroyed and this is accompanied by a loss of function, there must be a close relationship between this structure and the function that is lost. However, it is important to realize that these models are not adequate for surgical planning because lesion studies are compromised by several shortcomings.

An important drawback of lesion-derived models is that they are, for the larger part, based on data from stroke-damaged patients. In these patients, usually a relatively large cortical area is destroyed due to occlusion or haemorrhage in the territory of a major cerebral artery. Data from these brain-damaged patients generally, therefore, overestimate the size of critical language areas and are unable to differentiate between various smaller but different functional areas that lie within the same region. It is difficult to generalize findings in individual patients to a larger population as brain anatomy differs between normal subjects, whereas its morphology can be further affected by pathology[71,72]. Additional variability is introduced as some form of post-lesional recovery of function nearly always occurs, depending on the extent and severity of the lesion, age, co-morbidity, and functional state of remaining brain areas and the time elapsed since injury. Brain-damaged patients with aphasia usually recover part of their language function, indicating reorganization of function to former non-critical language areas. Evidence for plasticity of the language system also comes from children with early unilateral brain injury to either the left or right hemisphere who nevertheless can acquire language capabilities that are within the normal range[73–76]. Another confounding factor is that lesions might affect connections between structures. In this case, the core of the lesion is distant from the areas that are dysfunctional due to a lack of proper input.

In a substantial number of patients, language disorders do not conform with the classical language model and lesions or electrocortical stimulation do not result in the expected language deficits[1,77,78]. These findings, in combination with the development of functional imaging techniques and standardized instruments in neuropsychology, eventually led to the development of fundamentally different views on cerebral language representation. Although language models remain useful in understanding the majority of aphasic syndromes in clinical practice, surgical planning requires brain mapping techniques to elucidate each individual's variability in the topography of language function and to identify the critical regions.

3. Language lateralization

At the end of the 1990s, Petersen *et al.* were the first to show that functional neuroimaging techniques were capable of visualizing brain areas that were active during the processing of language tasks[66]. It was soon postulated that PET and, in particular, FMRI, could be used to predict cerebral language dominance in a clinical setting. In 1995, Desmond *et al.* showed a concordance in lateralization between FMRI and the amobarbital test in each of seven epilepsy patients, three of whom had atypical, right-sided language dominance. Since then, several papers have studied the use of FMRI for presurgical assessment of the language dominant hemisphere (see Table 3.1). However, despite the many advantages of BOLD FMRI over the amobarbital test, FMRI has not yet become a trusted tool in clinical practice for this purpose. There are some centres that advocate its use as a supplementary tool to existing invasive presurgical techniques, but actual replacement has not yet been reported. One of the major problems is the observed variability in obtained language activation maps between studies, despite the use of similar or identical experimental task designs, and the difficulty to extract only those areas that are considered truly relevant (i.e. 'critical') for language. In this section, we will review the FMRI literature on presurgical language lateralization and, in particular, focus on the requirements that have to be met for replacement of the language part of the amobarbital test.

Table 3.1 Characteristics of 15 studies in the literature that compared results from FMRI and the Wada test for assessment of hemispheric language dominance. Column 3 specifies whether the number of voxels (# voxels) or signal magnitude was used to calculate a lateralization index (LI). Column 6 specifies whether FMRI stimuli were visual (V) or auditory (A). Wada test results were usually categorized as left, right, or bilateral (column 8); three studies calculated the LI as a continuous value. Column 9 yields the total number of patients and the number of atypical patients (i.e. patients with bilateral or right-hemispheric language representation according to the Wada test). In columns 10–13, agreement between FMRI and the Wada test is given for patients with left (L), right (R), or bilateral (B) language representation. These data were not specified in all studies. Whenever possible (numbers in grey boxes), we calculated individual agreement between FMRI and the Wada test with cut-off values for FMRI of –25 and 25 (i.e. patients were classified as having right-hemispheric dominance when LI < –25, left hemispheric dominance when LI > 25, and bilateral language representation with a LI in between –25 and 25). (Abbreviations: ns = not specified; * based on visual judgement of FMRI activation maps; ** no explicit criterion for bilateral patients; LI <0 yields right-hemisphere dominance, LI >0 yields left-hemisphere dominance, no criterion specified for bilateral language; *** 'concordance in all cases determining the hemisphere with greater language representation'; **** 6 of 7 patients underwent FMRI after anterior temporal lobectomy.

1	2	3 fMRI LI	4 fMRI decision criterium	5 fMRI task	6 fMRI stimuli	7 fMRI control	8 Wada LI	9 nr patients total (atypical)	10 fMRI Wada overall match as mentioned in study	11 fMRI-L Wada-L agreement	12 fMRI-R Wada-R agreement	13 fMRI-B Wada-B agreement
author	year											
Desmond	1995	#voxels	ns	semantic decision of words	A	perceptual decision (letters)	discrete	7 (3)	7/7 (100%)****	4/4	3/3	0/0
Binder	1996	#voxels	ns	semantic decision of words	A	perceptual decision (tones)	continuous	20 (4)	***	18/18	1/3	1/1
Bahn[1]	1997	#voxels	ns	verbal fluency, rhyming	V	rest	discrete	7 (2)	7/7 (100%)	5/5	2/2	0/0
Hertt-Panniere	1997	#voxels and signal magnitude	ns	verbal fluency, (from letters)	A	rest	discrete	7 (1)	7/7 (100%)	6/6	0/0	1/1
Worthington[2]	1997	*	*	verbal fluency, (ns)	ns	rest	discrete	9 (ns)	5/6 (56%)	ns	ns	ns
Yetkin[3]	1998	#voxels	ns	verbal fluency, (from letters)	A	rest	continuous	13 (1)	13/13 (100%)	12/12	0/1	0/0
Benson	1999	#voxels and signal magnitude	**	verbal generation	V	fixating on crosshair	discrete	12 (3)	11/12 (92%)	9/9	2/2	0/1
Lehericy[4]	2000	#voxels	cut-off LI (-25/25)	verbal fluency, (from category)	A	rest	continuous	10 (1)	8/10 (80%) (frontal areas)	8/9	0/0	0/1
		#voxels	cut-off LI (-25/25)	story listening	A	listening to story story played backwards	continuous	10 (1)	9/10 (90%) (temporoparietal areas)	9/9	0/0	0/1
		#voxels	cut-off LI (-25/25)	sentence repetition	A		continuous	10 (1)	ns (low concordance)	ns	ns	ns
Carpentier	2001	#voxels	ns	sentence processing	V, A	perceptual decision (lines, tones)	discrete	10 (2)	8/10 (80%)	6/8	2/2	0/0
Rutten	2002	#voxels	cut-off LI (-25/25)	verb generation	V	looking at symbols	discrete	18 (7)	13/18 (72%)	10/11	2/3	1/4
		#voxels	cut-off LI (-25/25)	verbal fluency, (from letters)	V	rest	discrete	18 (7)	9/18 (50%)	8/11	1/3	0/4
		#voxels	cut-off LI (-25/25)	picture naming	V	looking at symbols	discrete	18 (7)	11/18 (61%)	7/11	2/3	2/4
		#voxels	cut-off LI (-25/25)	sentence comprehension	V	looking at symbols	discrete	18 (7)	12/18 (67%)	9/11	1/3	2/4
		#voxels	cut-off LI (-25/25)	conjoint analysis of four tasks	V		discrete	18 (7)	15/18 (83%)	10/11	2/3	3/4
Spreer	2002	#voxels	cut-off LI (-20/20)	semantic decision of words	V	perceptual decision (colours)	discrete	12 (4)	8/12 (75%) (whole brain)	6/8	2/3	1/1
		#voxels	cut-off LI (-20/20)	semantic decision of words	V	perceptual decision (colours)	discrete	12 (4)	12/12 (100%) (frontal areas)	8/8	3/3	1/1
		#voxels	cut-off LI (-20/20)	semantic decision of words	V	perceptual decision (colours)	discrete	12 (4)	10/12 (83%) (temporoparietal areas)	8/8	2/3	0/1
Adcock	2003	#voxels	cut-off LI (-29/29)	verbal fluency, (from letters)	V	rest	discrete	19 (4)	16/19 (84%)	14/15	0/1	2/3
		signal magnitude	cut-off LI (-27/27)	verbal fluency, (from letters)	V	rest	discrete	19 (4)	17/19 (89%)	15/15	1/1	1/3
Sabbah[5]	2003	#voxels	cut-off LI (-20/20)	verbal fluency, (from letters. from category)	A	rest	discrete	20 (8)	19/20 (95%)	12/12	7/8	0/0
Woermann[6]	2003	*	*	verbal fluency, (ns)	ns	rest	discrete	100 (29)	86/94 (91%)	ns	ns	ns
Gaillard	2004	*	*	verbal fluency	A	rest	discrete	25 (3)	ns	ns	ns	ns
		*	*	reading comprehension	V	looking at number of dots	discrete	25 (3)	ns	ns	ns	ns
		*	*	auditory comprehension	A	rest or reversed speech	discrete	25 (3)	ns	ns	ns	ns
		*	*	reading stories	V	looking at number of dots	discrete	25 (3)	ns	ns	ns	ns
		*	*	listening to stories	A	rest or reversed speech	discrete	25 (3)	ns	ns	ns	ns
		*	*	conjoint analysis of five tasks			discrete	25 (3)	21/25 (84%)	19/22	2/2	0/1

[1] Bahn MM *et al.*; *Localization of language cortices by functional MR imaging compared with intracarotid amobarbital hemispheric sedation.* AJNR (1997); **169**(2); pp 575–579. [2] Worthington C *et al.*; *Comparison of functional magnetic resonance imaging for language localization and intracarotid speech amytal testing in presurgical evaluation for intractable epilepsy. Preliminary results.* Stereotactic and Functional Neurosurgery (1997); **69**(1–4); pp 197–201. [3] Yetkin FZ *et al.*; *Functional MRI of frontal lobe activation: comparison with Wada test results.* ANJR (1998); **19**(6); pp 1095–1098. [4] Lehericy S *et al.*; *Functional MR evaluation of temporal and frontal language dominance compared with the Wada test.* Neurology (2000); **54**(8); pp 1625–1633. [5] Sabbah PS *et al.*; *Functional MR imaging in assessment of language dominance in epileptic patients.* Neuroimage (2003); **18**; pp 460–467. [6] Woermann FG *et al.*; *Language lateralization by Wada test and fMRI in one hundred patients with epilepsy.* Neurology (2003); **61**; pp 699–701.

3.1 The concept of language dominance

Within a few years after Broca's announcement that language areas were located in the left, hence dominant hemisphere, it gradually became clear that this was not the case for every patient. In some of the aphasic stroke patients, the lesion was found to be located in the right hemisphere. As it was noted that among these patients the incidence of left-handedness was larger than in the general population, the classical rule was formulated that the dominant hemisphere is contralateral to the dominant hand. Although this rule nicely restored the symmetry that was lost when the Broca–Wernicke model of language was proposed, it is not true. Only 20–30% of left handers develop aphasia after right-hemisphere damage (in right handers, the incidence is <2%) and are, therefore, in the majority of cases left-hemisphere dominant for language[79,80]. These data are comparable with results in Wada-tested patients.

FMRI studies have confirmed that, in the majority of both right- and left-handed subjects, the left hemisphere is language dominant. Pujol *et al.* studied frontal language areas with a word generation task in 50 left-handed and 50 right-handed subjects. They found that typical (i.e. left-sided) language lateralization occurred in 96% of right handers and in 76% of left handers[81]. Four per cent of right handers had a bilateral distribution of language function. Of the atypical left handers, 14% were bilateral, whereas 10% had language functions exclusively in the right hemisphere. Similar findings for 50 normal, right-handed subjects were found by Springer *et al.* with an auditory semantic decision task: 94% left-hemisphere dominance and 6% bilateral language representation[70].

There is now abundant evidence that atypical language organization is also found more often in patients with structural or functional damage in the left hemisphere (e.g. arteriovenous malformations or epilepsy)[56,82–84]. Reported incidences in Wada-tested patients vary from 4% to 55%. In these patients, the right hemisphere has taken over some, or even all of the language functions. In general, this recovery of language is more successful if the injury occurs in early childhood. Studies of children that underwent hemispherectomy suggest that both hemispheres may contribute to language functions until the age of about five years. Nevertheless, some form of lesion-induced language recovery frequently occurs at older age (e.g. in stroke patients), where it can involve redistribution of language functions to ipsilateral or contralateral brain areas[54].

Figure 3.1 illustrates the need for neurosurgeons to have routinely available techniques that can map language functions prior to surgery. This 14-year-old left-handed patient had a ten-year history of complex partial seizures. Further analysis revealed a tumour in the classical language area of Broca (i.e. the posterior part of the left inferior frontal gyrus), without any abnormalities on neuropsychological and neurological examinations. The Wada test showed left-hemisphere dominance, so intrahemispheric reorganization of frontal language areas had occurred. Given the risk of surgical damage to these language areas, it was decided to perform surgery with electrocortical language mapping. Remarkably, no language areas were found on the exposed cortical surface with ESM. After resection of the tumour, and guided by FMRI findings, Broca's area was found to be located in the depth of a sulcus, posteriorly and superiorly behind the tumour[85]. There were no postoperative deficits; pathological–anatomical analysis showed a ganglioglioma.

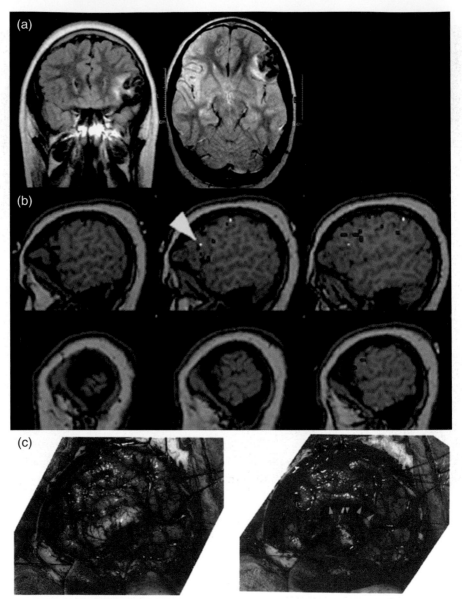

Fig. 3.1 (**a**) Left inferior frontal tumour (Broca's area) in a 14-year old left-handed epilepsy patient without neurological or neuropsychological deficit. (**b**) Composite results of multiple-task FMRI. Sagittal slices of the left hemisphere are shown. The most lateral slice is in the bottom left corner, the most medial slice is located in the upper right corner. Significant voxels (p<0.05, Bonferroni-corrected) are colored and superimposed on anatomical images (in-plane resolution, 2 mm). The red voxel (arrow) represents the area that is active during all four different language tasks (location corresponding to the sterile marker in shown in (**b**)).The blue voxels represent areas active during verb generation, the white voxels that are active during picture naming, and the green voxels during repetitive reciting of the days of the week. (Reproduced with permission of Rutten et al., 1999 (85)) (**c**) Photograph of the craniotomy before (left) and after (right) resection. The head of the patient is facing toward the left. The blue arrow on top of the sterile marker (white) points to the site where language errors were obtained with intraoperative electrocortical stimulation mapping. The yellow arrows indicate sites where mapping did not induce language errors.

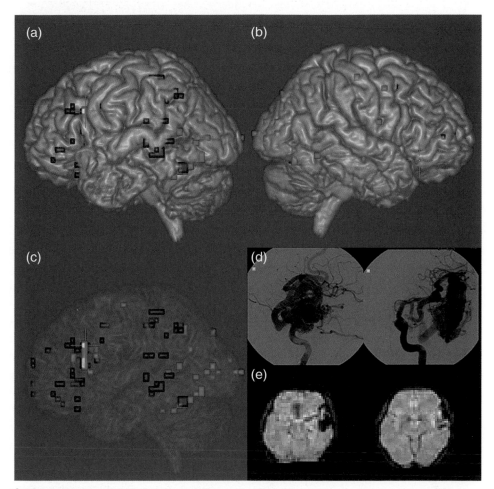

Fig. 3.2 Left temporal arteriovenous malformation (AVM) in a 35-year old left-handed patient with epilepsy. FMRI results are shown for verb generation (red voxels) and picture naming (green voxels), superimposed on a rendering of the left (**a**) and right (**b**) hemisphere. A considerable amount of FMRI activity is located within sulci and below the cortical surface. In figure (**c**), FMRI activation in made visible to approximately 10 to 15 mm beneath the cortical surface of the left hemisphere. In figure (**d**) (courtesy of GN Beute, Elisabeth Hospital, Tilburg, The Netherlands) the AVM is shown on lateral and anterior-posterior images from cerebral angiography. The axial slices (**e**) show the amount of BOLD signal that is measured (shown on a range from high (white) to low (black) signal). Note that in this patient, no reliable FMRI signal can be measured in the immediate vicinity of the AVM, due to flow and susceptibility effects.

Figure 3.2 shows another example where assessment of surgical risks is mandatory. The 35-year-old left-handed patient presented with epilepsy and postictal aphasia that related to a left temporal arteriovenous malformation (AVM). Perisylvian AVMs in the language-dominant hemisphere can be intimately related to language cortex and are even considered inoperable in some cases due to the associated high risks of postoperative language deficits[83,86]. In this patient, FMRI yielded strong left-hemisphere language dominance but also showed a margin of approximately 2cm between the posterior border of the

AVM and posterior temporal language areas. Following complete resection, there were language deficits that started two days after surgery and completely resolved within a few days. These deficits are best explained by postoperative oedema. Cannestra *et al.* recently studied 20 patients with dominant perisylvian AVMs with both FMRI and ESM[87]. They concluded that electrocortical language mapping is not necessary when the AVM is at least one gyrus located from FMRI activity. In their series, awake language mapping could be avoided in 75% of patients, based on presurgical FMRI findings.

These cases clearly demonstrate that FMRI has the potential to provide adequate presurgical functional information from a single non-invasive source that is currently only available through multiple invasive sources (Wada test and ESM). Judging from promising reports in the literature, one may expect replacement of the language part of the Wada test within the next few years. In general, these studies report a high but not perfect concordance between FMRI and the Wada test. As FMRI, unlike the Wada test, examines regional brain function in the presence of both functioning hemispheres, the results from both modalities may not completely agree. Besides differences in methodology, there is another important fundamental issue that may explain part of the observed incongruence in the literature. In current clinical and surgical practice, language representation is considered to be discrete (i.e. language is either present or is not present within an hemisphere). Consequently, neurosurgeons will ask whether or not surgery in an hemisphere has potential risks for language functioning. Most of the Wada test studies work with this assumption and classify language distribution as a categorical variable (i.e. left, right, or bilateral). FMRI language studies, on the other hand, consistently find activity in the 'non-dominant' hemisphere, even in healthy right-handed subjects that are generally considered left-hemisphere dominant. To match Wada test findings, FMRI studies, therefore, calculate a lateralization index (LI) that is usually based on the extent of activation in both hemispheres (LI = L-R/L+R, where L and R are the extent of activation in the left and right hemisphere, respectively). Arbitrarily chosen cut-off values for the LI then decide whether or not the extent of language-related FMRI activation in a hemisphere is sufficient to classify it as 'dominant' for language. These studies implicitly assume that the non-dominant hemisphere activation represents non-critical language processes.

Some authors have proposed a fundamentally different view on language representation and suggest that language dominance might be a continuous property of both hemispheres[70,88]. Springer *et al.* used FMRI to measure language lateralization in a group of 100 neurologically normal, right-handed subjects. A semantic language activation task was used relative to a non-linguistic, auditory discrimination task. Although, as expected, the greater majority of normal subjects was left-hemisphere dominant (94% had a LI >20), a continuous range of values for the LI was observed (see Fig. 3.3). In the same study, an even broader distribution for the LI was found for 50 right-handed epilepsy patients; this distribution was shifted towards lower LI values in accordance with the significant larger incidence of atypical language representation in epilepsy patients. A similar continuous distribution of the FMRI LI in epilepsy patients was found by Spreer and colleagues[88].

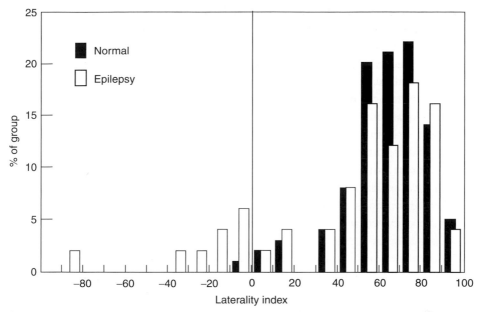

Fig. 3.3 Frequency distribution of the FMRI-determined lateralization index (LI) in 100 normal subjects and 50 epilepsy patients. The LI varies between −100 (all FMRI activity in right hemisphere) and 100 (all activity in left hemisphere). (Reprinted with permission from Springer et al.., 1999[70])

The notion of this language continuum assumes a degree of equipotentiality between hemispheres with respect to basic language processing functions and is supported by evidence from a number of Wada test studies[69,89,90]. In three of fifteen studies that compared FMRI to the Wada test (Table 3.1), Wada results were classified according to a graded scale instead of the classical categorization left/right/bilateral. These studies describe a significant correlation between the lateralization indexes from the Wada test and FMRI (despite the fact that different tests are used). This correlation even holds when only left-hemisphere dominant patients were considered. There are two mechanisms that could explain this concept of graded language representation: either the different linguistic components that make up language function (i.e. phonological, semantic, or attentional processes) are each represented in different hemispheres, or each component itself is to some extent represented in both hemispheres. Additional evidence for critical right-hemisphere language processing comes from lesion studies. It is now well recognized that right-hemisphere damage in previously healthy subjects can affect 'discourse' (i.e. the ability to tell a story or to understand a joke) and prosody.

3.2 The amobarbital (or Wada) test

The amobarbital test (or Wada test, named after its inventor Juhn Wada) is widely used in epilepsy surgery and, occasionally, tumour surgery, to probe whether a single hemisphere is capable of normal language (and memory) function[91,92]. It uses an ultrashort-acting barbiturate that is injected into either one of the internal carotid arteries, effectively disabling a large part of one hemisphere for approximately five minutes. During this period, the contralateral hemisphere is examined for language (and other functional) capacities. While the patient is asked to perform a series of language tasks (object naming, reading, picture describing, etc.), he is monitored for aphasic errors. The test is performed under EEG monitoring to document functional changes in the ipsilateral hemisphere and, as a result of possible overflow of amobarbital, the contralateral hemisphere. Validity of the test is based on two assumptions: first, the injected amobarbital can reach and anaesthetize all brain areas in the ipsilateral hemisphere that are involved in language function; second, during the testing period (i.e. the time that the amobarbital is effective), there is no substitution of language function by non-anaesthetized ipsilateral or contralateral brain areas.

There are several factors that may confound interpretation of the Wada test[93]. At times, agitation or somnolence make determination of language dominance problematic. Inadequate anaesthetization of brain regions may also lead to false-negative results on laterality of function. For instance, as the temporoparietal region receives blood from the middle and/or the posterior cerebral artery (these arteries originate from the carotid and vertebrobasilar system, respectively), the amobarbital that is injected via the carotid system may not always adequately deactivate some of the temporoparietal areas involved in speech comprehension[94]. Another possible confounder is that the amobarbital may cross-over to the other hemisphere via variations in vaculature; this can be anticipated with angiography.

Between different clinical centres, there is no standardized set of parameters in terms of which language functions are evaluated during the test. This accounts for at least some of the considerable variability in the reported incidences of typical (i.e. left-sided) and non-typical (i.e. right-sided or bilateral) language dominance. Most groups use naming or responses to verbal comments, but others have predominantly relied on the duration of speech arrest as an important parameter for hemispheric language dominance[91,95]. There is some concern that the Wada test underestimates the incidence of bilateral language dominance, as inconsistencies have been reported with clinical outcome[96] or the findings of ESM[97,98]. These arguments favour the notion that the Wada test may not be a highly independent measure of language dominance.

3.3 FMRI versus the Wada test: an overview of the literature

We found 15 studies that systematically compared FMRI against the Wada test for the purpose of language lateralization (Table 3.1). Only patients that underwent amobarbital anaesthetization of both hemispheres were included, as unilateral testing does not exclude possible bilateral language representation[99]. The total number of patients was 289 (median 12 patients, range 7–100 patients); the greater majority had intractable epilepsy. All FMRI tasks were covert (to avoid scanning artefacts) and block-designed. Most patients (75%) in these studies had typical language dominance according to the Wada test. In more recent studies, the number of atypical patients has increased, as it was realized that the predictive value of FMRI can only be calculated when large groups of typical as well as atypical patients are studied.

For the typical Wada patients, excellent agreement between FMRI and Wada test results is reported in every study. Overall agreement is 91% (median 100%, range 64–100%). The average agreement rises to 96% when only the best task per study is considered.

Somewhat lower rates of agreement are found for patients with right-hemisphere language dominance according to the Wada test. In cases of disagreement in these patients, FMRI mostly finds bilateral language representation. The agreement for FMRI and the Wada test is lowest for bilateral Wada patients; average agreement is approximately 50%.

There is a large variation across studies in data presentation (task design, stimulus presentation), data acquisition (scan technique, scanning equipment), and data analysis (single- versus multiple-task analysis, voxel-based analysis versus smoothing or clustering of voxels, parametric versus non-parametric statistics, various measures for the FMRI lateralization index). In some of the studies, particularly those from the earlier years, no specific FMRI criteria are mentioned for determination of individual hemispheric dominance (Desmond, Bahn, Binder). Some studies use independent raters to visually judge the FMRI activation maps (Worthington, Woermann, Gaillard), whereas a number of other studies use regression analysis to express the correlation between patients (Binder, Lehericy). Although such a correlation may be statistically significant, it does not suffice for clinical application where misdiagnosis can carry severe consequences. This requires quantitative assessment of the number of misdiagnosed subjects. Most studies, therefore, quantify the agreement between FMRI and Wada test results via a LI that is calculated for each patient. Despite the overall high agreement between FMRI and the Wada test that is reported across studies, there is a large variability in the LIs (and cut-off values) between different studies. For instance, average LIs (+/− standard deviation, SD) for typical Wada patients range from 69 +/− 23 (Rutten) to 14 +/− 6 (Benson). Note that, for instance, the average LI for typical patients in the study of Benson *et al.* is below the cut-off value of 20 that is used in the studies of Sabbah and Spreer to classify patients as having typical hemispheric language dominance.

In ten out of fifteen studies, a single language task design was used; six of these studies used a verbal fluency task (patients have to generate different words from a given letter or category), one study used a verb generation task (patient have to think of a verb that relates to a given noun e.g. shoe → walking). Tasks in these studies were contrasted with relative simple control conditions e.g. 'rest' (the instruction to 'do nothing') or looking at a fixation cross or symbols. Three studies (Desmond, Binder, Spreer) used a more elaborate semantic decision task where patients had to press a button to indicate their choice. These tasks were controlled with perceptual judgement tasks to optimize elimination of non-linguistic processes from the activation maps. Lehericy *et al.* used three different language tasks with auditory presentation: verbal fluency, story listening, and sentence repetition. The latter two tasks were included to focus more specifically on temporoparietal language areas, as most previous studies showed that classical language 'production' tasks (verbal fluency, verb generation, or semantic decision) predominantly activate frontal areas. In addition to global hemispheric Lis, they calculated regional indices for frontal and temporoparietal areas. This is important for identification of patients with bilateral language functions, where frontal and temporoparietal language areas do not necessarily reside in the same hemisphere. For example, Staudt *et al.* demonstrated that in patients with early left-hemisphere lesions, frontal language areas had shifted to opposite, undamaged homologue regions[90]. Similar findings were reported for epilepsy, tumour, and AVM patients in FMRI and Wada test studies[89,99–103]. Lehericy *et al.* found

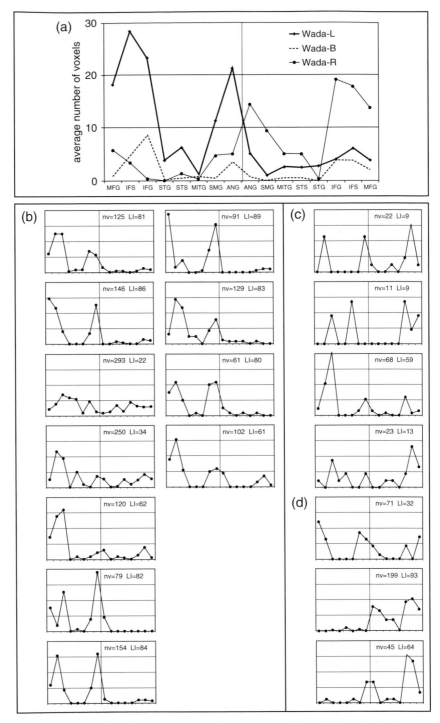

Fig. 3.4 (**a**) Average number of voxels for a combined analysis of four FMRI tasks (verb generation, verbal fluency, picture naming and sentence comprehension) in each of 16 volumes of interest (VOI) for patients with either left (n=11), right (n=3) or mixed (n=4) language dominance according to

that the asymmetry of frontal FMRI activation for the verbal fluency and story listening task was correlated with Wada test LIs. Although the sentence-repetition task, as well as the story-listening task, increased the sensitivity for detection of temporoparietal areas, it yielded no significant correlation with Wada test results. Temporal lobe activation was not significantly correlated with Wada test indices in any of the tasks, even though reversed speech was used as a control task for the story-listening task.

Spreer *et al.* also calculated regional LIs. They used a semantic decision task, where patients had to indicate (via a button press) the synonym for a given word among four other visually presented words. A colour discrimination task was used as control. As in the studies by Lehericy, Bahn, and Rutten, frontal LIs gave a better agreement with the Wada test than global or temporoparietal LIs. This suggests that global LIs, at least with the tasks that are presently used, may occasionally be misleading.

It is a general finding in FMRI studies that even subtle differences in task design can lead to substantial different activation patterns, in particular for tasks that target cognitive functions. Benson *et al.*, therefore, first tested a panel of three tasks in healthy volunteers to investigate their possible clinical use for assessment of hemispheric language dominance. Only a verb generation task yielded reliable left-lateralized activity, whereas a naming and a reading task did not. The verb-generation task was subsequently used in patients with a broad spectrum of different brain lesions for comparison with the Wada test, where they report good agreement with FMRI.

Five studies combined two or more tasks to increase detection power or to favour detection of areas that are commonly activated in different tasks (Bahn, Carpentier, Gaillard, Lehericy, Rutten). This latter conjoint task approach aims at a more selective detection of critical language areas[104]. Rutten *et al.* conjointly analysed four different language tasks: verbal fluency, verb generation, picture naming, and sentence processing. This approach gave a better concordance with Wada test results than the individual task approach, in particular for atypical patients (see Fig. 3.4 for details). Of the individual tasks, the verb-generation task yielded the best results, although no individual task was able to reliably predict atypical patients. Two remarkable differences in activation patterns between bilateral and unilateral language patients were observed. First, in three of four bilateral patients, there was a discordance between frontal (right hemispheric) and temporoparietal (left hemispheric) language representation, that was not observed for the left or right hemispheric dominant patients. Such a dissociation has occasionally

---

the Wada test (respectively, thick, thin and dotted lines). Left hemispheric VOIs are depicted on the left side of each figure, right hemispheric VOIs on the right. Graphs for the 18 individual patients are shown in figures (**b**),(**c**) and (**d**) (respectively the patients with left, mixed and bilateral language dominance) The vertical axis displays the percentage of FMRI activity (maximum is 40%) in each of the VOIs (i.e., the number of active voxels per VOI relative to the total number of voxels in all VOIs for that patient). For each patient, the number of voxels (nv) and the lateralization index (LI) are shown. Abbreviations: MFG – middle frontal gyrus, IFS = inferior frontal sulcus, IFG = inferior frontal gyrus, STG = superior temporal gyrus, STS = superior temporal sulcus, MITG = middle and inferior temporal gyrus, ANG = angular gyrus, and SMG = supramarginal gyrus. (Reprinted with permission from Rutten et al., 2002)[101].

been described, but the observed incidence in this study is relatively high[99]. Second, bilateral patients had significantly less brain activity than unilateral patients (see Fig. 3.4). Although the patient sample is too small to draw any conclusions, these results suggest that the use of only one language task and/or the acquisition of relatively short time series (few FMRI scans) lower the detection power for language areas in bilateral patients. The observed frontal versus temporoparietal dissociation in bilateral patients may have contributed to the poor results that were obtained with the individual task approaches, as some of the individual tasks rely more on activation in specific regions (e.g. frontal activation in the word-generation tasks). If indeed different linguistic functions are balanced between hemispheres in certain bilateral patients, one can imagine that the use of multiple different FMRI tasks gives a better approximation of the distribution of language components across hemispheres than the use of a single task. The combined task approach did also significantly increase detection power for language related activity and yielded frontal and temporoparietal language areas in every patient; LIs calculated from these two regions were significantly correlated.

In a recent paper, Gaillard *et al*[106]. found that concordance with Wada test results could be improved when a panel of FMRI tasks was used that target different aspects of language processing. Five tasks were used, both with auditory and visually presented stimuli. For analysis, tasks were clustered to verbal fluency, reading comprehension, and auditory comprehension. Three independent raters scored each cluster by visual inspection of images at different statistical thresholds. Agreement between FMRI and Wada test was found in 21 of 25 patients. The use of a panel of tasks also led to a better agreement among raters than when single task results had to be judged.

To what extent can FMRI already replace the Wada test for language lateralization? The abovementioned studies demonstrate that for patients with typical language dominance according to the Wada test, FMRI generally shows left-lateralized activation maps. With selected FMRI tasks, overall sensitivity of FMRI (i.e. how often are Wada test findings confirmed by FMRI?) for these patients is >90%. Combining different tasks seems mandatory to increase sensitivity and specificity, in particular for atypical patients. To be of clinical use, FMRI requires a high predictive value (i.e. how often are FMRI findings confirmed with the Wada test?) and reliable criteria to distinguish typical from atypical patients. As of yet, there are no FMRI protocols that agree with Wada test results for all patients. We found with the combined-task approach that all patients that had a LI >75 were classified as typical by the Wada test[101,105]. This suggests that the Wada test can be partially replaced with this specific FMRI protocol, as only the patients with a LI <75 need additional Wada testing to differentiate between typical or atypical language dominance. A similar strategy was proposed by Gaillard and colleagues; they also stress the use of multiple tasks to increase sensitivity and reliability of FMRI maps[106].

In conclusion, the use of FMRI for identification of language areas is not yet trusted in a clinical setting and this is mainly due to two reasons. First, replacement of existing techniques requires extensive testing and validation in large groups of patients. This not only requires comparison to results of the Wada test (that in itself can be disputed on methodological and practical grounds) but also, in particular, to the true gold standard — patient outcome. To date, this has rarely been done[107]. Clearly, the number of atypical patients that has been studied is too small to calculate predictive values for FMRI tasks. Second, FMRI findings are not very consistent across studies, tasks, patients, or healthy volunteers. The large number of variables that affect outcome in FMRI experiments requires standardization for objective use in clinical practice. In the following sections, we will discuss in more detail methodological drawbacks and possible solutions for the use of FMRI in a clinical setting.

4. Language localization

4.1 What do we need to know?

All teams involved in epilepsy or brain tumour surgery are confronted with the problem of localization of language function, although the term 'language' is imprecise by itself. As discussed before, this definition greatly depends on the question asked. Historically, neurosurgeons have used a rather restrictive but practical definition for 'language' based on clinical outcome and findings during awake language mapping with ESM. This method has become the gold standard for localizing language areas during neurosurgical procedures[108–110]. It is true that its methodology can vary across institutions and that some issues (e.g. intensity of stimulation) are still discussed, but the technique is safe, accurate, and has largely proven its usefulness in preventing postoperative aphasia[108–111]. No other brain-mapping technique has been used so intensively in this field. Following the works of Penfield (1959)[2] and Ojemann (1989)[37], object naming is most often used. Reasons are that it is simple to use, that naming deficits are common to all aphasic syndromes, and that is has yielded good postoperative language outcome.

Language is not only 'naming' however. Other language tasks have been used during direct cortical mapping, such as reading, writing, verb generation, repetition, or language comprehension. For these different language tasks, task-specific sites are found, in addition to cortical areas that are commonly shared (see Fig. 3.7 for an example)[109,112,113]. Similar observations are made in bilinguals; when two languages are tested with ESM, there are both specific as well as commonly activated temporoparietal[113] and frontal brain areas[112]. These findings suggest that an ESM-detected area is not necessarily involved in all aspects of critical language processing and have implications for use of the term 'critical language area'.

How do we know that the cortical areas that are found for instance with reading, repetition, or language comprehension tasks are really 'critical' for those particular functions? Do these areas really produce significant and persistent language impairments when they are removed? Despite good clinical outcome in large series of patients, there is no direct proof that ESM-detected language areas are critical for language function. To date, no large study has been conducted on this topic and it is easy to understand why: all cortical areas found are generally spared by the neurosurgeon that thinks, intuitively, that they need to be preserved. One of us showed, in a large study using specifically reading tasks during direct stimulation, that it was very difficult to evaluate the real impact of the use of reading tasks on postoperative language abilities[112].

It is tempting to already introduce FMRI for presurgical planning as the technique is non-invasive and relatively easy to use. However, despite some promising reports in the literature, significant uncertainties persist about the capabilities of language FMRI for this purpose[114–116]. If FMRI is to replace ESM, the fundamental issue for neurosurgeon and patient is to know whether FMRI is able: (1) to detect with accuracy all critical language areas in the surgical field and (2) to ensure that, when no FMRI activation is present, no critical language areas are present. In other words, to assume that if we remove these areas, the patient will not have symptoms of aphasia postoperatively. A difficulty is that when sites are qualified as 'silent' with either FMRI or ESM, it cannot be excluded that the use of other tasks will yield activation.

Whether FMRI data are clinically relevant requires a large prospective, statistically significant survey, testing not only the correlation between direct cortical mapping and FMRI but also the correlation between preoperative FMRI data and postoperative language deficits. To date, no such study has been undertaken. However, it is not illusory to think that this study is possible: similar studies have been done with other invasive methods[107]. To guide us in this, one could naturally use the established relation between naming sites detected by electrostimulation and the absence of postoperative deficits. So, some authors (including ourselves) have designed FMRI protocols that especially use confrontation naming tasks to test whether FMRI is able to detect the areas that are found with direct cortical stimulation. In the following paragraphs, we analyse the existing data on the correlation between language FMRI and direct cortical stimulation, and the methodological issues of the FMRI technique. Finally, we summarize how FMRI can be used in preoperative language evaluation.

4.2 Electrocortical stimulation: principles and pitfalls

Electrical stimulation of the cortex originates in the early observations made by Frisch and Hitzig in animals[117]. According to Beevor and Horsley, the first direct electrical stimulation of the cortex in man was carried out by Bartholow in 1874[118,119]. Penfield was the first who systematically used intraoperative ESM for localization of sensorimotor and language areas. He concluded in his *Speech and Brain-Mechanisms* that destruction of larger parts of the temporoparietal language area 'would certainly produce the gravest aphasia' but speculated that Broca's area was less indispensable. Still, he proclaimed that 'despite the suspicion of dispensability of the anterior speech area of Broca, we still advise that this area, which can be outlined so clearly by stimulation, should be carefully avoided during surgery' (p. 203)[2]. (See Devinsky (1993) for a detailed historical overview on ESM[33].)

ESM can either be performed intraoperatively, which is considered the gold standard, or extraoperatively. The latter requires an additional operation where arrays of grid electrodes are implanted a few days prior to the resection itself. The clinical strategy for localization of language functions with ESM resides on stimulation of multiple cortical sites in the planned area of resection. During each stimulation, which lasts 5–10 seconds, the patient performs a particular task. This short duration constrains the way in which language functions can be tested (e.g. one cannot test for more complex comprehension of sentences or text). When errors are reproducibly induced during stimulation at a particular cortical site, this site is thought to be critical for the particular function that is being tested and is not included in the resection. Negative stimulation responses are of equal importance, as these indicate that an area can be safely resected.

Application of an alternating electrical current to cortical tissue has a variety of excitatory and inhibitory effects, both locally and at a distance from the site of stimulation[120]. One of the main criticisms of the use of cortical stimulation in brain mapping is that electrical stimulation of the cortex could be considered far from normal physiological brain activity. Behaviourally, stimulation of the sensorimotor areas induces movements or sensory-like symptoms, suggesting predominantly excitatory activity, whereas stimulation of associative cortex usually has inhibitory effects (e.g. interference with language functions). Although the exact nature and extent of the neuronal disruption is not known, ESM is estimated to have a spatial resolution of 5–10mm[37,121]. The effects of bipolar stimulation are repeatable and can change dramatically over the course of a few millimetres, indicating the relatively small size of different functional areas. No permanent tissue damage or changes suggestive of kindling have been described with ESM[34,122]. In addition to its high spatial and temporal resolution, another advantage of the technique is the sudden onset of the effects and its immediate reversibility, which probably eliminates the possibility of compensatory reorganization of function.

ESM, however, has limitations and disadvantages, indicating that its status as a gold standard is not without controversy. As mentioned before, there is no direct proof that ESM-detected language areas are, per se, critical for normal language function. Haglund et al[125]. found an increase in postoperative aphasia when the resection encroached within 1cm of ESM-detected temporal language areas, thereby suggesting a causal relationship between loss of function and deficits found with ESM. On the other hand, other studies found evidence that not all language areas that are found with ESM are of equal importance for normal language function[123]. There is even some evidence that removal of a small ESM-detected language area in the anterior temporal lobe that is present in addition to a larger posterior language area, does not necessarily affect postoperative language function[124]. Occasionally, patients suffer from long-term postoperative dysphasia, even though ESM did not yield language errors in the area that was resected. One of the explanations for this finding is that intrasulcal language areas (i.e. language areas that are located in the depth of a sulcus) can go unnoticed with ESM[85].

An important limitation is that ESM is an invasive technique that can only be performed intraoperatively (within the limited territory that is exposed during surgery) or following surgical implantation of intracranial electrodes for stimulation. If performed during operation, it requires specific anaesthetic considerations and patient cooperation during awake language-mapping studies, which excludes younger children and part of the adult population. ESM is, therefore, restricted to a subset of patients who have a clinical indication for a neurosurgical operation, in particular patients with long-standing epilepsy or tumours in sensorimotor or language-related areas. As in these patients reorganization may have affected the distribution of functional areas, there is no normal reference population for ESM data[37,125–127]. There are also no reproducibility data for ESM, as there are no data on the location of ESM-derived sites in the same patients in between operations without intervening brain damage[34,128].

Several 'local' circumstances (e.g. the occurrence of liquor on the cortex) are likely to influence the effects of stimulation, which prevents reliable standardization of the technique[111]. The stimulating current should be large enough to alter cortical function, but not so large that it will evoke seizure activity (afterdischarges) in neighbouring cortical areas (as this distorts the localizing value of stimulation)[129]. There is also limited time in the operating room, which usually only allows for testing of one particular language task. Most studies have used an object-naming task for this purpose. As different language tasks in part yield different critical language areas, ESM should, and may, underestimate the number of areas that are critical for language[34].

4.3 FMRI versus cortical stimulation: an impossible match?

The validation stage of the FMRI technique in the language field is fundamental. The specific correlation between language FMRI data and direct cortical mapping has been seldom studied[87,116,130–133]. Although it seems natural to correlate both techniques by using a similar task, the conceptual and technical differences between direct brain mapping and FMRI must be acknowledged. FMRI can identify sites of neural activity associated with a particular function, but the ability to selectively show critical areas has not yet been established. When creating language maps for presurgical planning, non-critical language functions should not contaminate statistical maps. We have previously discussed the issue of critical versus non-critical involvement of brain regions and strategies for robust and selective detection of critical language areas (e.g. combined analysis of multiple tasks, stringent thresholding). Furthermore, the validation of intrasulcal activations is problematic (intrasulcal stimulation is normally not possible) and this could be considered a major drawback of this mode of correlation[85]. Direct cortical mapping has been validated by clinical results (i.e. if you respect ESM-detected language sites, the risk of permanent aphasia is low). From a neurosurgical point of view, FMRI should give similar information to be useful in presurgical planning.

How to correlate FMRI data and direct brain stimulation in practice? Both authors of this chapter conducted studies that evaluated the use of FMRI as an alternative to intra-operative direct brain mapping in patients with brain tumours and epilepsy[116,134]. One of us (F–E.R.) has chosen the 'site by site' correlation with FMRI data visualized in 3D reconstructions of the brain. In this study, we found an imperfect correlation between the results of FMRI and ESM for two specific tasks (naming and verb generation)[134]. The FMRI naming task had poor localization value for both frontal and temporoparietal areas. The FMRI verb-generation task was slightly better correlated with ESM. In this study, we also compared pre- and postoperative FMRI data; our experience was limited to eight patients. To our knowledge, the comparison between pre- and postoperative language FMRI studies and direct brain mapping had seldom been done. Complete agreement between pre- and postoperative FMRI studies and direct brain mapping was only observed in three of our eight patients. Although we should be cautious about drawing conclusions based on these individual cases, these results question, at least, the value of naming or verb-generation FMRI tasks (and their reproducibility) in patients with brain tumours. It has previously been shown, for motor FMRI data, that an absent or barely detectable preoperative signal can become detectable postoperatively, and this questions the ability of FMRI to detect reliable task-related activity near brain tumours[135,136].

In our other study, 13 epilepsy patients were included that underwent awake mapping in temporoparietal areas (see Fig. 3.8)[116]. ESM failed during surgery in two patients. FMRI information from four different tasks was read into a surgical guidance system. Given the potential inaccuracy of this technique due to effects of brain shift (e.g. after opening of the dura), we used a cortical rendering to fine tune the exact position of the FMRI areas. In our experience, a surface MRI rendering of the cortical anatomy allows for accurate and swift localization of sulci and gyri in patients. The ESM procedure (that used an object-naming task) was recorded on video and stimulated sites were digitized. A computer algorithm calculated whether or not significant FMRI activity was present within a radius of 6.4mm around ESM sites. In eight patients, ESM detected language areas. In seven of these eight patients, FMRI detected all these areas, but the results of at least three FMRI tasks had to be combined to achieve 100% sensitivity. In one patient, sensitivity was 38%; here, FMRI information was included in a larger area found with ESM. The *presence* of FMRI activity at negative ESM sites (i.e. sites where no language functions were disrupted with ESM) limited the predicted value of FMRI to 51%. Thus, on average, twice as many areas were found with FMRI than ESM. This precludes current replacement of ESM, as areas would be spared unnecessarily. On the other hand, FMRI could very reliably predict the *absence* of positive ESM sites, suggesting that these areas could have been safely resected without the use of ESM. This implies FMRI can be used to optimize the ESM procedure, as only a limited number of brain areas needs to be checked.

Overall, the correlation between FMRI and ESM has been less frequently studied for language than for motor function. Some authors have claimed that there was a good correlation between language FMRI data and ESM[130–133,137]. Using different tasks, consisting of picture naming and listening to recordings of spoken words, Ruge *et al.* have shown, for three patients, a high degree of correlation between FMRI and ESM[137]. Lurito *et al.*, also in three patients, showed that the correlation between both techniques in receptive language areas was high but not perfect, with a parietal language area detected by direct brain mapping that was not detected by FMRI[132]. Fitzgerald *et al.*, using five different activation tasks and correlating their results with electrostimulation to 11 patients (such as word reading, visual and auditory verb generation, listening to single words and text), found that FMRI data were very sensitive for detecting language areas but poorly specific[131]. Pouratian *et al.* studied ten patients with arteriovenous malformation and found a specificity of 66% and a sensitivity of 96% for FMRI-detected language areas compared with ESM[133]. Mueller *et al.*, testing two patients with tumours in frontal areas, found a good correspondence between FMRI-activated areas (word-generation task) and electrostimulation[108].

So what is the message of the literature about the correlation between FMRI and ESM? We think that the reported cases are too inconstant to draw definitive conclusions. One important issue is the significant variability of FMRI data across patients, tasks, and statistical thresholds. These variations have a large impact on the correlation between results from cortical mapping and FMRI. As of yet, we think that the use of language

FMRI in surgical planning is not feasible without additional use of ESM. Reasons for the observed discrepancies are probably multifactorial. The choice of paradigms of activation is of paramount importance in FMRI. A naming task is usually chosen, to mimic as closely as possible the task that is used during intraoperative ESM. In FMRI, this task has been said to produce poorly lateralized activity with important visual cortex activation[131]. Some authors have stated that a number of brain areas, including dorsolateral frontal and lateral temporal cortices, are more frequently activated with a verb-generation task than with a naming task.[138] In our studies, we had to combine different FMRI tasks to increase the sensitivity for ESM-detected language areas[85,116,131,139]. Single FMRI tasks were not sufficient for this purpose. When we assume that critical language areas are involved in all aspects of language function, it must be concluded that single FMRI tasks (at least the ones that are used in the literature) are not sensitive enough for this purpose. However, another more likely explanation is that different language functions are represented, in part, by different sets of critical language areas. This is supported by the fact that some FMRI tasks (e.g. verb generation) are more sensitive for critical frontal language areas, whereas other tasks (e.g. sentence comprehension) are more sensitive for critical temporoparietal language areas[140]. A similar conclusion can be drawn from the ESM literature, where different tasks can detect different language areas. This implies that the match between FMRI and ESM can be further optimized when multiple different tasks are used during ESM. This hypothesis can be tested in patients where grid electrodes are implanted before surgical resection, as there is more time in these patients to perform ESM. Ultimately, FMRI results should be compared to patient outcome.

5. **Methodological issues**

Besides validated and standardized FMRI protocols, clinical use, in particular, requires an easy-to-use and time-efficient investigation that can be performed by radiological personnel. FMRI results should be readily available (preferably via automated analyses available on the scanner) and allow for easy implementation in a surgical guidance system for use during surgery. Ideally, interpretation of FMRI maps should not require expert knowledge. Real-time FMRI and functional neuronavigation are already technically feasible and one may, therefore, expect that functional FMRI will become a commonplace tool in the near future[141,142]. Still, several methodological issues need to be solved.

5.1 **Task design**

Part of the differences in results between FMRI and the Wada test or ESM can be explained by the experimental design of the FMRI task (see Fig. 3.5 for an example). Current FMRI studies typically identify more language regions than existing clinical methods, suggesting that FMRI not only identifies areas that are critical for language processing, but also areas that participate in a less critical manner in networks that sustain language function. Neurosurgical use of FMRI requires very strict criteria, as both the presence and the absence of areas that harbour critical language functions need to be identified with sufficient spatial resolution. Although these criteria are somewhat less strict for language lateralization than for language localization, non-critical areas will

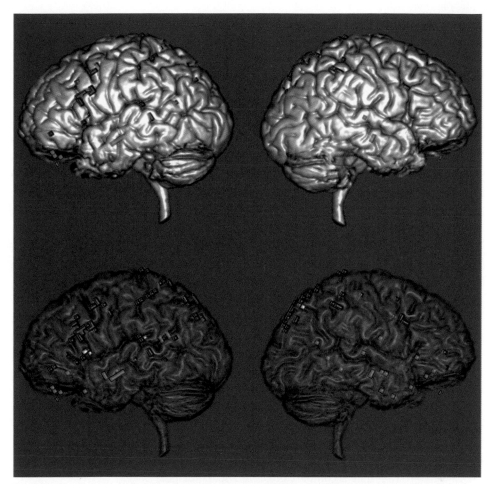

Fig. 3.5 Differences in regional brain activity between FMRI tasks that involve processing of single words or pictures (red voxels, combined results from 'classic' language tasks: verb generation, verbal fluency and picture naming) and a task that involves processing of sentences (green voxels). Yellow voxels are active in sentence processing and in one or more of the other tasks (i.e., 'red + green'). The patient had left hemispheric dominance according to a bilateral Wada test, in agreement with the distribution of activity from the classic language tasks that is predominantly seen in left inferior and middle frontal gyrus and left temporoparietal areas. In addition to activity in these areas, the sentence comprehension task yielded strong bilateral activation of the temporal lobes, and inferior frontal and orbitofrontal areas. Top row images show the cortical representation of FMRI activity, while in the bottom row images activation has been made visible beneath the cortical surface (< 10 – 15 mm).

affect the obtained measures for lateralization and can easily lead to false classification of hemispheric dominance. Thus, the task has to be constructed so as to extract only the function of interest (FOI) to the examiner (i.e. critical language function).

Most studies use a subtraction design, where an activation task engages the FOI, and a baseline task involves all other components except the FOI. Brain regions that are associated with the FOI are then identified by serial subtraction of activation and baseline scans.

Simple baseline tasks (e.g. a pure resting state) are not sufficient, as too many areas will remain in the activation maps that are not directly related to the FOI. One example is a verbal fluency task, that is often used in language lateralization studies, and where patients have to generate words that start with a particular letter or belong to a particular category. In addition to classical language areas, (left-sided) dorsolateral prefrontal areas are usually found in these studies[81]. But is this activation related to 'pure' language processing or is it, for instance, related to verbal memory processes that keep track of the words that have already been generated? Questions like these should be discussed before the experiment to construct a valid control task. On the other hand, care should be taken that control stimuli do not evoke (uncontrolled) language processing that will cancel out language areas in the activation maps. For instance, the use of a perceptual judgement task where a subject has to decide whether a word is represented in upper or lower case letters is likely to evoke some form of (automatic) language processing[68].

A problem with the subtraction task design is that it requires explicit identification of all cognitive and sensorimotor components in the tasks. Even if this were possible, for cognitive subtraction to work, one has to assume that these different components do not interact (this principle is known as *pure insertion*)[104]. In this case, new cognitive components can be added to a task without affecting existing ones. However, in language studies, the various components seem intricately intertwined. There are many linguistic and non-linguistic tasks that require neural systems that process visual or auditory sensory information or temporarily store this information. The extent to which some of these systems are specific for language is not known but it is likely that a particular brain area participates in multiple functions. Given this redundancy, the use of a subtraction design can lead to undesirable subtraction of language-related activation, even when control tasks are used that are considered non-linguistic on theoretical grounds. For instance, Binder *et al.* showed that many areas that are implicated in semantic processing are active even when a resting state is compared to a non-semantic task[60].

An alternative way to isolate the FOI is to construct multiple pairs of activation and baseline tasks, that are conjointly analysed[104,105]. A major advantage is that this conjunction approach does not require explicit formulation of the FOI and that baseline tasks need not be perfect (although they must not include the FOI). The underlying principle is that only the FOI is present in all (or most) of the subtraction pairs. This approach led to more robust and reliable language LIs in normal subjects than with the use of individual tasks[105]. It also found better results in patients, in particular for atypical patients[101,106]. An additional advantage is that detection power increases (as statistical power increases with an increase in the number of scans). There are other possible task designs (parametric, event-related), but these have been seldom used for clinical language mapping and are considered beyond the scope of this chapter[90].

5.2 Sensitivity

Sensitivity reflects the ability of FMRI to detect critical language functions. With BOLD FMRI, local neuronal activity is indirectly measured via local haemodynamic changes. Signal changes are small (typically 1–5%) and require repeated measurements and statistical criteria to obtain significant signal-to-noise contrast. Consequently, brain activation maps are influenced by many variables at all levels of the experiment. Head motion can significantly compromise sensitivity and needs to be anticipated, in particular in patients with cognitive disturbances or in a suboptimal clinical condition. We often repeat instructions to these patients or stay with them in the scanner room. A cine loop is useful for identification of severely distorted scans, whereas motion correction algorithms can reduce scan artefacts. It is essential to monitor patient performance during the task, as these patients may have language or attentional disturbances. Because overt responses still induce too many artefacts, tasks should include measurements of indirect responses (e.g. via button press). Little is known of how cognitive strategies or impaired performance effect (FMRI) language maps. Nevertheless, FMRI studies have shown that it is possible to detect patterns of language reorganization in stroke patients with mild or moderate aphasia. For obvious reasons, patients with a severe global aphasia have not been studied with current task designs.

Although several issues on the exact nature of BOLD signal remain to be solved, recent insights have shown a direct link between neural activity and BOLD contrast[143,144]. Signal changes in language FMRI are very small and less robust than those seen in motor FMRI. There are some reports in the literature that BOLD responses may vary across subjects or brain regions, and also within subjects across time[145]. For traditional block-design experiments, where relative long periods of neural activity are evoked, these variations will likely result in only small changes in activation maps. Still, when the amount of activation is compared across normal subjects with identical motor or language tasks, a large variability is observed. Similar variations in the pattern and the amount of FMRI activation are observed in patients (e.g. see Fig. 3.8). The exact reasons for this variability are unknown. Although intersubject variations will play a role (due to variations in structural and functional neuroanatomy), there is certainly also a significant within-subject variability. Repeating the experiment does not yield similar numbers of activated voxels — a fact that cannot be fully explained by learning effects or slight variations in scanner characteristics[146]. The extent of brain activity as measured with FMRI is, therefore, not a reliable correlate for brain function.

As clinical experience with FMRI is expanding, there is some evidence accumulating that the BOLD response does not always adequately reflect neuronal activity near cerebral lesions. Data indicates that lesions and oedema may alter neurovascular reactivity or induce susceptibility artefacts[147,148]. For instance, in the patient that is shown in Fig. 3.2, the BOLD FMRI signal could not be reliably measured within the AVM. This loss of signal is probably due to flow in the large and abnormal AVM vessels and to magnetic susceptibility artefacts (the patient had a history of bleeding from the AVM, leading to local hemosiderin deposits that affect susceptibility). In their series, Cannestra *et al.* also describe a varying ability of FMRI to detect function directly bordering or within an AVM.[87] Other factors that can potentially influence BOLD responses are age of the subject[149], sensorimotor or cognitive deficits[150,151], task performance[152], medication or drugs[153]. Although these issues do not automatically have clinical relevance, we must bear in mind the potential limitations or uncertainty of this technique for brain mapping.

Holodny *et al.* found a reduction in the amount of motor cortex activation near brain tumours (in particular glioblastomas) as compared to the ipsilateral side. They suggested that these differences were due to loss of autoregulation near tumour vasculature[154]. Ulmer *et al.* retrospectively reviewed preoperative FMRI mapping in 50 patients with cerebral lesions[155]. FMRI demonstrated motor or language activation in 97% of perilesional cortical areas and homotopic reorganization in 32% of cases. However, in seven patients (two AVMs, one encephalitis, four gliomas), FMRI suggested an interhemispheric shift of cortical function which later proved to be false (as compared to Wada testing, cortical mapping, or functional outcome). A postictal state may also influence sensitivity of FMRI. Jayaker *et al.* found right temporal activation in a first FMRI examination in a 14-year old patient, and predominant left temporal activation when the examination was repeated two weeks later[156]. These latter findings were confirmed with electrocortical stimulation. They suggested that the initial absence of activation was related to a cluster of seizures prior to the first FMRI examination, although the mechanism remains unexplained and neurological examination at the time was normal.

Typically, two approaches have been taken to quantify brain activation. Most studies determine the *extent* of activation (i.e. the number of voxels that survive a particular statistical criterion). For assessment of the relative contribution of each hemisphere, a LI is calculated. There are a number of problems with this approach (note the implicit assumption that larger activation patterns have greater functional significance). First, the number of active voxels and the LI are highly dependent on the statistical threshold (Fig. 3.6)[157–159]. With a decrease in threshold, the LI decreases. This is expected, as with lower threshold the amount of false-positive voxels increases equally in both hemispheres, effectively diminishing laterality. With an increase in threshold, the LI increases (in agreement with clinical findings that language areas are usually left-lateralized). Whereas specificity for language areas increases, the use of a more stringent threshold unfortunately diminishes detection power for critical language areas. We have found that in a group of patients where FMRI and ESM results were compared, that no single threshold could be set to obtain optimal results in every individual patient[116]. Other authors also noted that some patients need to be treated with more restrictive thresholds than others[131].

To date, the choice of the best analysis thresholds of language FMRI signals remains an unsolved issue, and thresholds are often chosen arbitrarily. Thus, the spatial extent and the number of activated FMRI areas strongly depend on the level of the threshold. Consequently, activation patterns for a given patient can vary between bilaterality and unilaterality. However, even with fixed statistical procedures, there are large differences in the LI between normal subjects or between patients with known hemispheric dominance. Some authors have used individually set thresholds to improve results, but this really assumes a priori knowledge and does not suffice when we want to use FMRI as a clinical tool[158,160]. Knecht *et al.* set the level of significance so that it corresponded to a similar amount of voxels in each subject. They reasoned that similar subject performance will engage similar amount of brain tissue[158]. There are, however, no physiological justifications for these assumptions. Another approach to quantify brain activation is to use the *magnitude* of language-related signal changes. Some authors found more reliable and

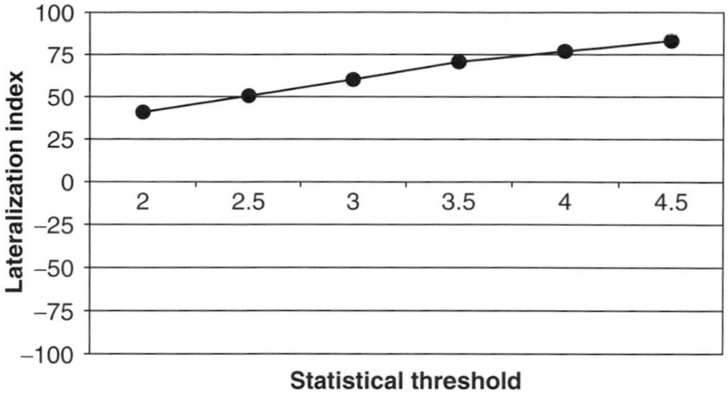

Fig. 3.6 Graph showing the dependency of the language lateralization index and the statistical threshold in a group of nine normal, right-handed subjects. Average lateralization indices are displayed; the results of three language tasks were combined (verb generation, antonym generation and picture naming). A voxel-based analysis was used. Horizontal axis shows cut-off T-values.

robust results when this method was compared to voxel counting[161,162]; others found no differences[163]. The advantage is that no threshold is involved in the calculation of laterality indices; the disadvantage is that predefined regions have to be selected, and this requires presumptions about the areas that are activated. This seems particularly problematic for patients as, in fact, this is what you want to test.

5.3 Spatial accuracy

Precise definition of the activation boundaries of FMRI areas is necessary in order to safely maximize surgical resection. Many parameters determine BOLD contrast and the spatial resolution of FMRI images: magnetic field strength, duration of the FMRI session, type of FMRI pulse sequence, temporal resolution, or slice thickness[164]. Figures 3.7 and 3.8 show two different 'types' of activation patterns that are, to some unknown extent, related to the various differences in data acquisition and analyses that were used in both studies. Note, in particular, the larger areas of activation and the absence of small areas of activation in Fig. 3.7 as compared to Fig. 3.8.

The eventual choice of parameters always depends on the question that needs to be answered by the FMRI experiment and requires a trade-off between these values. High spatial resolution is not necessarily advantageous for studies where a language lateralization index is calculated, or where data are normalized and averaged across subjects for group-wise analyses. In these cases, FMRI images are sometimes smoothed to facilitate detection of brain activity at the cost of higher spatial imprecision. With ESM, it has been shown that language areas can be as small as one voxel (e.g. 4mm^3). Smoothing reduces the ability to distinguish between separate but closely positioned active brain areas and might, therefore, compromise detection of language areas in individual patients. On the other hand, an increase of the spatial resolution reduces signal-to-noise contrast and this will decrease detection power for brain activity. It is beyond the scope of this chapter to discuss all these issues but it is important to understand the potential importance of these factors in

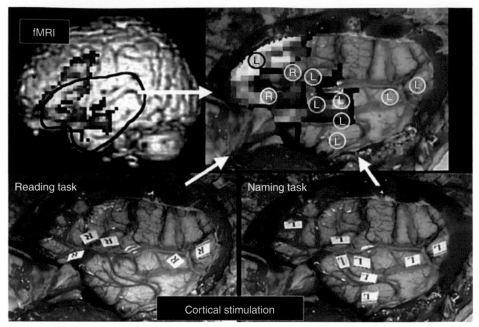

Fig. 3.7 Sixty years old woman with a metastasis from a melanoma in the temporal lobe. The results of various EPI-FMRI tasks are combined (naming, word reading and writing) and projected on a 3D model of the patients brain. Data were smoothed. Intraoperative cortical stimulation was done with both reading (lower left figure) and naming (lower right figure) tasks. "R" and "L" represented reading and naming interferences. When both reading and writing interferences were found at the same site, in the upper right figure only "L" marks were noted. Although some FMRI activations were correlated to cortical stimulation results, correlation between cortical stimulation and FMRI was not perfect in this case.

clinical practice. A spatial resolution of 3 or 4mm^3 seems adequate (and is feasible) for neurosurgical application, where precise gyrus localization is the minimum requirement[116].

The use of a neuronavigational system with integrated FMRI data is important for clinical use because it is easy to use and allows for 3D visualization of surgical planning. Neuronavigational devices, however, can have inaccuracies of up to 1cm[165]. Also, we showed in a study on motor FMRI[151] that the registration of FMRI data in anatomic slices can lead to functional mislocalizations. To be used for neurosurgical purposes, FMRI echo-planar images (EPI) must be matched to corresponding anatomical images. EPI introduces geometrical distortions into the images, which can complicate anatomical coregistration of EPI data. A number of groups have, therefore, used the PRESTO technique to obtain fast 3D volumes of the brain without significant geometric distortions[166,167]. Differences in pixel size between FMRI and MRI images, anatomic distortion of echoplanar images, and errors due to reformatting of FMRI data for implementation in the neuronavigational system are also potential sources of mislocalization.

Finally, there is the so-called 'draining vein effect'. Part of the FMRI activation comes from large extraparenchymatous veins that are not directly involved in the activation

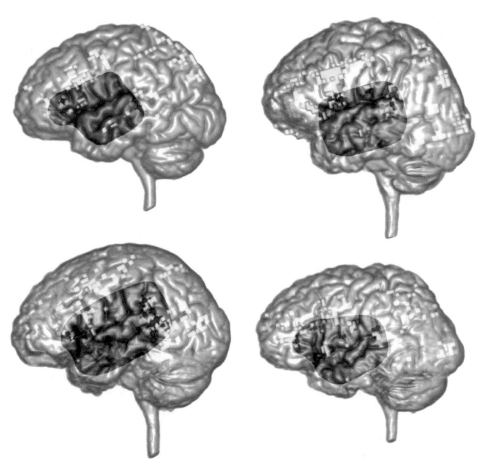

Fig. 3.8 Language areas detected with PRESTO- FMRI (yellow, results of four different language tasks combined) and intraoperative cortical stimulation (red, picture naming), shown in a cortical rendering for four patients. The surgically exposed part of the cortex is indicated with the brighter area. In the patient that is shown in the lower left corner, a large arteriovenous malformation was present at the cortical surface of the anterior temporal lobe, which accounts for the locally disturbed view of the rendered cortex. (Reprinted with permission from Rutten et al., 2002)[116]

process[168,169]. Some authors have claimed that this could be a serious limitation to accurate detection of neuronally active areas. At least, it poses the question of what a sensible resolution of FMRI images might be.

5.4 Reliability

Reliability of a technique is the ability to yield reproducible results in repeated investigations. Several studies have addressed reproducibility of FMRI for various sensorimotor and cognitive tasks[157,160,170–173]. In general, reproducibility of the extent of FMRI activation is not very good and is highly variable both between and within subjects[146]. Rutten *et al.* found that for individual language tasks, the average proportion of active voxels that were active in different experiments was only 25% but this number could be significantly increased when tasks were conjointly analysed[157]. In contrast, the *relative* amount of active voxels (as expressed by the LI) was significantly reproducible across different experiments. Of a set of individual tasks, verb generation yielded highest correlation across sessions (0.70). The most robust effects were observed when tasks were analysed in combination (correlation > 0.79). Interestingly, correlations were independent of the level of statistical thresholding. This is important for clinical applications where many of the earlier discussed sources of error can introduce variability of the activation maps and compromise reliability. Fernandez *et al.* yielded similar reproducible results for a synonym judgement task[160]. They found test-retest reliability higher for a LI in frontal areas than for temporoparietal areas. As they used spatially normalized data, no conclusions on a voxel-by-voxel basis could be drawn.

5.5 **Validity**

Validity reflects the correspondence between a function of interest and a standard to which results can be compared. For clinical language mapping, 'critical language function' is of interest. As was previously discussed, there is no clear definition for this concept, nor a definite neural substrate. Sabsevitz *et al.* recently published a study where (mild) naming decline after left anterior temporal lobectomy correlated with a preoperative language lateralization index measured with FMRI[107]. Patients underwent the Wada test and, in case of a language-dominant hemisphere, electrocortical mapping to tailor the surgical resection. Both FMRI and, to a lesser extent, the Wada test predicted postoperative naming outcome. Remarkably, naming decline was not prevented by the use of ESM that is considered the gold standard for this purpose. This is probably explained by the fact that the observed naming decline was not always clinically significant. Hunter *et al.* reported a patient who showed left-hemisphere dominance with PET, whereas the Wada test yielded right-hemisphere dominance[96]. After left temporal lobectomy, the patient had language impairments that persisted for six months. Wyllie *et al.* found that in two of nine patients that were right-hemisphere dominant according to the Wada test, ESM found language areas in the left hemisphere[97]. We observed a similar case, where language activation was found with FMRI and ESM in the left inferior frontal cortex in a right-sided Wada patient[98]. These studies provide additional reason to doubt the validity of the current clinical standards and underline the fact that FMRI studies, ultimately, should compare results to patient outcome.

5.6 **Other factors**

Several other factors limit the use of language FMRI in neurosurgical practice. First, FMRI is very sensitive to changes in cortical areas but not in subcortical areas like white matter tracts. Detection and the sparing of these white matter tracts can be very important during tumour removal[174]. Larger white matter tracts can be visualized with new diffusion-tensor imaging (DTI) techniques, that seem a promising future alternative for subcortical electrical stimulation. The combination of FMRI and DTI has been found beneficial in presurgical planning of both 'functional' gray and white matter[175]. A second limitation is that current clinical FMRI protocols still require the expertise of several persons (neurosurgeons, radiologists, and computer engineers), although a similar statement can be made for ESM.

Another unsolved issue is detection of language areas in children. Direct electrical stimulation mapping is used in epileptic children where epileptic foci and abnormal cortex or neoplasms are located near language areas[176]. Our teams consider that intraoperative brain mapping can be done in children older than nine years of age; in younger children, extraoperative brain mapping via subdural grids is used. On the other hand, language FMRI can be done in children from six years of age. In particular for these patients, FMRI is beneficial.

Finally, FMRI is restricted to patients who have no significant language deficits because the validity of FMRI language maps in aphasic patients is, as of yet, unknown. Similar reservations should however be made for ESM, as even subtle language deficits can compromise straightforward interpretation of results.

6. Conclusions: the current role of language FMRI in presurgical planning

There is now abundant evidence that existing clinical language models are inadequate for use in neurosurgery. Modern research supports the view that various language functions are sustained by relatively large overlapping networks that are organized around a variable number of small cortical regions that are somehow critical for normal language function. This variability requires tools that can identify language areas in the individual patient.

FMRI has the fundamental advantage that functional information can be obtained prior to an invasive investigation or an operation, potentially allowing for risk management, patient selection, and surgical strategies. An additional advantage is that FMRI information can be relatively easily integrated in existing surgical guidance systems, offering both structural and functional information to the surgeon during the operation. This integration can now be done with commercially available software. Although we know of no institute where FMRI has completely replaced invasive techniques for presurgical planning, FMRI is already used as an adjunct to existing techniques in various fields of neurosurgery for brain tumours[150,151,177–180], epilepsy[116], and pain[151,181]. FMRI shows good overall concordance with Wada test findings for evaluation of hemispheric language dominance and recent studies suggest that the Wada test can at least be partially replaced by FMRI[101,106]. Still, we have found no evidence that language FMRI can already make critical surgical decisions in the absence of direct cortical mapping. We think that FMRI and direct brain mapping should be used as complementary techniques that do not exclude each other in language area detection, at least not in the near future.

There are a number of prerequisites for clinical use of FMRI that need further refinement, in particular high detection power for both the presence and absence of critical language functions and development of user-independent protocols. Detection power of FMRI seems at least similar to that of the current clinical standards (the Wada test and ESM) when the results of different FMRI tasks are combined; individual tasks are usually not sufficient for this purpose. In contrast, FMRI finds more language-related areas, and for definite implementation of FMRI in surgical practice, the precise functional role of these additional areas needs to be investigated in future studies. Most importantly, more studies are needed, as the overall number of patients that has been studied is too small. Given the variability in language maps between different studies, patients, or tasks, research should focus on development of robust and reliable FMRI protocols. As both the Wada test and ESM have their own practical and methodological drawbacks, future studies should include pre- and postoperative functional outcome of patients to evaluate the real usefulness of language FMRI. Ultimately, this should lead to development of protocols that can predict both direct and late effects of surgery on language abilities of the individual patient.

Acknowledgements

The authors thank Dr Isabelle Berry, Dr Jean–Albert Lotterie, and Dr Nick Ramsey for their cooperation and help with FMRI protocols.

References

1. Willmes K, Poeck K. To what extent can aphasic syndromes be localized? *Brain* 1993; **116**:1527–40.
2. Penfield WP, Roberts L. *Speech and brain mechanisms.* Princeton: Princeton University Press, 1959.
3. Damasio AR. Aphasia. *New England Journal of Medicine* 1992; **326**(8):531–9.
4. Damasio AR, Damasio H. Aphasia and the neural basis of language. In: (ed. MM Mesulam) *Principles of behavioral and cognitive neurology.* New York: Oxford University Press, 2000: p. 294–315.
5. Nobre AC, Plunkett K. The neural system of language: structure and development. *Current Opinion in Neurobiology* 1997; **7**(2):262–8.
6. Ellis AW, Young AW. *Human cognitive neuropsychology.* Psychology Press, 1996.
7. Goodglass H, Klein B, Carey P, Jones K. Specific semantic word categories in aphasias. *Cortex* 1966; **2**:74–89.
8. Damasio AR, Tranel D. Nouns and verbs are retrieved with differently distributed neural systems. *Proceedings of the National Academy of Sciences USA* 1993; **90**(11):4957–60.
9. Daniele A, Giustolisi L, Silveri MC, Colosimo C, Gianotti G. Evidence for a possible neuroanatomical basis for lexical processing of nouns and verbs. *Neuropsychologia* 1994; **32**:1325–41.
10. Wernicke C. *Der aphasische symptomencomplex.* Breslau, Germany: Cohn and Weigert, 1874.
11. Lichtheim L. On aphasia. *Brain* 1885; **7**:433–84.
12. Geschwind N. Disconnexion syndromes in animals and man. *Brain* 1965; **88**:237–94.
13. Dejerine J. Contribution a l'étude anatomo-pathologique et clinique des différentes varietés de cécité verbale. *Mém Soc Biol Fév* 1892; 27.
14. Dejerine J. Sur un cas de cecite verbale avec agraphie, suivi d'autopsie. *Mémoires de la Société Biologique* 1891;(3):197–201.
15. Young RM. *Mind, brain and adaptation in the nineteenth century* (2nd edn). New York: Oxford University Press, 1970.
16. Doody RS. A reappraisal of localization theory with reference to aphasia. Part 1: Historical considerations. *Brain and Language* 1993; **44**(3):296–326.
17. Marie P. Revision de la question de l'aphasie. *Sem Med* 1906; 2.
18. Dejerine J, Roussy G. Le syndrome thalamique. *Revue Neurologique* 1906; **12**:521.

19. Ojemann G. Subcortical language mechanisms. *Studies in neurolinguistics* 1976; **1**:103–38.

20. Luria AR. On quasi-aphasic speech disturbance in lesions of deep structures in the brain. *Brain and Language* 1977; **4**:359–432.

21. Brown CM, Hagoort P. *The neurocognition of language*. New York: Oxford University Press, 1998.

22. Linebarger MC, Schwartz MF, Saffran EM. Sensitivity to grammatical structure in so-called agrammatic patients. *Cognition* 1983; **13**:361–92.

23. Ross ED. Affective prosody and the aprosodias. In: (ed. MM Mesulam) *Principles of behavioral and cognitive neurology*. New York: Oxford University Press, 2000: p. 316–31.

24. Ross ED, Mesulam MM. Dominant language functions in the right hemisphere? Prosody and emotional gesturing. *Archives of Neurology* 1979; **36**:144–8.

25. Schwartz MF, Marin OSM, Saffran EM. Dissociation of language function in dementia: a case study. *Brain and Language* 1979; **7**:277–306.

26. Damasio H, Grabowski TJ, Tranel D, Hichwa RD, Damasio AR. A neural basis for lexical retrieval. *Nature* 1996; **380**:499–505.

27. Coltheart M, Curtis.B, Atkins P, Haller M. Models of reading aloud: dual-route and parallel-distributed processing approaches. *Psychological Review* 1993; **100**:589–608.

28. Marshall JC, Newcombe F. Patterns of paralexia: a neurolinguistic approach. *Journal of Psycholinguistic Research* 1973; **2**:175–99.

29. Simos PG, Breier JI, Wheless JW, Maggio WW, Fletcher JM, Castillo E, *et al.* Brain mechanisms for reading: the role of the superior temporal gyrus in word and pseudoword naming. *Neuroreport* 2000; **11**(11):2443–7.

30. McClelland JL, Rumelhart DE. An interactive activation model of context effects in letter perception. I. An account of basic findings. *Psychological Reviews* 1981; **88**:375–407.

31. Shallice T. *Language operations: are input and output processes separate? From neuropsychology to mental structure*. Cambridge: Cambridge University Press, 1988: p. 158–83.

32. Foerster O. The motor cortex in man in the light of Hughlings Jackson's doctrines. *Brain* 1936; **59**:135–59.

33. Devinsky O, Beric A, Dogali M. *Electrical and magnetic stimulation of the brain and spinal cord*. New York: Raven Press, 1993.

34. Ojemann GA. Brain organization for language from the perspective of electrical stimulation mapping. *Behavioral and Brain Sciences* 1983;(2):189–230.

35. Whitaker HA, Ojemann GA. Graded localisation of naming from electrical stimulation mapping of left cerebral cortex. *Nature* 1977; **270**(5632):50–1.

36. Van Buren JM, Fedio P, Frederick GC. Mechanism and localization of speech in the parietotemporal cortex. *Neurosurgery* 1978; **2**(3):233–9.

37. Ojemann GA, Ojemann JG, Lettich E, Berger MS. Cortical language localization in left, dominant hemisphere: an electrical stimulation mapping investigation in 117 patients. *Journal of Neurosurgery* 1989; **71**:316–26.

38. Krainik A, Lehericy S, Duffau H, Vlaicu M, Poupon F, Capelle L, *et al.* Role of the supplementary motor area in motor deficit following medial frontal lobe surgery. *Neurology* 2001; **57**:871–8.

39. Luders H, Lesser RP, Hahn J, Dinner DS, Morris HH, Resor S. Basal temporal language area as demonstrated by electrical stimulation. *Neurology* 1996; **36**:505–10.

40. Burnstine TH, Lesser RP, Hart J, Jr. Characterization of the basal temporal language areas in patients with left temporal lobe epilepsy. *Neurology* 1990; **40**:966–70.

41. Guiot G, Herzog E, Rondot P, Molina P. Arrest or acceleration of speech evoked by thalamic stimulation in the course of stereotactic procedures for Parkinsonism. *Brain* 1961; **84**:363–79.

42. Ojemann G, Fedio P, Van Buren JM. Anomia from pulvinar and subcortical parietal stimulation. *Brain* 1968; **91**:99–116.

43. Toth S. Effects of electrical stimulation of subcortical sites on speech and consciousness. In: (ed. G. Somjen) *Neurophysiology studied in man*. Amsterdam: Excerpta Medica, 1972: p. 40–6.

44. Duffau H, Capelle L, Denvil D, Gatignol P, Sichez N, Lopes M, *et al*. The role of dominant premotor cortex in language: a study using intraoperative functional mapping in awake patients. *Neuroimage* 2003; **20**(4):1903–14.

45. Duffau H, Capelle L, Lopes M, Faillot T, Sichez JP, Fohanno D. The insular lobe: physiopathological and surgical considerations. *Neurosurgery* 2000; **47**:801–11.

46. Duffau H, Bauchet L, Lehericy S, Capelle L. Functional compensation of the left insula dominant for language. *Neuroreport* 2001; **12**:2159–63.

47. Bittar RG, Ptito A, Reutens DC. Somatosensory representation in patients who have undergone hemispherectomy: a functional magnetic resonance imaging study. *Journal of Neurosurgery* 2000; **92**(1):45–51.

48. Chugani HT, Muller RA, Chugani DC. Functional brain reorganization in children. *Brain and Development* 1996; **18**(5):347–56.

49. Graveline C, Hwang P, Bone G, Shikolka C, Wade S, Crawley A, *et al*. Evaluation of gross and fine motor functions in children with hemidecortication: predictors of outcomes and timing of surgery (published erratum appears in *J Child Neurol* 1999 Aug;14(8):following table of contents). *J Child Neurol* 1999; **14**(5):304–15.

50. Holloway V, Gadian DG, Vargha–Khadem F, Porter DA, Boyd SG, Connelly A. The reorganization of sensorimotor function in children after hemispherectomy: A functional MRI and somatosensory evoked potential study. *Brain* 2000; **123**(Pt 12):2432–44.

51. Muller RA, Rothermel RD, Behen ME, Muzik O, Chakraborty PK, Chugani HT. Plasticity of motor organization in children and adults. *Neuroreport* 1997; **8**(14):3103–8.

52. Muller RA, Rothermel RD, Behen ME, Muzik O, Mangner TJ, Chugani HT. Differential patterns of language and motor reorganization following early left hemisphere lesion: a PET study. *Archives of Neurology* 1998; **55**(8):1113–19.

53. Staudt M, Grodd W, Niemann G, Wildgruber D, Erb M, Kräheloh–Mann I. Early left periventricular brain lesions induce right hemisphere organization of speech. *Neurology* 2001; **57**(1):122–5.

54. Weiller C, Isensee C, Rijntjes M, Huber W, Muller S, Bier D, *et al*. Recovery from Wernicke's aphasia: a positron emission tomographic study. *Annals of Neurology* 1995; **37**(6):723–32.

55. Hertz–Pannier L, Chiron C, Jambaqué I, Renaux–Kieffer V, Van de Moortele P–F, Delalande O, *et al*. Late plasticity for language in a child's non-dominant hemisphere. *Brain* 2002; **125**:361–72.

56. Thiel A, Herholz K, Koyuncu A, Ghaemi M, Kracht LW, Habedank B, *et al*. Plasticity of language networks in patients with brain tumors: a positron emission tomography activation study. *Annals of Neurology* 2001; **50**(620):629.

57. Price CJ. The anatomy of language: contributions from functional neuroimaging. *Journal of Anatomy* 2000; **197**(Pt 3):335–59.

58. Price CJ, Indefrey P, van Turenhout M. The neural architecture underlying the processing of written and spoken word forms. In: (eds. CT Moonen, PA Bandettini PA) *Functional MRI*. Berlin–Heidelberg: Springer–Verlag, 1999: p. 211–40.

59. Mesulam MM. From sensation to cognition. *Brain* 1998; **121**(Pt 6):1013–52.

60. Binder JR. Functional MRI of the language system. In: (eds. CT Moonen, PA Bandettini PA) *Functional MRI*. Berlin–Heidelberg: Springer–Verlag, 1999: p. 407–19.

61. Giraud AL, Price CJ. The constraints functional neuroimaging places on classical models of auditory word processing. *Journal of Cognitive Neuroscience* 2001; **13**(6):754–65.

62. Fiez JA. Phonology, semantics, and the role of the left inferior prefrontal cortex [editorial]. *Human Brain Mapping* 1997; **5**(2):79–83.

63. Raichle ME, Fiez JA, Videen TO, MacLeod AM, Pardo JV, Fox PT, *et al*. Practice-related changes in human brain functional anatomy during nonmotor learning. *Cerebral Cortex* 1994; **4**:8–26.

imaging data in a surgical guidance system for intraoperative identification of motor and language cortices. Technical note and illustrative case. *Neurosurgical Focus* 2003; 15(1) (see *www.neuro-surgery.org/focus*).

143. Logothetis NK, Pauls J, Augath M, Trinath T, Oeltermann A. Neurophysiological investigations of the basis of the FMRI signal. *Nature* 2001; **412**:150–7.

144. Bandettini PA, Ungerleider LG. From neuron to BOLD: new connections. *Nat Neurosci* 2001; **4**(9):864–66.

145. Aguirre GK, Zarahn E, D'Esposito M. The variability of human, BOLD hemodynamic responses. *Neuroimage* 1998; **8**(4):360–9.

146. McGonigle DJ, Howseman AM, Athwal BS, Friston KJ, Frackowiak RS, Holmes AP. Variability in FMRI: an examination of intersession differences. *Neuroimage* 2000; **11**(6 Pt 1):708–34.

147. Ojemann JG, Neil JM, MacLeod AM, Silbergeld DL, Dacey RG, Petersen SE, *et al.* Increased functional vascular response in the region of a glioma. *Journal of Cerebral Blood Flow and Metabolism* 1998; **18**(2):148–53.

148. Carpentier AC, Constable RT, Schlosser MJ, de Lotbiniere A, Piepmeier JM, Spencer DD, *et al.* Patterns of functional magnetic resonance imaging activation in association with structural lesions in the rolandic region: a classification system. *J Neurosurg* 2001; **94**(6):946–54.

149. Hesselmann V, Zaro WO, Wedekind C, Krings T, Schulte O, Kugel H, *et al.* Age related signal decrease in functional magnetic resonance imaging during motor stimulation in humans. *Neurosci Lett* 2001; **308**(3):141–4.

150. Atlas SW, Howard RS2, Maldjian J, Alsop D, Detre JA, Listerud J, *et al.* Functional magnetic resonance imaging of regional brain activity in patients with intracerebral gliomas: findings and implications for clinical management. *Neurosurgery* 1996; **38**(2):329–38.

151. Roux FE, Ibarrola D, Tremoulet M, Lazorthes Y, Henry P, Sol JC, *et al.* Methodological and technical issues for integrating functional magnetic resonance imaging data in a neuronavigational system. *Neurosurgery* 2001; **49**(5):1145–56.

152. Sergent J. Brain-imaging studies of cognitive functions. *Trends Neurosci* 1994; **17**(6):221–7.

153. Laurienti PJ, Field AS, Burdette JH, Maldjian JA, Yen YF, Moody DM. Dietary caffeine consumption modulates FMRI measures. *Neuroimage* 2002; **17**(2):751–7.

154. Holodny AI, Schulder M, Liu WC, Wolko J, Maldjian JA, Kalnin AJ. The effect of brain tumors on BOLD functional MR imaging activation in the adjacent motor cortex: implications for image-guided neurosurgery. *AJNR Am J Neuroradiol* 2000; **21**(8):1415–22.

155. Ulmer JL, Hacein–Bey L, Mathews VP, Mueller WM, DeYoe EA, Prost RW, *et al.* Lesion-induced pseudo-dominance at Functional magnetic resonance imaging: implications for preoperative assessments. *Neurosurgery* 2004; **55**(3):569–81.

156. Jayaker P, Bernal B, Medina LS, Altman N. False lateralization of language cortex on functional MRI after a cluster of focal seizures. *Neurology* 2002; **58**:490–2.

157. Rutten GJ, Ramsey NF, van Rijen PC, van Veelen CW. Reproducibility of FMRI-determined language lateralization in individual subjects. *Brain and Language* 2002; **80**:421–37.

158. Knecht S, Jansen A, Frank A, van Randenborgh J, Sommer J, Kanowski M, *et al.* How atypical is atypical language dominance? *Neuroimage* 2003; **18**(4):917–27.

159. Liégeois F, Connelly A, Salmond CH, Gadian DG, Vargha–Khadem F, Baldeweg T. A direct test of lateralization of language activation using FMRI: comparison with invasive assessments in children with epilepsy. *Neuroimage* 2002; **17**:1861–7.

160. Fernández G, Specht K, Weis S, Tendolkar I, Reuber M, Fell J, *et al.* Intrasubject reproducibility of presurgical language lateralization and mapping using FMRI. *Neurology* 2003; **60**:969–75.

161. Chee MW, Lee HL, Soon CS, Westphal C, Venkatraman V. Reproducibility of the word frequency effect: comparison of signal change and voxel counting. *Neuroimage* 2003; **18**:468–82.

162. Cohen MS, DuBois RM. Stability, repeatability, and the expression of signal magnitude in functional magnetic resonance imaging. *Journal of Magnetic Resonance Imaging* 1999; **10**(1):33–40.

163. Adcock JE, Wise RG, Oxbury JM, Oxbury SM, Matthews PM. Quantitative FMRI assessment of the differences in lateralization of language-related brain activation in patients with temporal lobe epilepsy. *Neuroimage* 2003; **18**:423–38.

164. Yoo SS, Talos IF, Golby AJ, Black PM, Panych LP. Evaluating requirements for spatial resolution of FMRI for neurosurgical planning. *Human Brain Mapping* 2004; **21**(1):34–43.

165. Roberts DW, Hartov A, Kennedy FE, Miga MI, Paulsen KD. Intraoperative brain shift and deformation: a quantitative analysis of cortical displacement in 28 cases. *Neurosurgery* 1998; **43**(4):749–58.

166. Liu G, Sobering G, Duyn J, Moonen CT. A functional MRI technique combining principles of echo-shifting with a train of observations (PRESTO). *Magnetic Resonance in Medicine* 1993; **30**:764–68.

167. Van Gelderen P, Ramsey NF, Liu G, Duyn JH, Frank JA, Weinberger DR, *et al.* Three-dimensional functional magnetic resonance imaging of human brain on a clinical 1.5-T scanner. *Proceedings of the National Academy of Sciences USA* 1995; **92**(15):6906–10.

168. Segebarth C, Belle V, Delon C, Massarelli R, Decety J, Le Bas JF, *et al.* Functional MRI of the human brain: predominance of signals from extracerebral veins. *Neuroreport* 1994; **5**(7):813–16.

169. Jezzard P, Ramsey NF. Quantitative functional MRI. In: (ed. PS Tofts PS) *Quantitive magnetic resonance imaging in the brain: monitoring disease progression and treatment response.* Wiley, 2003: p. 413–53.

170. Casey BJ, Cohen JD, O'Craven K, Davidson RJ, Irwin W, Nelson CA, *et al.* Reproducibility of FMRI results across four institutions using a spatial working memory task. *Neuroimage* 1998; **8**(3):249–61.

171. Machielsen WC, Rombouts SA, Barkhof F, Scheltens P, Witter MP. FMRI of visual encoding: reproducibility of activation. *Human Brain Mapping* 2000; **9**:156–64.

172. Ramsey NF, Tallent K, Van Gelderen P, Frank JA, Moonen CT, Weinberger DR. Reproducibility of human 3D FMRI brain maps acquired during a motor task. *Human Brain Mapping* 1996; **4**:113–21.

173. Brannen JH, Badie B, Moritz CH, Quigley M, Meyerand ME, Haughton VM. Reliability of functional MR imaging with word-generation tasks for mapping Broca's area. *AJNR Am J Neuroradiol* 2001; **22**:1711–18.

174. Duffau H, Capelle L, Sichez N, Denvil D, Lopes M, Sichez JP, *et al.* Intraoperative mapping of the subcortical language pathways using direct stimulations. An anatomo-functional study. *Brain* 2002; **125**:199–214.

175. Hendler T, Pianka P, Sigal M, Kafri M, Ben Bashat D, Constantini S, *et al.* Delineating gray and white matter involvement in brain lesions: three-dimensional alignment of functional magnetic resonance and diffusion-tensor imaging. *J Neurosurg* 2003; **99**(6):1018–27.

176. Ojemann SG, Berger MS, Lettich E, Ojemann GA. Localization of language function in children: results of electrical stimulation mapping. *J Neurosurg* 2003; **98**(3):465–70.

177. Lehericy S, Duffau H, Cornu P, Capelle L, Pidoux B, Carpentier A, *et al.* Correspondance between functional magnetic resonance imaging somatotopy and individual brain anatomy of the central region: comparison with intraoperative stimulation in patients with brain tumors. *J Neurosurg* 2000; **92**:589–98.

178. Roux FE, Ibarrola D, Lotterie J, Berry I. Perimetric visual field and functional MRI correlation: implications for image-guided surgery in occipital brain tumours. *J Neurol Neurosurg Psychiatry* 2001; **71**:505–14.

179. Schulder M, Maldjian JA, Liu WC, Holodny AI, Kalnin AT, Mun IK, *et al.* Functional image-guided surgery of intracranial tumors located in or near the sensorimotor cortex. *J Neurosurg* 1998; **89**(3):412–18.

180. Yousry TA, Schmid UD, Jassoy AG, Schmidt D, Eisner WE, Reulen HJ, *et al.* Topography of the cortical motor hand area: prospective study with functional MR imaging and direct motor mapping at surgery. *Radiology* 1995; **195**(1):23–9.

181. Latchaw RE, Hu X. Functional MR imaging in the evaluation of the patient with epilepsy. Functional localization. *Neuroimaging Clin N Am* 1995; **5**(4):683–93.

4

Ageing: age-related changes in episodic and working memory

Sander Daselaar, Nancy Dennis, and Roberto Cabeza

1. **Introduction**

Ageing is associated with ongoing deterioration of not only the anatomy and physiology of our brain, but our cognitive abilities as well. As our brain shrinks and its functions decline, cognitive processes become slower and start to fail. Deficits in memory function are among the most-heard complaints in older adults, and cognitive research generally agrees with these self-observations. Modest difficulties in learning and memory can be found, to some extent, in all older adults. Understanding age-associated deficits in memory is important for two reasons. First, in view of the growing number of older adults in today's society, cognitive ageing is increasingly becoming a problem in general health care, and effective therapeutic intervention methods can only be developed on the basis of knowledge obtained through fundamental research. Second, there is a subgroup of elderly whose memory impairments are more severe, preventing normal functioning in their environment. In these persons, such memory impairments can be the earliest manifestation of pathological age-related conditions such as Alzheimer's dementia (AD). Particularly in the early stages of this disease, the differentiation from normal, age-related memory impairments is very difficult. Thus, it is important to outline which memory impairments can be regarded as a correlate of normal ageing and which are associated with age-related pathology.

The two forms of memory that are most affected by ageing are working memory and episodic memory. Working memory (WM) refers to the short-term memory maintenance and simultaneous manipulation of information. Clinical and functional neuroimaging evidence indicates that WM is particularly dependent on the functions of the prefrontal cortex (PFC) and the parietal cortex[1]. Episodic memory (EM) refers to the encoding and retrieval of personally experienced events[2,3]. Clinical studies have shown that EM is primarily dependent on the integrity of the medial temporal lobe (MTL) memory system[4,5]. However, functional neuroimaging studies have also emphasized the contributions of PFC to EM processes[6].

Due to increased access to functional brain imaging techniques such as FMRI, ageing research has now started to focus on the relation between age-related changes in memory and changes in brain function. FMRI provides the ideal method to investigate patterns of neurocognitive decline because changes in brain activity can be directly linked to the effects of ageing on behavioural measures, providing a bridge between cerebral ageing and cognitive ageing. One popular neurocognitive view is that the decline in memory associated with healthy ageing results from a selective decline in frontal regions, whereas degradation of other brain regions, such as the MTL, is a hallmark of pathological age-related conditions[7–9]. In this chapter, we examine this idea by reviewing findings from FMRI studies of healthy ageing and memory with a focus on age-related changes in pre-frontal cortex (PFC) and MTL regions. In our review, we also include studies that used an alternative brain imaging technique based on cerebral blood flow, namely positron emission tomography (PET). Although the field has generally shifted toward the use of FMRI, because of its high temporal and spatial resolution and its non-invasive character, the early landmark studies of ageing and memory have primarily used PET.

In relation to these findings, we will also address two major cognitive accounts of age-related memory decline, the *resource deficit theory*[10] and the *associative deficit theory*[11]. The *resource deficit theory* of cognitive ageing posits that ageing reduces the availability of certain cognitive resources such as attention. In turn, older adults perform poorer on cognitive tasks with increased cognitive load, requiring greater self-initiated processing. The *associative deficit theory* posits that age-related deficits in binding underlie age-related memory decline. Binding or co-joining two pieces of information into one cohesive unit is a cognitive process that underlies many basic cognitive functions — and can require significant cognitive resources to execute[11].

The chapter has four main parts. In the first part, we begin with a brief overview of behavioural evidence indicating how WM and EM functions change as we age, and also discuss the brain changes that accompany the ageing process. In the second part, we take an in-depth look at functional neuroimaging studies of WM and EM that revealed age-related changes in MTL and/or PFC regions. In the third part, we discuss different interpretations of age-related memory decline that have emerged from these findings and how they relate to the resource and associative deficit theories of ageing. We also discuss the possible implications for clinical applications of FMRI aimed at an earlier diagnosis of age-related pathological conditions. Finally, we discuss some current issues and future directions.

2. Age-related changes in brain and behaviour

2.1 Behavioural changes

2.1.1 Working memory

WM is considered to operate as a mental blackboard for computations that subserve higher-level processing such as language, problem solving, and reasoning[12,13]. Within WM, a dissociation has been proposed between two different maintenance systems, a subvocal rehearsal system for verbal and phonological information (phonological loop), and a visuospatial storage system (visuospatial sketchpad). These two systems are under the control of a central processing unit, termed the central executive[13].

In general, behavioural studies have indicated that age differences in WM become larger with increasing task difficulty, presumably because of a greater reliance on executive processes. Increases in complexity include additional processing of information held in working memory[14,15], manipulations of divided attention[16,17], and proactive interference[18]. For instance, a consistent finding is that simple maintenance abilities are relatively spared in older adults, while performance is affected disproportionally when WM tasks require additional processing of information[19,20]. Dobbs and Rule[14] compared performance on several WM tasks that differed in their maintenance and processing requirements in five groups ranging in age between 30 and 70+ years. They reported little differences on simple forward and backward digit span tasks, but substantial age deficits on an auditory version of the N-back task, which required maintenance of target information and simultaneous processing of new information. Salthouse and colleagues[21] also performed a large-scale WM experiment involving 120 males ranging in age from 20 to 79 years. Age differences in performance between younger and older adults increased with both task complexity and increased demands on processing resources. Similarly, Wiegersma and Meertse[14] found no age-related deficits on WM tasks involving simple reproduction of sequenced items, but age-related decline in performance when the tasks required subjective re-ordering of the sequenced items.

Older adults are also more susceptible to divided attention manipulations during WM performance than are younger adults[19,20]. For example, in a study by West[16], young and older adults performed a version of the N-back task both with and without distracters. He found that older adults were much more impaired by distraction. Similar results were obtained in an event-related brain potential study by Chao and Knight[17]. They compared young and older adults on an auditory WM task, which required the short-term maintenance of a single tone both with and without distracting tones. They found that older adults showed larger auditory evoked responses to the distracters, and also showed greater interference from these distracters, resulting in poorer performance in older than in younger adults.

Finally, older adults are also more susceptible to effects of proactive interference (PI) in WM tasks[18]. Bowles and Salthouse (2003) found that, on two separate WM tasks, older adults demonstrated increased difficulty across the second half of trials. Results were interpreted as reflecting greater susceptibility in ageing to PI, and that this type of interference contributes significantly to age-related decline in WM. Furthermore, when interference is removed from WM span tasks, older adults demonstrate improvements in overall span scores[22] and improved recall in cognitive tasks (e.g. prose recall)[23].

Although behavioural evidence suggests that age deficits in WM are most pronounced on tasks that put a greater demand on executive processes, the possibility of age-related deficits in 'simple' WM tasks should not be ignored. It has been suggested that deficits in maintenance tasks of WM may just be undetectable at the behavioural level[20,24]. Reuter–Lorenz proposes that rote maintenance and involved processing operations decline with age, but an increased reliance on executive processes can mask declines in the former in older adults. As a result, older adults are left with less executive resources to meet increased task demands. Furthermore, this increase in activation necessary for maintenance and storage operations acts as a compensatory mechanism, reducing age-related behavioural differences on 'simple' WM tasks (see below).

2.1.2 Episodic memory

Age-related deficits in EM may reflect difficulties in the incorporation of new information into the episodic memory store, or *episodic encoding* (EE), and/or in recovery of stored information, or *episodic retrieval* (ER). Behavioural work has tried to separate the contributions of deficits in EE and ER to age-related EM decline by applying separate manipulations to each phase. Behavioural studies have indicated that age-related decline in EM is associated with deficits in both EE and ER phases. Like studies of WM, age deficits generally become greater when there is more demand on executive functions or little environmental support. We discuss some findings on EE and ER in the following sections.

Episodic encoding It has been proposed that age-related decline in EM is associated primarily with problems during the encoding phase of EM tasks. This idea is based on the finding that interference during EE compared to ER results in disproportionate age differences in memory[25,26]. For instance, in a study by Park et al.[26], young and older adults studied categorized words while performing a number-monitoring task during encoding, retrieval, or at both times. Older adults' memory performance was disproportionately impaired when attention was divided at EE, but there was a similar effect of divided attention on both groups during ER.

Age deficits in EE are most pronounced when there is little environmental support to help encoding. For instance, age differences tend to be larger when young and older adults intentionally try to encode a list of study items than when a deep semantic processing task is used to guide encoding. In a study by Craik and colleagues[27], young and older adults encoded a list of words either with or without an associative, short descriptive phrase. Age deficits were less pronounced when the encoded words were accompanied by the descriptive phrases. Similarly, age differences in the encoding of associations between study items are much greater when there is no apparent link between the elements. For example, Smith et al.[28] found that age differences in recall of a target picture to a context picture was better when sentences were generated that integrated the pictures or when there was already a pre-existing relationship between the pictures. They interpreted these findings in terms of age differences in self-initiated processing.

As mentioned, an alternative interpretation of age deficits in encoding of contextual information is that older adults show selective deficits in associative memory or *binding*, which may be related to reduced MTL function[11]. Evidence for a deficit in binding comes from studies showing that older adults consistently exhibit age-related deficits on tasks requiring binding, even when memory for individual features is intact[29–31]. Chalfonte and Johnson (1996) tested age differences in encoding of both colour and item information across three experiments. While no effect of age was found for individual features, older adults exhibited significant deficits in recognition for combined features compared to younger adults. Additionally, age differences in memory for bound features persisted across various encoding instructions. Similar results were reported by Mitchell et al.[31] who also interpreted results as an age-related deficit in co-joining/binding features in memory. Recent studies have indicated that this associative deficit is not limited to arbitrary associations (e.g. word–colour, item–location), but also more ecologically valid/meaningful pairings such as name–face associations[11,32]. Thus, available evidence suggests that, even though older adults show deficits in general memory performance, this deficit is greater for associative memory.

Episodic retrieval Despite the evidence suggesting greater deficits in EE, age-related memory deficits are present during ER as well. In line with the findings on WM, age differences in retrieval become larger on tasks that put a greater demand on executive functions. Older adults experience more difficulties on free recall and source memory tasks, which require a completely self-initiated search, than on recognition tasks, in which the study item is provided and one merely has to decide whether it was part of a previously studied list or not[33–35]. One explanation for this finding is that older adults do not spontaneously produce retrieval cues to guide the search process.

In line with this idea, several studies have found that age deficits reduced when cues are provided. That is, older adults benefit when provided with environmental support at retrieval[27,36]. In the Park et al. study, older adults showed no age deficit following incidental word encoding when retrieval involved an implicit word–stem completion task. Given the first 2–4 letters of the studied word, older adults showed equivalent performance to young when asked to complete the word–stem. The benefit of increased environmental support leads to the distinction between differential decline of familiarity and recollection processes.

According to dual-process models, recognition memory can be based on the recovery of specific contextual details (recollection) or on the feeling that an event is old or new in the absence of confirmatory information (familiarity). Several studies have reported an increased reliance on familiarity processes in older adults during item recognition[37,38]. For example, Parkin and Walter[39] used the remember/know (R/K) paradigm in which participants indicate whether their recognition judgement was based on recollection (R) or familiarity (K). They found that older adults made fewer R responses and more K responses than younger adults. Furthermore, the extent to which older adults relied on familiarity-based recognition correlated with neuropsychological indices of frontal lobe dysfunction.

In line with the aforementioned deficits in associative encoding, older adults are also less accurate in recalling information associated with the context in which an item was encoded, including item colour, case, or font of words[40], domain presentation (e.g. auditory or visual)[41], and speaker gender[42]. For example, when given a list of made-up facts (e.g. 'Bob Hope's father was a fireman') and tested on them a week later, both younger and older adults can successfully recall the items, but older adults are impaired at knowing where they had first learned the information[43]. Similarly, older adults are impaired at knowing where on a computer screen an item was presented, though they have little problem in recognition of items themselves[44]. Thus, impaired memory for context appears to exceed memory impairments for individual items. A prevailing theory accounting for these context deficits involves age-related difficulties in binding pieces of information in memory.

2.2 Brain changes

The effects of ageing on the brain occur at many levels, from genes to gross anatomy. Reviewing this large research domain is beyond the scope of this chapter. Here, we only mention two examples of cerebral ageing measures that have been directly related to cognitive decline: brain atrophy and dopamine deficits.

2.2.1 Brain atrophy

In post-mortem and *in vivo* studies, the brains of older adults tend to have lower volumes of gray matter than young adult brains[45]. These volume declines are not only related to a loss of cells, but can also be ascribed to lower synaptic densities in older adults[46]. Cross-sectional studies suggest that the volume of gray matter declines linearly with ageing, whereas white matter volume increases during young age, plateaus during young adulthood and middle age, and declines during old age — an inverted U function[47].

Apart from differential age effects on gray and white matter volume, the relation between age and brain volume is also not uniform across different brain regions. The region most affected is the PFC, whereas other regions, such as the occipital cortex, are relatively unaffected by the ageing process[48].

PFC volume has been seen to decrease at an average rate of 5% per decade beginning in the 20s[47], largely due to decreases in synaptic density. The disproportional effect of ageing on PFC volume, together with the finding that age differences tend to be larger on tasks assumed to depend on PFC function, has led to the proposal that age deficits are primarily the result of frontal decline (for a review, see[9]). However, other brain regions, including the basal ganglia[49,50] and the thalamus [51–53] also show a pronounced decline in brain volume with increasing age. In fact, in the last decades of normal life, volumetric changes in PFC do not differ from those in other neocortical areas[54,55].

Furthermore, MTL volume also declines with age, even though not all structures are equally affected. The hippocampus exhibits a significant volume loss of 2–3% per decade, whereas the rhinal cortex appears to be much less affected by healthy ageing[56]. For instance, a recent cross-sectional study by Raz and colleagues[56] found substantial age-related shrinkage not only in the prefrontal cortex (Fig. 1a) but also in the hippocampus (Fig. 1b), which was greatest in individuals with hypertension. In contrast, mean age-related shrinkage of the rhinal cortex was minimal (Fig. 1c).

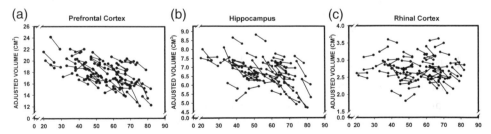

Fig. 4.1 Longitudinal changes in volumes of prefrontal cortex (**a**), hippocampus (**b**), and rhinal cortex (**c**) as a function of baseline age. (Reproduced with permission from Oxford University Press [56].)

Several studies have suggested that the decline in hippocampal volume contributes to age deficits in EM[57–60]. For instance, Golomb et al.[57] investigated the link between hippocampal atrophy and memory performance in a group of healthy older adults. They found that, after controlling for such factors as age, education, and vocabulary skills, individuals with hippocampal atrophy performed more poorly on memory tests, compared to those with no decline. Furthermore, as part of a longitudinal study on memory function, Golomb et al.[61] found a significant correlation between hippocampal atrophy across a 3.8 year span and decline in memory performance in a group of older adults (mean age = 68.4 years).

2.2.2 Dopamine deficits

Ageing affects not only brain anatomy but also brain physiology, including the function of neurotransmitter systems such as serotonin, acetylcholine, and dopamine[62]. Associated with volume decrements in PFC are decreases in dopamine (DA) concentration and transporter availability[63]. Additionally, dopamine D2 receptor density declines at a rate of 8% per decade beginning in the 40s. There is abundant evidence that dopamine (DA) systems play an important role not only in motor but also in higher-order cognitive functions. DA function can be measured *in vivo* using PET[64]. There is strong evidence of age-related losses in post- and presynaptic DA markers, which may reflect decreases in the number of neurons, the number of synapses per neurons, and/or the expression of receptor proteins in each neuron. D1 and D2 receptor binding declines from early adulthood at a rate of 4–10% per decade, and this decline is correlated with the decline of dopamine transporter, possibly reflecting a common causal mechanism.

DA deficits in Parkinson's disease (within the fronto-striatal system) are accompanied by reduction in processing speed, affecting WM[65]. Thus, it has been argued that this form of pathological ageing may be integral in composing a model for fronto-striatal cognitive deficits observed in normal ageing[8]. In support of this idea, cognitive performance on a wide range of tasks has been shown to correlate with DA functioning, exhibiting a critical role of DA in cognitive processes. In tasks involving episodic memory and perceptual speed, decreased performance with ageing was significantly correlated with D2 receptor availability and binding[66–68]. For instance, Volkow and colleagues used PET to examine the relationship between brain dopamine activity and tasks of motor and cognitive functioning across healthy individuals ranging in age between 24 and 86 years. Availability of D2 receptor correlated with tasks mediated by frontal brain regions (e.g. Wisconsin Card Sorting Test, Stroop Colour–Word Test). While the availability of D2 receptors declined with age, these correlations remained significant after controlling for age effects, suggesting that DA may influence cognition irrespective of age[66].

3. Functional neuroimaging studies of WM and EM

Cognitive ageing studies have described the effects of ageing on behavioural performance, and neurobiological studies have characterized the effects of ageing on the brain. Functional neuroimaging studies provide a bridge between these two domains by directly measuring age-related differences in brain activity during the performance of cognitive tasks. In general, these studies find brain regions that show weaker activiy in older than in younger adults, as well as regions that are recruited by older adults to a greater extent than young adults. Whereas age-related decreases in activation are usually attributed to cognitive deficits in older adults, age-related increases in activation are often interpreted as reflecting compensatory mechanisms in the ageing brain.

Regarding WM and EM functions, the most critical regions are PFC and MTL. Functional neuroimaging studies of cognitive ageing frequently find age-related changes in these two regions. In the case of PFC, the most consistent finding has been an age-related reduction in lateralization. This evidence has been conceptualized in a model called *Hemispheric Asymmetry Reduction in Older Adults* (HAROLD) which states that, under similar conditions, PFC activity tends to be less lateralized in older than in younger adults[69]. This model is supported by functional neuroimaging, electrophysiological, and behavioural evidence in the domains of episodic memory, semantic memory, working memory, perception, and inhibitory control[70]. In the case of MTL, the most consistent finding has been an age-related reduction in activity, particularly during EM studies. However, recent studies suggest that not all MTL regions show reduced activity in older adults. Actually, some MTL regions show preserved or increased activity in older adults, possibly reflecting differential age effects on various EM processes.

In this section, we first review the effects of ageing on PFC activation for both WM and EM tasks. Then, we turn to the effects of ageing on MTL activation as it relates to these cognitive processes. Although the number of studies is still too scarce to identify clear patterns in the data and a considerable amount of variability still remains unexplained, we try to emphasize the most consistent findings across studies. Table 4.1 presents an overview of reported age differences in PFC and MTL activity grouped by memory domain and ordered by place of discussion in this review section.

3.1 Prefrontal cortex

3.1.1 Working memory

Imaging studies of ageing and WM function have shown altered patterns of activation in older compared to younger adults, particularly in frontal regions. Generally, ageing is associated with increases in task-related PFC activity, which is in turn associated with better performance [71,72]. Hence, increases in PFC activation during WM tasks have been usually interpreted as compensatory. Additionally, PFC activity in older adults is not only greater overall but is often more bilateral, exhibiting the aforementioned HAROLD pattern.

Age-related increases in PFC activity were found by Grossman *et al.*[73] in a study of sentence comprehension that manipulated verbal WM demands (short vs. long antecedent noun — gap linkage). Despite similar recruitment of a semantic network across age groups, there were age differences in recruitment of areas associated with a verbal WM network. Compared to younger adults, older adults showed less activation in the left parietal cortex, but increased activation in the left premotor cortex and dorsal portions of left inferior PFC. This up-regulation of PFC areas within the verbal WM network was viewed as compensatory for older adults, whose performance did not differ from that of younger participants.

Table 4.1 Age differences in PFC and MTL activity during working memory, episodic encoding, and retrieval.

Cognitive function			PFC																				MTL			
			LEFT										RIGHT										LEFT		RIGHT	
Mod	Study	Contrast	4	8	6	44	45	47	11	46	9	10	10	9	46	11	47	45	44	6	8	4	PHG	HC	HC	PHG
WORKING MEMORY																										
F	Grossman 02	sentence compreh. - bl		○	○						○	○	○	○			●	●					●			
F	Rypma 00	letter: WM Enc, main, retr									●	●			●	●										
F	Rypma 01	letter: WM: 6-1 letter load		●							●	●	○	●	●	●		●	●							
P	Reuter-L. 00	letter: WM - bl (VOIs)									○	○						○								
P	Reuter-L. 00	locat: WM - bl (VOIs)	○	○							○	○														
F	Park 03	scenes: maint or probe					○	○										○	○				●			
F	Cabeza 04	word: WM - base	●	○							○	○	○					○	○	○	●		●		●	
F	Mitchell 00	objects.: combo > obj / loc											●										●			
P	Grady 98	face: WM - bl					●				○						●						●			
P	Grady 98	incr w/ long delays											●				●						●			
EPISODIC MEMORY ENCODING																										
P	Cabeza 97	word pair: Enc - Rn/Rc	●	●							●															
P	Anderson 00	word pairs: FA Enc - FA Rc		●	●	●	●				●		○	○	○			●	●	●						
F	Stebbins 02	word: deep - shall.		●		●	●	●			●															
F	Rosen 02	Old-high, word: deep - shall.															○	○								
F	Daselaar 03b	Old-low, word: rem - bl																					●	●		
F	Morcom 03	words Dm										○	○													
F	Gutchess 05	picture Dm	○	○									○							○			●			●
P	Grady 02	face: Enc - Rn					●																			
P	Grady 95	face: Enc - 2 bl					●	●							○											●
F	Logan 02 exp 1	words: intent enc - bl					●	●											○	○						
F	Logan 02 exp 2	word: deep - shallow																	○	○						
F	Daselaar 03b	word: deep - shallow											●											●		
EPISODIC MEMORY RETRIEVAL																										
P	Cabeza 97	word pair: Rn - Enc									●															
P	Madden 99	word: Rn - bl	○	○				○				○	○	○					○							
P	Cabeza 00	word: Rn - recEncy										○														
F	Daselaar 03b	Old-high, word: Rn - bl						○																		
F	Daselaar 03b	Old-low, word: Rn - bl						○																		
P	Schacter 96	stem Rc: low - high				○							●	●												
P	Schacter 96	stem Rc: high - low																								
P	Bäckman 97	stem Rc: Rc - bl							○	○													○		○	
P	Cabeza 00	word: Context - Rn											●	○												
P	Anderson 00	pair Rc: FA - FA Enc					○	○		○		●	●	●					○							
P	Cabeza 02	Old-high: Context - Recall										●	●	○			○									
F	Maguire 03	autobio events - publ event																								○
F	Cabeza 04	Rn - bl	●	○								○					○	○			●	○	●	●	
F	Daselaar 06	Recollection (exp. increase)																						●	●	
F	Daselaar 06	Familiarity (linear decrease)																						○		

Symbols: ● = regions more activated or activated only by young adults; ○ = regions more activated or activated only by old adults
Abbreviations: bl = baseline; Dm = Subsequent memory effect; Enc = Encoding; F = fMRI; FA = full attention; HC = hippocampus; intent = intentional; lex dec = lexical decision; loc = location; Mod = scanner modality; obj = object; PHG = parahippocampal gyrus; P = PET; Rc = recall; Reuter-L = Reuter-Lorenz; Rn = recognition; VOIs = volumes of interest

Age-related increases in PFC activity were also found in studies by Rypma and colleagues. In one study, Rypma and D'Esposito[72] differentiated the effects of ageing on encoding, maintenance, and retrieval phases of WM using event-related FMRI. The main result was that older adults showed reduced dorsolateral PFC activity during the retrieval phase but ventrolateral PFC activity was similar to young adults during all three phases. These results suggest that the retrieval phase of WM is more sensitive to ageing than encoding and maintenance phases.

In another study, Rypma et al.[74] examined verbal WM for different memory loads (one vs. six letters). This contrast yielded three main findings. First, left-lateralized ventrolateral PFC activity was similar in younger adults and older adults. Second, right-lateralized dorsolateral PFC activity was weaker in older than in younger adults. Finally, a left anterior PFC region was more activated in older adults than in younger adults. The authors suggested that ageing impairs executive aspects of WM mediated by dorsolateral PFC but not maintenance operations (e.g. phonological loop) mediated by left ventrolateral PFC. Results are consistent with the aforementioned dissociation between dorsolateral and ventrolateral PFC. Additionally, the age-related increase in left PFC activity was attributed to functional compensation.

As noted, several imaging studies have not only identified increased PFC activations in healthy ageing but, more specifically, an age-related reduction in hemispheric asymmetry (HAROLD). For example, Reuter–Lorenz et al.[71] used a maintenance task in which participants maintained four letters in WM and then compared them to a probe letter. As shown in Fig. 4.2, young adults showed left-lateralized activity, while older adults showed bilateral activity. They interpreted this HAROLD pattern as compensatory. Consistent with this interpretation, the older adults showing the bilateral activation pattern were faster in the verbal WM task than those that did not. In addition to the verbal WM condition, they also included a spatial WM task. In this task, younger adults activated right PFC and older adults additionally recruited left PFC. Thus, even though age-related increases were in opposite hemispheres, both verbal and spatial WM conditions yielded the HAROLD pattern (Fig. 4.2). This finding supports the generalizability of the HAROLD model to different kinds of stimuli. A follow-up study including additional participants[75] found bilateral activations in older adults not only in PFC but also in parietal regions.

Park et al.[76] found similar age-related bilateral PFC activity in a study involving processing of complex visual scenes. Participants maintained scenes in working memory or viewed

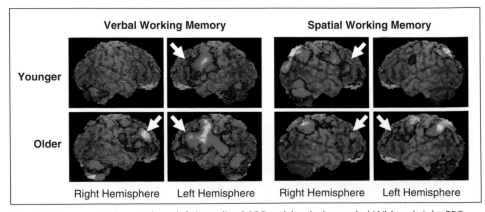

Fig. 4.2 Young participants show left-lateralized PFC activity during verbal WM and right PFC activity during spatial WM, whereas older adults show bilateral PFC activity in both tasks: the HAROLD pattern.[137] (Reproduced with permission from MIT Press)

them continuously. During the probe, older adults showed greater ventral PFC activity than younger adults, bilaterally. Although there was a trend for PFC activity to be more bilateral in older adults (i.e. HAROLD), the difference was not significant. The age-related increase in ventral PFC activity was attributed to compensation and/or retrieval effort.

Cabeza et al.[77] also found more bilateral PFC activation in older adults during verbal WM compared to left-lateralized activation in younger adults using a word delayed–response test. Interestingly, the older adults additionally showed a decrease in occipital activity, which was correlated with an increase in right PFC activity. They interpreted the occipital reduction as a visual processing deficit, whereas the increase in right PFC (HAROLD) was suggested to reflect compensation for the visual deficit.

In summary, WM studies often found that older adults show reduced activity in the PFC regions engaged by younger adults but greater activity in other PFC regions, such as contralateral PFC regions (i.e. the PFC hemisphere less engaged by younger adults). In some cases[71], contralateral recruitment led to a more bilateral pattern of PFC activity in older adults (i.e. HAROLD). In general, age-related increases in PFC activity were attributed to compensatory mechanisms.

3.1.2 Episodic encoding

Functional imaging studies of EE and ageing have used both incidental and intentional encoding tasks and a wide variety of stimuli. Despite this variability in methods and stimuli, PFC findings have been quite consistent: older adults typically show reduced left PFC activity compared to younger adults. We first discuss studies investigating intentional encoding of material. Then we will focus on studies that examine the influence encoding instruction has on activation differences in ageing.

In a study examining the intentional encoding of word pairs, Cabeza et al.[78] found that older adults showed less activity in the left PFC compared to younger adults. Importantly, they also noted the younger adults selectively recruited the left PFC whereas older adults showed equivalent activity in left and right PFC (i.e. HAROLD). Since younger adults and older adults had similar memory scores, they interpreted the additional recruitment of the right PFC by older adults as compensatory. Similarly, Anderson et al.[79] studied intentional encoding of moderately associated word pairs under conditions of full and divided attention. During full attention, the older adults showed reduced activity in the left PFC as well as increased activity in the right PFC, leading to bilateral frontal activity in older adults (i.e. HAROLD).

Age differences in PFC activation have also been shown when investigating levels of processing at encoding. When comparing deep and shallow encoding of words, Stebbins et al.[80] reported greater activity in both younger adults and older adults for the deep relative to the shallow encoding condition. However, the older adults showed decreased activation in the left PFC. Furthermore, decreased performance on neuropsychological tests correlated with reduced PFC activity. As a result of the reduced left PFC activity, PFC activity in older adults was more symmetric than in younger adults, again in accord with the HAROLD model.

Rosen et al.[81] also studied deep and shallow encoding of words in younger adults and older adults. However, they distinguished between older adults with high and low memory scores based on a neuropsychological test battery. They reported equivalent left PFC activity and greater right PFC activity in the old-high group relative to younger adults. In contrast, the old-low group showed reduced activity in both the left and right PFC. As a result, the old-high group showed a more bilateral pattern of PFC activity than younger adults (HAROLD).

Similarly, Daselaar et al.[82] compared groups of high- and low-performing old adults on a verbal encoding/recognition task, who were divided, post hoc, based on their memory scores. During the semantic encoding task (pleasant/unpleasant decisions) all groups showed left lateralized activations patterns, but PFC activity was slightly less lateralized in the low-performing elderly, and even less so in the high-performing elderly. Consistent with the results of Cabeza et al.[69], these findings support the compensatory interpretation of HAROLD.

Morcom et al.[83] used event-related FMRI to study subsequent memory for semantically encoded words. Recognition memory for these words was tested after a short and a longer delay. At the short delay, performance in older adults was equal to that of younger adults at the long delay. Under these conditions, activity in the left inferior PFC was greater for subsequently recognized than forgotten words in both age groups. Conversely, older adults showed greater right PFC activity than younger adults resulting in a more bilateral pattern of frontal activity (HAROLD).

Finally, Gutchess et al.[84] studied subsequent picture memory using a deep processing task. The older adults showed increased activity in the left PFC. Since picture encoding in younger adults was associated with bilateral PFC activity, these findings suggest a selective recruitment of the left PFC, which may be compensatory.

One question arises from these studies: What effect, if any, does encoding strategy play in age-altered PFC activations? The following three studies addressed this issue by directly comparing incidental to intentional instructions at encoding.

Grady and colleagues (not included in Table 4.1)[85] compared intentional versus incidental encoding conditions across various stimuli (e.g. words, pictures). They scanned participants during shallow (uppercase/lowercase, picture size), deep (living/non-living), and intentional encoding conditions. Overall, picture encoding resulted in greater activity in visual and MTL regions, while word encoding yielded greater activity in the left PFC and left lateral temporal cortex. However, deep encoding produced greater left PFC activity, while intentional encoding yielded greater right PFC activity. Though older adults showed the same patterns, the overall level of activity was reduced. Interestingly, they did not find a difference in deep versus intentional encoding of pictures, indicating that age differences were greater for words than for pictures.

The same research group performed another study comparing intentional and incidental encoding conditions, this time using faces as study items[86]. Convergent with their earlier study investigating intentional face encoding[87], older adults showed decreased activity in the left PFC compared to younger adults and diminished connectivity between frontal and MTL areas during both encoding conditions.

However, despite the lack of activation differences across encoding instructions mentioned above, a more recent study did find age-related frontal differences for intentional encoding instructions. During self-initiated encoding instructions, Logan et al.[88] reported that older adults compared to younger adults showed less activity in the left PFC, but greater activity in the right PFC, resulting in a more bilateral activity pattern (HAROLD). Results were similar for intentional encoding of both verbal and non-verbal material. Interestingly, further exploratory analyses revealed that this pattern was present in a group of old-older adults (mean age = 80), but not in a group of young-older adults (mean age = 67), suggesting that contralateral recruitment occurs very late in life (Fig. 4.3).

To summarize encoding studies, the most consistent finding was an age-related reduction in left PFC activity. This finding was more frequent for intentional than for incidental encoding studies suggesting that the environmental support provided by a deep semantic encoding task may attenuate the age-related decrease in left PFC activity. This effect was found within subjects in the study by Logan et al.[88]. The difference between intentional versus incidental encoding conditions suggests an important strategic component in age-related memory decline. The reduction in left PFC activity was often coupled with an increase in right PFC activity, leading to a bilateral pattern of PFC activity in older adults (HAROLD). Importantly, extending to encoding a finding originally reported for retrieval[69], two studies that divided older adults into high and low performers found the HAROLD pattern only in the high-performing group[81,82]. These findings provide direct support for the compensation account of HAROLD.

3.1.3 Episodic retrieval

As noted previously, age-related deficits in episodic retrieval tend to be more pronounced for recall and context memory tasks than for recognition tasks[89]. However, considerable differences in activity have also been observed during simple recognition tasks. We will

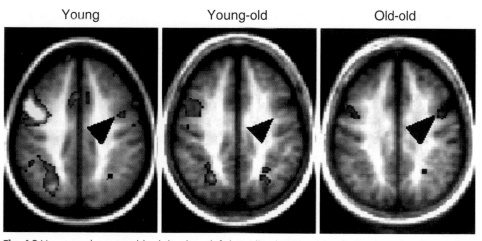

Fig. 4.3 Young and young-old adults show left-lateralized PFC activity during intentional encoding of words, whereas old-old adults show bilateral PFC activity (HAROLD) (Reproduced with permission from Elsevier Publishers[138].)

first review studies looking at recognition processes and then examine those that focus on recall and different forms of context memory.

The face encoding study by Grady et al.[87] included also a face recognition test. During this task, older adults showed reduced activity in parietal and occipital regions but equivalent activity to young adults in the right PFC. This last finding contrasts with the age-related reduction in left PFC activity found in the same study during face encoding. Based on these results, the authors suggested that age effects are more pronounced on encoding than on retrieval. As noted below, however, many subsequent PET and FMRI studies have found reliable age-related changes in PFC activity during episodic retrieval.

The word-pair encoding study by Cabeza et al.[78] included also a word-pair recognition task. During this task, older adults showed reduced activity in the right PFC but increased activity in other brain regions, such as the precuneus. The age-related reduction in the right PFC contrasts with the lack of age effects in this region's activity in Grady et al.'s (1995) study. This inconsistency could reflect differences in stimuli (faces vs. words) or retrieval processes (recognition of items vs. recognition of pairs).

The age-related reduction in right PFC activity during recognition was replicated by Madden et al.[90] using a single-word recognition task. Additionally, this study found an age-related increase in the left PFC. This age-related increase extended to recognition, a finding previously reported for recall by Cabeza et al.[91] which is reviewed below. As in the previous recall study, the age-related increase in the left PFC led to a more bilateral pattern in older adults (i.e. HAROLD). In a subsequent study, Madden et al.[90] re-analysed the recognition data using a stepwise regression method that distinguished between exponential (tau) and Gaussian (mu) components of RT distributions. Young adults showed a correlation between mu and right PFC activity, whereas the older adults showed correlations in left and right PFC regions related to both mu and tau. Since tau is associated with task-specific decision processes, and mu, with residual sensory coding and response processes, the authors concluded that attentional demands were greater for older adults, leading to the recruitment of additional regions. These findings suggest that the retrieval network is more widely distributed in older adults.

Daselaar et al.[82] used event-related FMRI to study recognition of words in younger adults and older adults. Based on recognition performance (high/low) in the scanner, older adults were divided into old-high and old-low groups. During recognition compared to baseline, the old-low group showed much increased activity throughout the brain relative to the other groups. In addition, the old-low group and younger adults showed bilateral PFC activity, whereas the old-high group showed a more left lateralized pattern of frontal activity. In other words, the old-low group showed a non-selective increase in global brain activity, whereas the old-high group showed selective recruitment of the left PFC. The authors interpreted these findings in terms of strategic retrieval differences. Interestingly, when correctly recognized old words were compared to correctly rejected new words, these group differences disappeared. The difference in activity between these two trial types is generally considered to be a correlate of retrieval success. Hence, these findings suggest that age differences in episodic recognition reflect strategic differences rather than a change in the processes supporting the actual recovery of information.

Like recognition, memory studies employing cued and free recall tasks have seen a difference in activation patterns across age. Age differences exist for both single item recall and recall of multiple items and/or features. During recall of a previously studied word list, Schacter et al.[92] scanned young and old subjects under different levels of performance. High and low levels of recall were produced by varying encoding conditions. In the high-minus-low contrast, both groups showed similar hippocampal activations. In the low-minus-high contrast, bilateral anterior PFC regions were more activated in younger than in older adults, whereas left posterior PFC areas were more activated in older adults. These findings support the idea that elderly use different functional networks at retrieval than younger adults.

The aforementioned word-pair study by Cabeza et al.[78] included not only a recognition test but also a cued-recall test. During recall, older adults showed weaker activity in the anterior cingulate and left temporal cortex. In addition, consistent with Schacter et al., older adults showed weaker activations in the right PFC than the younger adults. Conversely, older adults showed greater activity than younger adults in the left PFC. The net result was that PFC activity during recall was right lateralized in younger adults but bilateral in older adults. The authors noted this change in hemispheric asymmetry and interpreted it as compensatory. This was the first study identifying the HAROLD pattern and the first one suggesting the compensatory interpretation of this finding. This study also compared age-related changes in activity during recall and recognition. These changes were more pronounced during recall than during recognition, consistent with behavioural evidence that recall is more sensitive to ageing.

Bäckman et al.[93] found a similar result as Cabeza et al.[78] using word-stem cued recall instead of word-pair cued recall: younger adults activated the right PFC whereas older adults activated both the left and right PFC (HAROLD). Also using word pairs, Anderson et al.[79] investigated the effects of divided attention on cued recall. They reported negligible effects of divided attention in both groups. However, under full attention conditions, older adults showed weaker activations primarily in the right PFC but stronger activations primarily in the left PFC, suggesting an attenuation of the right-lateralized pattern shown by younger adults (HAROLD).

Cabeza et al.[94] investigated item and temporal-order memory tasks. In the item task, a word pair was presented consisting of one studied word and one new word, and participants indicated which word was studied. In the temporal-order task, both words were studied, and participants indicated which of the two words appeared later in the study list. They reported that younger adults showed increased activation in the right PFC for temporal-order compared to item memory, whereas older adults did not. In contrast, the activations during item memory were relatively unaffected by age. These findings are in line with the hypothesis that memory deficits in older adults are due to PFC dysfunction, and that context memory is more heavily dependent on the frontal lobes than item memory.

In another study of context memory by Cabeza and colleagues[69], younger adults, high-performing older adults (old-high), and low-performing older adults (old-low) studied words presented auditorily or visually. During scanning, they were presented with words visually and made either old/new decisions (item memory) or heard/seen decisions (context memory). Consistent with their previous results, younger adults showed right PFC activity for context trials, whereas older adults showed bilateral PFC activity (HAROLD). Importantly, however, this pattern was only seen for the old-high adults, supporting a compensation account of the HAROLD pattern (Fig. 4.4).

Summarizing the studies on retrieval, the HAROLD pattern has been found more frequently in studies using more challenging recall and context memory tasks than during simple item recognition. These findings suggest a three-way interaction between age, task difficulty, and frontal laterality. Importantly, distinguishing between old-high and old-low adults, the study by Cabeza et al.[69] provided direct evidence for the compensation account of HAROLD.

3.2 Medial temporal lobes

Frontal activations in ageing show both reductions and increases across ageing, as well as shifts in lateralization of activation. On the other hand, activation within the MTL generally shows age-related decreases compared to that seen in younger adults. However, some studies show a shift in the foci of activation from the hippocampus proper to more parahippocampal regions in ageing. Evidence for such a shift will be presented below where appropriate and discussed further in the conclusions.

3.2.1 Working memory

In WM tasks, older adults tend to show reductions in hippocampal activity associated with maintenance operations. Mitchell et al.[95] investigated a WM paradigm with an important episodic encoding component. In each trial, participants were presented with an object in a particular screen location and had to hold in WM the object, its location, or both (combination trials). Combination trials can be assumed to involve not only

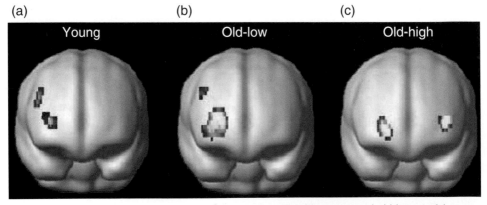

Fig. 4.4 PFC activity during memory retrieval is right-lateralized in young and old-low participants, but bilateral in old-high subjects (HAROLD). (Reproduced with permission from Elsevier Publishers[69].)

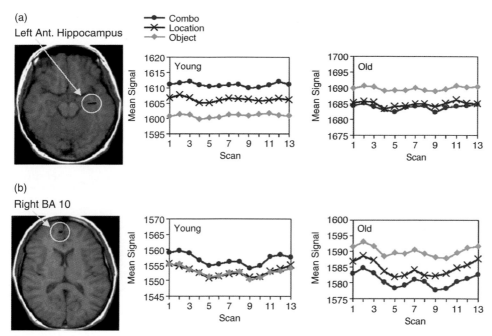

Fig. 4.5 (a) The left hippocampus showed an age x condition interaction. In young adults, hippocampal activity was greater in combination trials (object + location) than in the object only and location only conditions. In older adults, activation was lower in the combination trials than in the object only condition. **(b)** Right anterior PFC also showed an age x condition interaction. In young adults, activation was greater in the combination than in the location only condition. In older adults, activation in both combination and location only conditions was lower than in the object only condition. (Reproduced with permission from Elsevier Publishers[31].)

WM maintenance but also the binding of different information into an integrated memory trace (associative memory encoding). Older adults showed a deficit in accuracy in the combination condition but not in the object and location conditions. Two regions were differentially involved in the combination condition in younger adults but not in older adults: a left anterior hippocampal region and an anteromedial PFC region (right BA 10) (Fig. 4.5). According to the authors, a disruption of a hippocampal–PFC circuit may underlie binding deficits in older adults.

Older adults also exhibit difficulty maintaining hippocampal activation across long delays. Grady et al.[96] investigated a face WM task with varied intervals of item maintenance (1–21 secs). As the delay extended from 1 to 6 sec, left hippocampal activity increased in younger adults but decreased in older adults, which implies that older adults have difficulties initiating memory strategies mediated by MTL or sustaining MTL activity beyond very short retention intervals.

In addition to showing greater ventral PFC activation while maintaining faces in WM, older adults in the aforementioned Park et al. study[76] also showed an age-related reduction in hippocampal activity. The left hippocampus was more activated in the viewing than in the maintenance condition in younger adults, but not in older adults. As in Mitchell et al.'s[95] study, the age-related reduction in hippocampal activity was attributed to deficits in associative encoding.

Three nonverbal working memory studies[76,95,96] found age-related decreases in hippocampus activity, whereas no verbal working memory study found such decreases. It is possible that nonverbal tasks were more dependent on hippocampal-mediated relational memory processing and, hence, more sensitive to age-related deficits in these regions. Additionally, age-related differences in activation during maintenance tasks support the theory that age differences in 'simple' WM do exist and are indeed undetectable at the behavioural level.

3.2.2 Episodic encoding

In their study examining face encoding, Grady et al.[87] found that older adults showed less activity in the left PFC and MTL than younger adults. Furthermore, they found a highly significant correlation in younger adults, but not in older adults, between hippocampus and left PFC activity. Based on these results, they concluded that encoding in older adults is accompanied by reduced neural activity and diminished connectivity between PFC and MTL areas.

Daselaar et al.[97] investigated levels of processing in ageing using a deep (living/nonliving) vs. shallow (uppercase/lowercase) encoding task. Despite seeing common activation of regions involved in a semantic network across both age groups, activation differences were seen when comparing levels of processing. Older adults revealed significantly less activation in the left anterior hippocampus during deep relative to shallow classification. Researchers concluded that under-recruitment of MTL regions contribute, at least in part, to age-related impairments in encoding.

Similarly, the same group showed decreased activity in the MTL for poor-performing older adults compared to young and high-performing elderly. Despite the equivalent activation that was shown in PFC activation in their verbal encoding/recognition task, Daselaar et al.[82] found that the older adults showed decreased activity in the left hippocampus\parahippocampal cortex during successful encoding of words (Fig. 4.6). Based on these findings, they concluded that MTL dysfunction during encoding is an important factor in age-related memory decline.

Similar to Daselaar et al.[82], Gutchess et al.'s[84] study of subsequent picture memory observed reduced activity in the MTL for subsequently remembered items, even when older adults were not divided into high- and low-memory groups. Additionally, older adults exhibited a significant negative correlation between inferior frontal and parahippocampal activity, whereas younger adults did not. Results suggest that those older adults exhibiting the least involvement of the parahippocampus conversely activated inferior frontal areas the most. Data suggest that prefrontal regions could be activated to compensate for declines in MTL activations in older adults.

Age-related reductions in MTL activity[82,84,97] indicate that, besides frontal changes, reduced MTL function also contributes to age-related memory decline. Increased PFC activity in older adults may be compensatory, offsetting reduction in MTL activation.[84]

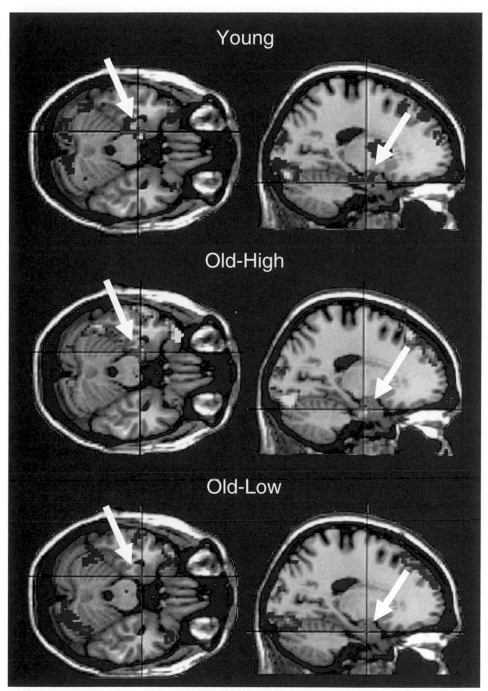

Fig. 4.6 Young adults and older adults with high memory performance (old-high) exhibit similar activation in the hippocampus/parahippocampal cortex, while older adults with low memory performance (old-low) exhibit less hippocampal/parahippocampal activation during successful encoding. (Reproduced with permission from Oxford University Press[82].)

3.2.3 Episodic memory retrieval

Cabeza *et al.*[77] investigated the effects of ageing on several cognitive tasks including a verbal recognition task. Within the medial temporal lobes, they found a dissociation between a hippocampal region which showed weaker activity in older adults than in younger adults and a cortical MTL region, which showed the converse pattern. Given evidence that hippocampal and parahippocampal regions are respectively more involved in recollection vs. familiarity[98,99], this finding is consistent with the notion that older adults are more impaired in recollection than in familiarity[39,100]. Actually, the age-related increase in parahippocampal cortex suggests that older adults may be compensating for recollection deficits by relying more on familiarity. Supporting this idea, older adults had a larger number of 'know' responses than younger adults and these responses were positively correlated with the parahippocampal activation.

A recent follow-up study by the same group showed a similar pattern of results[101]. Young and older adults made old/new judgements about previously studied words followed by a confidence judgement from low to high. These responses were then combined into a three-point *perceived oldness* scale (level 1 = 'new', level 2 = 'probably old', level 3 = 'definitely old'). There is a considerable amount of evidence that familiarity-based responses increase gradually as a function of perceived oldness, whereas recollection-based responses are primarily associated with the highest level of perceived oldness[102]. For example, the probability of 'know' responses increases monotonically from 'new' to 'definitely old' trials, whereas the vast majority of 'remember' responses are clustered around 'definitely old' trials[103]. Accordingly, using parametric FMRI analyses with perceived oldness as a covariate, *recollection-related activity* was defined as an exponential function in which activity remains low for levels 1 and 2 and increases sharply for level 3 (i.e. definitely old trials). In contrast, familiarity was defined as a linear *increase* or *decrease* as a function of perceived oldness. The results revealed a double dissociation within MTL. Recollection-related activity in the hippocampus was reduced in older adults as indicated by a sharper exponential increase of the perceived oldness function in young adults (Fig. 4.7a). In contrast, familiarity-related activity (linear decrease) in the rhinal cortex was augmented in older adults as indicated by the steeper *negative* slope of the perceived oldness function (Fig. 4.7b). In addition, age dissociations regarding recollection and familiarity were found within parietal and posterior midline regions. Finally, ageing reduced functional connectivity within a hippocampal-retrosplenial/parietotemporal network, but increased connectivity within a rhinal-frontal network. These findings indicate that older adults compensate for hippocampal deficits by relying more on the rhinal cortex, possibly through a top–down frontal modulation. Hence, consistent with their previous findings, these results suggest a greater reliance on familiarity-based recognition in older adults.

In addition to increases in activity in the left PFC during word-stem cued recall, Bäckman and colleagues[93] found increased MTL activation in older adults. Just as the increased left PFC activation resulted in more bilateral frontal activation for older adults, increased activation in the left MTL had the same effect. Compared to younger adults,

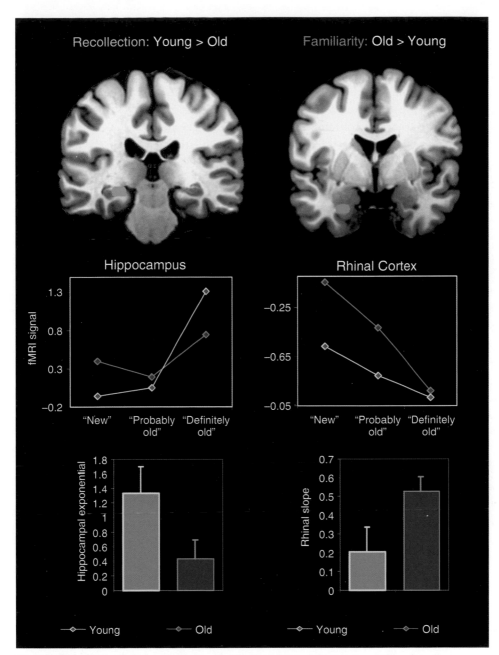

Fig. 4.7 The effects of ageing yielded a double dissociation between two MTL sub-regions: whereas recollection-related activity (exponential increase) in the hippocampus was attenuated by ageing, familiarity-related activity (linear decrease) in the rhinal cortex was enhanced by ageing. The hippocampal exponential rate parameter (λ) provides a measure of the sharpness of the exponential increase of the perceived oldness function in the hippocampus. The rhinal slope parameter provides a measure of the steepness of the perceived oldness function in the rhinal cortex. (Reproduced with permission from Oxford University Press[101].)

older adults showed more bilateral MTL activity. It should be noted that this bilateral activation was not accompanied by increased performance — older adults recalled only about half as many words as did younger adults.

This HAROLD pattern within MTL was also observed in a recent study using event-related FMRI. Maguire and Frith[104] investigated the recall of autobiographical events gathered in a pre-scan interview. Although the groups activated largely the same regions, they observed a striking difference in the MTL. Younger adults showed left-lateralized hippocampal activity, whereas older adults showed bilateral activity in the MTL. These findings suggest that HAROLD extends beyond the PFC not only to other cortical regions (as shown by several studies) but also to subcortical areas.

In sum, retrieval studies have found both increases and decreases in MTL activity. The findings by Cabeza and colleagues suggest that some of these increases reflect a shift from recollection (hippocampus) to familiarity-based retrieval (parahippocampal cortex).

3.3 Discussion

In summary, our review of functional neuroimaging studies of cognitive ageing has identified considerable age-related changes in activity during WM, EE, and ER tasks not only in the PFC, but also in the MTL. These findings suggest that functional changes in both PFC and MTL play a role in age-related memory deficits. Focussing first on PFC findings, the studies indicated both age-related reductions and increases in PFC activity. During WM tasks, older adults show reduced activity in the PFC regions engaged by young adults, but greater activity in other regions, such as contralateral PFC regions. The latter changes often resulted in the more bilateral pattern of PFC activity in older than younger adults known as HAROLD[71,76,77,105]. In general, age-related PFC increases and HAROLD findings have been attributed to functional compensation in the ageing brain. During EE tasks, the most consistent finding has been a reduction in left PFC activity. This finding is more frequent for intentional than for incidental encoding tasks. The age-related reduction in left PFC activity was often coupled with an age-related increase in right PFC activity (i.e. HAROLD). Finally, ER was also associated with HAROLD, and this pattern was found more often in studies using more challenging recall and context memory tasks than during simple item recognition tasks.

Age-related changes in PFC activity are generally in line with the *resource deficit theory* of cognitive ageing[10]. As described at the beginning of the chapter, this theory postulates that ageing reduces attentional resources and, as a result, older adults have greater difficulties with cognitive tasks that provide less environmental support and, hence, require greater self-initiated processing. Given the critical role of the PFC in managing attentional resources, this view predicts that age-related changes in PFC activity will be larger for tasks involving greater self-initiated processing and/or less environmental support. The results are generally consistent with this prediction. During EE, age-related decreases in left PFC activation were found frequently during intentional encoding conditions (which provide less environmental support) but rarely during incidental encoding conditions (which provide greater environmental support). Similarly, during ER, age-related differences in PFC activity were usually larger for recall and context memory tasks (which require greater cognitive resources) than for recognition memory tasks (which require less cognitive resources). Thus, in general, age effects on PFC activity tend to increase as a function of the demands placed on cognitive resources. This finding is in keeping with aforementioned evidence that the anatomical integrity of the frontal lobes, as well as the dopamine modulation of this region, show significant decline with ageing.

However, not all age-related changes on PFC activity suggested decline; on the contrary, many studies found age-related increases in PFC that suggested compensatory mechanisms in the ageing brain. In particular, several studies found, in older adults, activations in contralateral PFC regions not activated by young adults. Activitynbehaviour correlations[71] and experimental comparisons between high- and low-performing older adults[81,82] demonstrated the beneficial contribution of these regions to memory performance in older adults. In this respect, it is important to note that resource deficit and compensatory interpretations are not incompatible. Actually, it is reasonable to assume that the recruitment of additional brain regions (e.g. in the contralateral PFC hemisphere) reflects an attempt to compensate for reduced cognitive resources. Moreover, age-related decreases suggestive of resource deficits and age-related increases suggestive of compensation have been often found in the same conditions. For example, EE studies have shown age-related decreases in left PFC activity coupled with age-related increases in right PFC activity. These changes often lead to a dramatic reduction in hemispheric asymmetry in older adults (i.e. HAROLD)[93] which is, overall, the most consistent finding across different memory domains.

Turning to MTL findings, several studies have found age-related decreases in hippocampal and parahippocampal regions. During WM, older adults demonstrate decline in hippocampal activation during encoding of multiple features[76,95]. During EE, however, declines in hippocampal activation are also seen for encoding of individual features in healthy older adults[82,84,87,97,106]. Finally, during ER, some studies found decreases in hippocampal activity[77,101] but also greater activity in older than younger adults in parahippocampal[77], rhinal[101], or contralateral MTL[93,107] regions, which may be compensatory.

In general, age-related changes in MTL activity are consistent with the *associative deficit theory*[11,30]. As noted in the first part of the chapter, this hypothesis postulates that age-related memory deficits are primarily the results of difficulties in encoding and retrieving novel associations between items. Given that relational memory has been strongly associated with the hippocampus[108], this hypothesis predicts that older adults will show decreased hippocampal activity during memory tasks, particularly when they involve associations. Consistent with this hypothesis, age-related reductions in hippocampal activity were found in WM tasks involving maintenance of complex visual scenes[76] and objects paired with specific locations[95]. Also, EE studies found these reductions during the encoding of complex scenes, which involve associations among picture elements[76], and during deep encoding of words, which involve identification of semantic associations[82,97]. Finally, a recent study specifically associated age-related reductions in hippocampal activity to recollection, which involves recovery of item-context associations (see Fig. 4.7)[101]. Yet, it should be noted that age-related changes in MTL activity were often accompanied by concomitant changes in PFC activity. Hence, in these cases, it is unclear whether such changes signal MTL dysfunction or whether they are the result of a decline in efficient memory strategies mediated by PFC regions. However, studies using incidental encoding tasks with minimal strategic requirements have also identified age differences in MTL activity without significant changes in PFC activity (see Fig. 4.6)[82,97].

As in the case of PFC, not all age-related changes in MTL activity suggest decline; several findings suggest compensation. First, similar to the bilateral pattern frequently observed in PFC, older adults have also demonstrated bilateral hippocampal recruitment while performing memory retrieval tasks[104]. Second, during ER, older adults have been found to show reduced activity in the hippocampus but increased activity in other brain regions such as the parahippocampal gyrus[77] and the rhinal cortex[101]. These results were interpreted as a recruitment of familiarity processes mediated by parahippocampal regions in order to compensate for the decline of recollection processes that are dependent on the hippocampus proper.

As mentioned at the beginning of this chapter, one of the biggest challenges in cognitive ageing research is to isolate the effects of healthy ageing from those of pathological ageing (e.g. AD). A general review of the structural neuroimaging literature suggests that healthy ageing is accompanied by greater declines in frontal regions compared to the MTL[47]. In contrast, pathological ageing is characterized by greater decline in the MTL than in frontal regions [109,110]. In fact, functional neuroimaging evidence suggests that prefrontal activity tends to be maintained or even increased in early AD[111]. Thus, these findings suggest that memory decline in healthy ageing is more dependent on frontal than MTL deficits, whereas the opposite pattern is more characteristic of pathological ageing[7,9]. In view of these findings, clinical studies aimed at an early diagnosis of age-related pathology have mainly targeted changes in the MTL[112]. Yet, the studies reviewed in this chapter clearly indicate that healthy older adults are also prone to MTL decline. Hence, rather than focussing on MTL deficits alone, diagnosis of age-related pathology may be improved by employing some type of composite score reflecting the ratio between MTL and frontal decline.

In terms of MTL dysfunction in healthy and pathological ageing, it is also critical to assess the specific type or loci of MTL dysfunction. As noted, a decline in hippocampal function can be seen in both healthy ageing and AD. Thus, even though hippocampal volume decline is an excellent marker of concurrent AD[113,114], it is not a reliable measure for distinguishing normal ageing from early stages of the disease[47]. In contrast, substantial changes in the rhinal cortex are present in early AD patients with only mild impairments[115–118], but not in healthy ageing (see Fig. 4.1c)[56]. In a discriminant analysis, Pennanen and colleagues[119] showed that, although hippocampal volume is indeed the best marker to discriminate AD patients from normal controls, the volume of the rhinal cortex is much better in distinguishing between incipient AD (mild cognitive impairment — MCI) and healthy ageing. Finally, it should be noted that, despite the rigorous screening procedures typical of functional neuroimaging studies of healthy ageing, it remains possible that early symptoms of age-related pathology went undetected in some of the studies reviewed in this chapter.

4. **Issues**

4.1 **Tasks and design**

One issue with regards to assessing age-related deficits in performance and activation is the fact of what one is testing. Cognitive tasks are never 'pure'; they always involve a complex blend of different cognitive operations. For example, as noted above, WM tasks can involve both encoding and retrieval operations. And within those operations are levels of maintenance, processing, etc. The same is true for all cognitive functions. Thus, when an age-related difference in activation is found, it is important to determine which component of the task is responsible for the difference. This type of task analysis could help explain some inconsistencies in the literature. For example, Cabeza *et al.*[78] found a significant age-related reduction in PFC activity during verbal recognition, whereas Madden *et al.*[90] did not. Given that recognition memory involves both recollection and familiarity[98], and that recollection is sensitive to ageing [100], the inconsistent findings could reflect a greater recollection component in the recognition task investigated by Cabeza *et al.* (associative recognition) than in the one studied by Madden *et al.* (item recognition).

The standard solution to the problem of task complexity is the subtraction method, which compares target and control conditions assumed to differ primarily in the process of interest. There are two main problems with this method, and both are magnified by group contrasts. First, activations reflect both the target condition and control condition employed. Thus, older adults may show weaker activations than young adults not because they did not engage a region during the target task but because they also engaged it during the control task[120]. This problem is attenuated, but not eliminated, by using low-level baselines (e.g. the fixation period in event-related FMRI studies) which may also show age-related differences. For example, Lustig *et al.*[121] scanned younger adults and older adults during a semantic classification task, which was intermixed with blocks of passive rest. They found that older adults showed less activity during rest (task-related deactivation) in posterior midline regions. These regions are commonly activated in younger adults during low-level baseline conditions[122–124]. Lustig *et al.* proposed that age differences in rest activity reflect a less efficient allocation in older adults of available resources to task-relevant processes.

Second, the subtraction method rests on the assumption that the extra component of the target condition does not affect the components shared with the control condition pure insertion assumption[125]. This assumption is problematic (e.g. see[126]) and may be further violated when the inserted task components interact with limitations in cognitive resources in older adults. To address this problem, future studies should complement subtraction analyses with other methods such as parametric manipulations, multivariate analyses, and activity–performance correlations.

4.2 **Subjects**

One important aspect of study design is the selection of older adults. On the one hand, one would like to select older adults who are perfectly healthy and who are matched to younger adults in all possible variables except age. One the other hand, one would like to investigate a sample of older adults that is representative of the general population. This is a general problem of cognitive ageing research, but some aspects of it are particularly thorny in functional neuroimaging studies, such as screening criteria and the sub-population of older adults investigated.

Regarding health screening, not all researchers agree on concrete inclusion/exclusion criteria. Most do agree that participants with high blood pressure should be excluded; hypertension may not only alter blood flow measures but it is also associated with covert cerebrovascular damage[127]. Also, while most studies exclude participants taking medications that could alter blood flow, there are no clear guidelines about which drugs to exclude for. Likewise, participants are usually excluded if they show pronounced atrophy or white-matter damage in MRI scans, but the boundary between normal and abnormal structural changes is not clear. Thus, there is an urgent need for studies assessing the effect of the various subject-related factors on haemodynamic measures — as this could lead to greater variability in activation. For example, Jennings et al.[128] found, during a WM task, hypertensive older adults showed different activation patterns than normotensive older adults.

There is also a wide range within older adults, both quantitatively and qualitatively. Quantitatively, older adults may differ in level of cognitive performance, with some older adults performing as well as younger adults and others showing significant deficits. This variability in age-related cognitive decline difference may account for some inconsistencies in the imaging literature (see discussion about performance differences below). Qualitatively, older adults may differ regarding the particular neurocognitive component in which they are most impaired. As shown by Glisky and collaborators[129,130], some older adults may be more affected on PFC-mediated executive functions, whereas other older adults may be more affected in MTL-mediated memory functions. Obviously, the proportion of these two patterns in the sample investigated is likely to affect what age effects one finds. Thus, future studies should try to characterize different levels of performance and ageing patterns and investigate their effect on brain activation patterns.

4.3 Performance

Brain activity can vary as a function of performance measures (e.g. accuracy[131], reaction time[72]). Therefore, in functional neuroimaging studies, if older adults perform more poorly than younger adults, it is unclear whether differences in activation between older adults and younger adults reflect the age effects or dissimilarities in performance. This is a typical 'chicken and egg' problem: do older adults perform poorly because their brain activity is different, or is their brain activity different because they perform poorly?

One approach to this problem is to match performance in young and old groups by manipulating tasks[83,101] or by scanning high-functioning elderly who naturally perform as well as young adults (e.g. see[78]). When cognitive performance is similar in the young and old groups, group differences in brain activity can be safely attributed to ageing. The main problem of this approach is that when performance differences are eliminated, it becomes more difficult to relate activation findings to the cognitive deficits typically displayed by older adults. A possible solution to this problem is to have an 'easy' and a 'difficult' version of the task, and compare younger adults and older adults both when performance is matched (e.g. young adults-difficult vs. old adults-easy) and when an age-related deficit is present (e.g. young adults-difficult vs. old adults-difficult or young adults-easy vs. old adults-easy)[94].

Another way to address the problem of performance differences is to use event-related FMRI designs and analyse only correct trials in both groups. This method does not eliminate differences in RTs, unless the number of trials is sufficiently large to allow selecting trials with similar RTs in the two groups. An alternative solution is to enter RTs as a covariate in the analyses, but risks eliminating activity associated with processes of interest (which are usually correlated with RTs).

4.4 Activations

After subjects have been appropriately selected, task components suitably analysed, and performance differences properly controlled, researchers are still faced with the fundamental problem of interpreting the age-related differences in activation they have found. This more general issue can actually be divided into three tasks: determining what kind of age-related activation differences were found; interpreting ageing effects on a particular brain region; and evaluating global network changes.

Determining the kind of age-related activity difference found is not a trivial problem. First, one must determine whether younger adults and older adults engage the same region to different degrees (quantitative difference) or different brain regions (qualitative difference). The interpretation of these two patterns is different but distinguishing between them is not easy. For example, quantitative differences may appear as qualitative due to threshold effects. Also, when younger adults and older adults activate adjacent areas (e.g. BA 9 vs. BA 46), the finding may be described as the 'same' activation in different locations or as 'different' activations. Second, another knotty problem is whether age-related differences in activation reflect changes in neural architecture or changes in cognitive architecture[132]. In other words, did younger adults and older adults engage different regions to perform the same cognitive operations or did they recruit different regions to perform different cognitive operations? If one wants to know if the neural correlates of process A change with age, it is critical that both groups engage process A to the same extent. At the same time, if ageing is associated with a shift from process A to process B, then the neural correlates of *both* processes should be investigated in *both* groups. The main problem, of course, is how to determine exactly the processes engaged by human subjects, since cognitive tasks can be performed in many different ways and introspective reports provide very limited information about the actual operations performed by the subjects.

Interpreting age-related differences in activation is also complex. In general, age-related decreases in activation have been interpreted as detrimental and age-related increases as beneficial. Unfortunately, the relation between neural activity and cognitive performance is not so simple; less activity may reflect more efficient processing[133,134], and more activity may reflect unnecessary or even disruptive processes[78]. Correlations could help interpret activation differences if one assumes that activations positively correlated with performance are beneficial and those negatively correlated with performance are detrimental. However, an activation may be beneficial for performance but be negatively correlated with performance *across subjects* when the region is recruited by participants who have difficulty with the task. To explain using an analogy, a walking-stick helps walking performance but its use is negatively correlated with walking performance (because it is used by those who have difficulty walking). Event-related designs can also help distinguish between beneficial and detrimental interpretations if one assumes that activity during successful trials is beneficial and activity during unsuccessful trials is detrimental. Yet, again, a region may be beneficial for performance but only for demanding trials, which have a greater chance of being unsuccessful.

Finally, although most studies have interpreted age-related differences in terms of local changes (e.g. PFC dysfunction), these differences may also reflect global network changes. For example, using structural equation modelling, we have found that age-related changes in the activity of a left PFC region during episodic encoding and retrieval were partly due to age-related changes in the interactions between this region and other components of the episodic memory network[78]. Thus, one of the main challenges for future imaging studies of cognitive ageing is to investigate not only local changes but also changes in functional connectivity.

Acknowledgements

This work was supported by a grant from the National Institute of Aging (R01AG19731; R. Cabeza, primary investigator) and partial support from NIA grant (T32 AG00029; Nancy Dennis)

References

1. Wager TD, Smith EE. Neuroimaging studies of working memory: a meta-analysis. *Cogn Affect Behav Neurosci* 2003;**3**(4):255–74.

2. Tulving E. *Elements of episodic memory*. Oxford: Clarendon Press, 1983.

3. Gabrieli JD. Cognitive neuroscience of human memory. *Annu Rev Psychol* 1998;**49**:87–115.

4. Milner B. Disorders of learning and memory after temporal lobe lesions in man. *Clinical Neurosurgery* 1972;**19**:421–446.

5. Squire LR, Schmolck H, Stark SM. Impaired auditory recognition memory in amnesic patients with medial temporal lobe lesions. *Learn Mem* 2001;**8**(5):252–6.

6. Simons JS, Spiers HJ. Prefrontal and medial temporal lobe interactions in long-term memory. *Nat Rev Neurosci* 2003;**4**(8):637–48.

7. Buckner RL. Memory and executive function in aging and AD: multiple factors that cause decline and reserve factors that compensate. *Neuron* 2004;**44**(1):195–208.

8. Hedden T, Gabrieli JD. Insights into the ageing mind: a view from cognitive neuroscience. *Nat Rev Neurosci* 2004;**5**(2):87–96.

9. West RL. An application of prefrontal cortex function theory to cognitive aging. *Psychol Bull* 1996;**120**(2):272–92.

10. Craik FIM, Byrd M. Aging and cognitive deficits: The role of attentional resources. In: Craik FIM, Trehub S, eds. *Aging and cognitive processes*. New York: Plenum, 1982: 191–211.

11. Naveh–Benjamin M. Adult age differences in memory performance: tests of an associative deficit hypothesis. *Journal of Experimental Psychology: Learning, Memory and Cognition* 2000;**26**(5):1170–87.

12. Baddeley A. The concept of working memory: a view of its current state and probable future development. *Cognition* 1981;**10**(1–3):17–23.

13. Baddeley A. Working memory: looking back and looking forward. *Nat Rev Neurosci* 2003;**4**(10):829–39.

14. Dobbs AR, Rule BG. Adult age differences in working memory. *Psychol Aging* 1989;**4**(4):500–3.

15. Wiegersma S, Meertse K. Subjective ordering, working memory, and aging. *Exp Aging Res* 1990;**16**(1–2):73–7.

16. West R. Visual distraction, working memory, and aging. *Mem Cognit* 1999;**27**(6):1064–72.

17. Chao LL, Knight RT. Prefrontal deficits in attention and inhibitory control with aging. *Cereb Cortex* 1997;**7**(1):63–9.

18. Bowles RP, Salthouse TA. Assessing the age-related effects of proactive interference on working memory tasks using the Rasch model. *Psychol Aging* 2003;**18**(3):608–15.

19. Craik FIM. Age differences in human memory. In: Birren JE, Schaie KW, eds. *Handbook of the psychology of aging*. New York: Van Nostrand Reinhold, 1977.

20. Reuter–Lorenz P, Sylvester CY. *The cognitive neuroscience of working memory and aging*. New York: Oxford University Press, 2005: p. 186–217.

21. Salthouse TA, Mitchell DR, Skovronek E, Babcock RL. Effects of adult age and working memory on reasoning and spatial abilities. *J Exp Psychol Learn Mem Cogn* 1989;**15**(3):507–16.

22. May CP, Hasher L, Kane MJ. The role of interference in memory span. *Mem Cognit* 1999;**27**(5):759–67.

23. Lustig C, Hasher L. Implicit memory is vulnerable to proactive interference. *Psychol Sci* 2001;**12**(5):408–12.

24. Reuter–Lorenz P. New visions of the aging mind and brain. *Trends Cogn Sci* 2002;**6**(9):394.

25. Anderson ND, Craik FI, Naveh–Benjamin M. The attentional demands of encoding and retrieval in younger and older adults: 1. Evidence from divided attention costs. *Psychol Aging* 1998;**13**(3):405–23.

26. Park DC, Smith AD, Dudley WN, Lafronza VN. Effects of age and a divided attention task presented during encoding and retrieval on memory. *J Exp Psychol Learn Mem Cogn* 1989;**15**(6):1185–91.

27. Craik FI, Byrd M, Swanson JM. Patterns of memory loss in three elderly samples. *Psychol Aging* 1987;**2**(1):79–86.

28. Smith AD, Park DC, Earles JL, Shaw RJ, Whiting WLt. Age differences in context integration in memory. *Psychol Aging* 1998;**13**(1):21–8.

29. Schacter DL, Osowiecki D, Kaszniak AW, Kihlstrom JF, Valdiserri M. Source memory: extending the boundaries of age-related deficits. *Psychol Aging* 1994;**9**(1):81–9.

30. Chalfonte BL, Johnson MK. Feature memory and binding in young and older adults. *Memory and Cognition* 1996;**24**(4):403–16.

31. Mitchell KJ, Johnson MK, Raye CL, Mather M, D'Esposito M. Aging and reflective processes of working memory: binding and test load deficits. *Psychology and Aging* 2000;**15**(3):527–41.

32. Naveh–Benjamin M, Guez J, Kilb A, Reedy S. The associative memory deficit of older adults: further support using face-name associations. *Psychol Aging* 2004;**19**(3):541–6.

33. Craik FIM, McDowd JM. Age differences in recall and recognition. *Journal Of Experimental Psychology-Learning Memory And Cognition* 1987;**13**:474–9.

34. Rabinowitz JC, Craik FI. Prior retrieval effects in young and old adults. *J Gerontol* 1986;**41**(3):368–75.

35. Rabinowitz JC. Aging and recognition failure. *J Gerontol* 1984;**39**(1):65–71.

36. Park DC, Shaw RJ. Effect of environmental support on implicit and explicit memory in younger and older adults. *Psychol Aging* 1992;**7**(4):632–42.

37. Bastin C, Van der Linden M. The contribution of recollection and familiarity to recognition memory: a study of the effects of test format and aging. *Neuropsychology* 2003;**17**(1):14–24.

38. Clarys D, Isingrini M, Gana K. Mediators of age-related differences in recollective experience in recognition memory. *Acta Psychol (Amst)* 2002;**109**(3):315–29.

39. Parkin AJ, Walter BM. Recollective experience, normal aging, and frontal dysfunction. *Psychology and Aging* 1992;**7**:290–298.

40. Park DC, Puglisi JT. Older adults' memory for the color of pictures and words. *J Gerontol* 1985;**40**(2):198–204.

41. Light LL, LaVoie D, Valencia–Laver D, Owens SA, Mead G. Direct and indirect measures of memory for modality in young and older adults. *J Exp Psychol Learn Mem Cogn* 1992;**18**(6):1284–97.

42. Kausler DH, Puckett JM. Adult age differences in memory for sex of voice. *J Gerontol* 1981;**36**(1):44–50.

43. McIntyre JS, Craik FI. Age differences in memory for item and source information. *Can J Psychol* 1987;**41**(2):175–92.

44. Parkin AJ, Walker BM, Hunkin NM. Relationships between normal aging, frontal lobe function, and memory for temporal and spatial information. *Neuropsychology* 1995;**9**:304–12.

45. Resnick SM, Pham DL, Kraut MA, Zonderman AB, Davatzikos C. Longitudinal magnetic resonance imaging studies of older adults: a shrinking brain. *J Neurosci* 2003;**23**(8):3295–301.

46. erry RD. Cell death or synaptic loss in Alzheimer disease. *J Neuropathol Exp Neurol* 2000;**59**(12):1118–9.

47. Raz N. The aging brain observed in vivo: differential changes and their modifiers. In: Cabeza R, Nyberg L, Park D, ed. *Cognitive Neuroscience of Aging*. New York: Oxford University Press, 2005: p. 19–57.

48. Raz N, Gunning FM, Head D, *et al*. Selective aging of the human cerebral cortex observed in vivo: Differential vulnerability of the prefrontal gray matter. *Cerebral Cortex* 1997;**7**(3):268–82.

49. Bugiani O, Salvarani S, Perdelli F, Mancardi GL, Leonardi A. Nerve cell loss with aging in the putamen. *Eur Neurol* 1978;**17**(5):286–91.

50. Schwartz M, Creasey H, Grady CL, et al. Computed tomographic analysis of brain morphometrics in 30 healthy men, aged 21 to 81 years. *Ann Neurol* 1985;**17**(2):146–57.

51. Xu Y, Jack CR, Jr., O'Brien PC, *et al*. Usefulness of MRI measures of entorhinal cortex versus hippocampus in AD. *Neurology* 2000;**54**(9):1760–7.

52. Sullivan EV, Rosenbloom M, Serventi KL, Pfefferbaum A. Effects of age and sex on volumes of the thalamus, pons, and cortex. *Neurobiol Aging* 2004;**25**(2):185–92.

53. Van Der Werf YD, Tisserand DJ, Visser PJ, *et al*. Thalamic volume predicts performance on tests of cognitive speed and decreases in healthy aging. A magnetic resonance imaging-based volumetric analysis. *Brain Res Cogn Brain Res* 2001;**11**(3):377–85.

54. Resnick SM, Goldszal AF, Davatzikos C, *et al*. One-year age changes in MRI brain volumes in older adults. *Cereb Cortex* 2000;**10**(5):464–72.

55. Salat DH, Kaye JA, Janowsky JS. Prefrontal gray and white matter volumes in healthy aging and Alzheimer disease. *Arch Neurol* 1999;**56**(3):338–44.

56. Raz N, Lindenberger U, Rodrigue KM, *et al*. Regional brain changes in aging healthy adults: general trends, individual differences and modifiers. *Cereb Cortex* 2005.

57. Golomb J, de Leon MJ, Kluger A, George AE, Tarshish C, Ferris SH. Hippocampal atrophy in normal aging. An association with recent memory impairment. *Arch Neurol* 1993;**50**(9):967–73.

58. Golomb J, Kluger A, de Leon MJ, *et al*. Hippocampal formation size in normal human aging: a correlate of delayed secondary memory performance. *Learn Mem* 1994;**1**(1):45–54.

59. Rosen AC, Prull MW, Gabrieli JD, *et al*. Differential associations between entorhinal and hippocampal volumes and memory performance in older adults. *Behav Neurosci* 2003;**117**(6):1150–60.

60. Lupien SJ, de Leon M, de Santi S, *et al*. Cortisol levels during human aging predict hippocampal atrophy and memory deficits. *Nat Neurosci* 1998;**1**(1):69–73.

61. Golomb J, Kluger A, de Leon MJ, *et al*. Hippocampal formation size predicts declining memory performance in normal aging. *Neurology* 1996;**47**(3):810–3.

62. Strong R. Neurochemical changes in the aging human brain: implications for behavioral impairment and neurodegenerative disease. *Geriatrics* 1998;**53 Suppl 1**:S9–12.

63. Volkow ND, Logan J, Fowler JS, *et al*. Association between age-related decline in brain dopamine activity and impairment in frontal and cingulate metabolism. *Am J Psychiatry* 2000;**157**(1):75–80.

64. Backman L, Farde L. The role of dopamine systems in cognitive aging. In: Cabeza R, Nyberg L, Park DC, eds. *Cognitive Neuroscience of Aging*. New York: Oxford University Press, 2005: p. 58–84.

65. Owen AM, James M, Leigh PN, *et al*. Fronto-striatal cognitive deficits at different stages of Parkinson's disease. *Brain* 1992;**115 (Pt 6)**:1727–51.

66. Backman L, Ginovart N, Dixon RA, *et al*. Age-related cognitive deficits mMediated by changes in the striatal dopamine system. *Am J Psychiatry* 2000;**157**(4):635–7.

67. Volkow ND, Gur RC, Wang GJ, *et al*. Association between decline in brain dopamine activity with age and cognitive and motor impairment in healthy individuals. *Am J Psychiatry* 1998;**155**(3):344–9.

68. Erixon–Lindroth N, Farde L, Wahlin TB, Sovago J, Halldin C, Backman L. The role of the striatal dopamine transporter in cognitive aging. *Psychiatry Res* 2005;**138**(1):1–12.

69. Cabeza R, Anderson ND, Locantore JK, McIntosh AR. Aging gracefully: compensatory brain activity in high-performing older adults. *Neuroimage* 2002;**17**(3):1394–402.

70. Cabeza R. Hemispheric asymmetry reduction in older adults: the HAROLD model. *Psychol Aging* 2002;**17**(1):85–100.

71. Reuter–Lorenz P, Jonides J, Smith ES, *et al*. Age differences in the frontal lateralization of verbal and spatial working memory revealed by PET. *J Cogn Neurosci* 2000;**12**:174–87.

72. Rypma B, D'Esposito M. Isolating the neural mechanisms of age-related changes in human working memory. *Nat Neurosci* 2000;**3**(5):509–15.

73. Grossman M, Cooke A, DeVita C, *et al*. Age-related changes in working memory during sentence comprehension: an FMRI study. *Neuroimage* 2002;**15**(2):302–17.

74. Rypma B, Prabhakaran V, Desmond JD, Gabrieli JDE. Age differences in prefrontal cortical activity in working memory. *Psychology and Aging* 2001;**16**:371–84.

75. Reuter–Lorenz P, Marshuetz C, Jonides J, Smith ES, Hartley A, Koeppe RA. Neurocognitive ageing of storage and executive processes. *European Journal of Cognitive Psychology* 2001;**13**:257–78.

76. Park DC, Welsh RC, Marshuetz C, *et al*. Working memory for complex scenes: age differences in fFrontal and hippocampal activations. *J Cogn Neurosci*. 2003;**15**(8):1122–34.

77. Cabeza R, Daselaar SM, Dolcos F, Prince SE, Budde M, Nyberg L. Task-independent and task-specific age effects on brain activity during working memory, visual attention and episodic retrieval. *Cereb Cortex* 2004;**14**(4):364–75.

78. Cabeza R, Grady CL, Nyberg L, et al. Age-related differences in neural activity during memory encoding and retrieval: A positron emission tomography study. *J Neurosci* 1997;**17**:391–400.

79. Anderson ND, Iidaka T, McIntosh AR, Kapur S, Cabeza R, Craik FIM. The effects of divided attention on encoding- and retrieval related brain activity: A PET study of yournger and older adults. *J Cogn Neurosci* 2000;**12**:775–92.

80. Stebbins GT, Carrillo MC, Dorman J, *et al*. Aging effects on memory encoding in the frontal lobes. *Psychology and Aging* 2002;**17**:44–55.

81. Rosen AC, Prull MW, O'Hara R, *et al*. Variable effects of aging on frontal lobe contributions to memory. *Neuroreport* 2002;**13**:2425–8.

82. Daselaar SM, Veltman DJ, Rombouts SA, Raaijmakers JG, Jonker C. Neuroanatomical correlates of episodic encoding and retrieval in young and elderly subjects. *Brain* 2003;**126**(Pt 1):43–56.

83. Morcom AM, Good CD, Frackowiak RSJ, Rugg MD. Age effects on the neural correlates of successful memory encoding. *Brain* 2003;**126**(1):213–29.

84. Gutchess AH, Welsh RC, Hedden T, *et al.* Aging and the neural correlates of successful picture encoding: frontal activations compensate for decreased medial-temporal activity. *J Cogn Neurosci* 2005;**17**(1):84–96.

85. Grady CL, McIntosh AR, Raja MN, Beig S, Craik FIM. The effects of age on the neural correlates of episodic encoding. *Cerebral Cortex* 1999;**9**:805–814.

86. Grady CL, Bernstein LJ, Beig S, Siegenthaler AL. The effects of encoding strategy on age-related changes in the functional neuroanatomy of face memory. *Psychology and Aging* 2002;**17**:7–23.

87. Grady CL, McIntosh AR, Horwitz B, et al. Age-related reductions in human recognition memory due to impaired encoding. *Science* 1995;**269**(5221):218–21.

88. Logan JM, Sanders AL, Snyder AZ, Morris JC, Buckner RL. Under-recruitment and nonselective recruitment: Dissociable neural mechanisms associated with aging. *Neuron* 2002;**33**:827–840.

89. Spencer WD, Raz N. Differential effects of aging on memory for content and context: a meta-analysis. *Psychology and Aging* 1995;**10**(4):527–39.

90. Madden DJ, Turkington TG, Provenzale JM, *et al.* Adult age differences in functional neuroanatomy of verbal recognition memory. *Human Brain Mapping* 1999;**7**:115–35.

91. Cabeza R, Grady C, *et al.* Age-related differences in neural activity during memory encoding and retrieval: A positron emission tomography study. *J Neurosci* 1997;**17**(1):391–400.

92. Schacter DL, Savage CR, Alpert NM, Rauch SL, Albert MS. The role of hippocampus and frontal cortex in age-related memory changes: A PET study. *Neuroreport* 1996;**7**:1165–9.

93. Backman L, Almkvist O, Andersson J, Nordberg A. Brain activation in young and older adults during implicit and explicit retrieval. *J Cogn Neurosci* 1997;**9**(3):378–91.

94. Cabeza R, Anderson ND, Houle S, Mangels JA, Nyberg L. Age-related differences in neural activity during item and temporal-order memory retrieval: a positron emission tomography study. *J Cogn Neurosci* 2000;**12**:1–10.

95. Mitchell KJ, Johnson MK, Raye CL, D'Esposito M. FMRI evidence of age-related hippocampal dysfunction in feature binding in working memory. *Brain Res Cogn Brain Res* 2000;**10**(1–2):197–206.

96. Grady CL, McIntosh AR, Bookstein F, Horwitz B, Rapoport SI, Haxby JV. Age-related changes in regional cerebral blood flow during working memory for faces. *Neuroimage* 1998;**8**(4):409–25.

97. Daselaar SM, Veltman DJ, Rombouts SA, Raaijmakers JG, Jonker C. Deep processing activates the medial temporal lobe in young but not in old adults. *Neurobiol Aging* 2003;**24**(7):1005–11.

98. Yonelinas AP. The nature of recollection and familiarity: a review of 30 years of research. *Memory and Language* 2002;**46**:441–517.

99. ggleton JP, Brown MW. Episodic memory, amnesia, and the hippocampal-anterior thalamic axis. *Behavioral and Brain Sciences* 1999;**22**:425–89.

100. Jennings JM, Jacoby LL. Automatic versus intentional uses of memory: aging, attention, and control. *Psychology and Aging* 1993;**8**(2):283–93.

101. Daselaar SM, Fleck MS, Dobbins IG, Madden DJ, Cabeza R. Effects of healthy aging on hippocampal and rhinal memory functions. *Cerebral cortex* 2006; **16**(12):1771–1782.

102. Yonelinas AP. The nature of recollection and familiarity: a review of 30 years of research. *Journal of Memory and Language* 2002;**46**(3):441–517.

103. Yonelinas AP. Components of episodic memory: the contribution of recollection and familiarity. *Philos Trans R Soc Lond B Biol Sci* 2001;**356**(1413):1363–74.

104. Maguire EA, Frith CD. Aging affects the engagement of the hippocampus during autobiographical memory retrieval. *Brain* 2003;**126**(7):1511–23.

105. Reuter–Lorenz PA, Marshuetz C, Jonides J, Smith EE, Hartley A, Koeppe R. Neurocognitive ageing of storage and executive processes. *European Journal of Cognitive Psychology* 2001;**13**(1–2):257–78.

106. Schiavetto A, Kohler S, Grady CL, Winocur G, Moscovitch M. Neural correlates of memory for object identity and object location: effects of aging. *Neuropsychologia* 2002;**40**(8):1428–42.

107. Maguire EA, Frith CD. Aging affects the engagement of the hippocampus during autobiographical memory retrieval. *Brain* 2003;**126**(Pt 7):1511–23.

108. Eichenbaum H, Otto T, Cohen NJ. Two functional components of the hippocampal memory system. *Behavioral and Brain Sciences* 1994;**17**(3):449–72.

109. Braak H, Braak E, Bohl J. Staging of Alzheimer-related cortical destruction. *Eur Neurol* 1993;**33**(6):403–8.

110. Kemper TL. Neuroanatomical and neuropathological changes during aging and in dementia. In: Knoepfel M, ed. *Clinical Neurology of Aging*. 2nd edn. New York: Oxford University Press, 1994: p. 3–67.

111. Grady CL. Functional connectivity during memory tasks in healthy aging and dementia. In: Cabeza R, Nyberg L, Park D, ed. *Cognitive Neuroscience of Aging*. New York: Oxford University Press, 2005: p. 286–308.

112. Scheltens P, Fox N, Barkhof F, De Carli C. Structural magnetic resonance imaging in the practical assessment of dementia: beyond exclusion. *Lancet Neurol* 2002;**1**(1):13–21.

113. Jack CR, Jr., Petersen RC, O'Brien PC, Tangalos EG. MR-based hippocampal volumetry in the diagnosis of Alzheimer's disease. *Neurology* 1992;**42**(1):183–8.

114. Laakso MP, Lehtovirta M, Partanen K, Riekkinen PJ, Soininen H. Hippocampus in Alzheimer's disease: a 3-year follow-up MRI study. *Biol Psychiatry* 2000;**47**(6):557–61.

115. Small SA, Tsai WY, DeLaPaz R, Mayeux R, Stern Y. Imaging hippocampal function across the human life span: is memory decline normal or not? *Ann Neurol* 2002;**51**(3):290–5.

116. Du AT, Schuff N, Amend D, *et al.* Magnetic resonance imaging of the entorhinal cortex and hippocampus in mild cognitive impairment and Alzheimer's disease. *J Neurol Neurosurg Psychiatry* 2001;**71**(4):441–7.

117. deToledo–Morrell L, Stoub TR, Bulgakova M, *et al.* MRI-derived entorhinal volume is a good predictor of conversion from MCI to AD. *Neurobiol Aging* 2004;**25**(9):1197–203.

118. Dickerson BC, Goncharova I, Sullivan MP, *et al.* MRI-derived entorhinal and hippocampal atrophy in incipient and very mild Alzheimer's disease. *Neurobiol Aging* 2001;**22**(5):747–54.

119. Pennanen C, Kivipelto M, Tuomainen S, *et al.* Hippocampus and entorhinal cortex in mild cognitive impairment and early AD. *Neurobiology of Aging* 2004;**25**(3):303–10.

120. DiGirolamo GJ, Kramer AF, Barad V, *et al.* General and task specific frontal lobe recruitment in older adults during executive processes: a FMRI investigation of task-switching. *Neuro Report.* 2001;**12**(9):2065–71.

121. Lustig C, Snyder AZ, Bhakta M, *et al.* Functional deactivations: change with age and dementia of the Alzheimer type. *Proc Natl Acad Sci U S A* 2003;**100**(24):14504–9.

122. Shulman GL, Corbetta M, Buckner RL, *et al.* Common blood flow changes across visual tasks.1. Increases in subcortical structures and cerebellum but not in nonvisual cortex. *J Cogn Neurosci* 1997;**9**(5):624–47.

123. McKiernan KA, Kaufman JN, Kucera–Thompson J, Binder JR. A parametric manipulation of factors affecting task-induced deactivation in functional neuroimaging. *J Cogn Neurosci* 2003;**15**(3):394–408.

124. Daselaar SM, Prince SE, Cabeza R. When less means more: deactivations during encoding that predict subsequent memory. *Neuroimage* 2004;**23**(3):921–7.

125. Friston KJ, Price CJ, Fletcher P, Moore C, Frackowiak RS, Dolan RJ. The trouble with cognitive subtraction. *Neuroimage* 1996;**4**:97–104.

126. Jennings JM, McIntosh AR, Kapur S, Tulving E, Houle S. Cognitive subtractions may not add up: the interaction between semantic processing and response mode. *Neuroimage* 1997;**5**(3):229–39.

127. Skoog I. Status of risk factors for vascular dementia. *Neuroepidemiology* 1998;**17**:2–9.

128. Jennings JR, Muldoon MF, Ryan CM, *et al.* Cerebral blood flow in hypertensive patients: An initial report of reduced and compensatory blood flow responses during performance of two cognitive tasks. *Hypertension* 1998;**31**:1216–22.

129. Glisky EL, Polster MR, Routhieaux BC. Double dissociation between item and source memory. *Neuropsychology* 1995;**9**:229–35.

130. Glisky EL, Rubin SR, Davidson PSR. Source memory in oder adults: an encoding or retrieval problem? *Journal of Experimental Psychology: Learning, Memory, and Cognition* 2001;**27**:1131–46.

131. Prince SE, Daselaar SM, Cabeza R. Neural correlates of relational memory: successful encoding and retrieval of semantic and perceptual associations. *J Neurosci* 2005; **25**(5):1203–1210.

132. Price CJ, Friston KJ. Scanning patients with tasks they can perform. *Human Brain Mapping* 1999;**8**(2–3):102–8.

133. Karni A, Meyer G, Jezzard P, Adams MM, *et al.* Functional MRI evidence for adult motor cortex plasticity during motor skill learning. *Nature* 1995;**377**(6545):155–8.

134. Raichle ME, Fiez JA, Videen TO, *et al.* Practice-related changes in human brain functional anatomy during nonmotor learning. *Cerebral Cortex* 1994;**4**(1):8–26.

5

Dementia: mild cognitive impairment and Alzheimer's disease

Bradford C. Dickerson and Reisa A. Sperling

1. Introduction

Alzheimer's disease (AD) is the most common cause of dementia[1]. In most individuals, the symptoms of the disease begin with mild memory difficulties after the sixth decade of life. Symptoms progress slowly, leading to significant impairment in memory, language, executive function, and other domains of cognition. Eventually, impaired cognitive abilities interfere with complex activities of daily life and ultimately result in the loss of independent function. The diagnosis is typically made in this context on the basis of clinical evidence of dementia with progressive impairment in multiple domains of cognition. Structural neuroimaging is often used in the clinical setting to evaluate for the presence of other pathologies (e.g. cerebrovascular or neoplastic disease). Functional neuroimaging, such as PET or SPECT, may be employed clinically to assist in the discrimination of different types of dementia (e.g. frontotemporal vs. Alzheimer's dementia). Current treatments are primarily symptomatic, in that clinical trials demonstrate short-term stabilization of cognitive function but not a slowing of the rate of decline[2]. Increasing emphasis is being placed on the development of disease modifying therapies — drugs that impede the underlying pathophysiologic process of neurodegeneration in AD and, thereby, slow the rate of cognitive decline.

By the time AD is typically diagnosed, substantial neuronal loss and neuropathologic change have damaged many brain regions. Although it may be possible to reverse some aspects of this damage, it would be ideal to initiate treatment with neuroprotective medications at a time when, or even before, AD is mildly symptomatic[3]. To approach this goal, our capability needs to be improved to identify individuals with prodromal AD — the earliest symptomatic phase of AD prior to dementia. Currently, individuals are categorized as having mild cognitive impairment (MCI) when symptoms suggestive of AD are present but mild enough that traditional diagnostic criteria (which require functional impairment consistent with dementia) are not fulfilled. This gradual transitional state may last for a number of years and diagnostic criteria have been developed[4] and operationalized[5]. Presymptomatic AD is the phase of the disease when pathologic alterations are developing but cognitive impairment is not yet apparent. This is likely best studied through the identification of cohorts with particular risk factors, such as genetic determinants (e.g. Down's syndrome or mutations in amyloid precursor protein (APP) or presenilin) or susceptibility factors (e.g. apolipoprotein E (*ApoE*) ε4).

Since AD involves the progressive neurodegeneration of particular brain regions, repeatable *in vivo* neuroimaging measures of brain anatomy, chemistry, physiology, and pathology hold promise as methods to provide novel insights into the fundamental pathophysiologic processs of the disease. In the clinic, imaging tools may provide markers to assist in early detection and differential diagnosis or to indicate the slowing of disease progression by therapeutic agents. One promising technique for both purposes is FMRI, which is thought to provide an *in vivo* correlate of neural activity. Given the growing body of evidence that alterations in synaptic function are present very early in the disease process, possibly long before the development of clinical symptoms and even significant neuropathology[6,7], FMRI may be particularly useful in detecting alterations in brain function that may be present very early in the course of AD. In this chapter, we will review the use of FMRI in MCI and AD, but will first briefly discuss other imaging modalities.

2. Imaging of brain anatomy, chemistry, and pathology in AD

2.1 Structural MRI

As expected from its role in memory function, the medial temporal lobe is the brain region most prominently affected early in AD. Many MCI patients have early-stage AD neuropathology in the medial temporal lobe[8]. The disease then spreads throughout limbic and paralimbic regions, affecting adjacent trans-entorhinal and inferior temporal neocortical regions, as well as the HF and the basal forebrain. Finally, neuronal loss and plaques and tangles can be found throughout neocortical association areas in frontal, parietal, and occipital lobes, and likely relate to the appearance of disturbances in other higher cortical functions.

Neuroimaging techniques that provide measures of brain structure can be useful in identifying individuals with structural alterations consistent with AD[9] and in following the degenerative changes in those regions over time. In the past 15 years, the quantitative measurement of brain-region volumes from MRI based on manual delineation by trained operators has consistently demonstrated atrophy of hippocampal, entorhinal, and other brain regions in patients with a clinical diagnosis of AD[10,11]. Similar, though milder findings, are present in MCI (see Fig. 5.1). Hippocampal volume derived from MRI correlates strongly with histological HF volume and neuronal loss[12] and severity of AD pathology[13,14], as well as with memory impairment in AD patients[15,16]. The rate of hippocampal atrophy measured from serial MRI scans relates to progression of clinical impairment in AD[17,18].

Longitudinal follow-up of MCI patients has revealed that diminished baseline hippocampal and/or entorhinal volume is associated with an increased likelihood of progressing to clinical dementia. The ability of volumetric MRI markers to predict AD in MCI improves with the addition of measurements of neocortical regions, such as the superior or middle-inferior temporal gyrus or portions of the cingulate gyrus[10].

Depending on the question of interest, one or more of a variety of methodologic approaches can be used to quantitatively measure aspects of brain structure, including

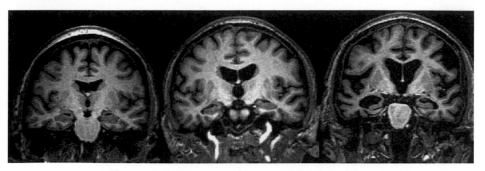

Fig. 5.1 Coronal MRI sections from individual subjects (control, MCI, and AD – left to right respectively), illustrating mild degree of atrophy in MCI and greater atrophy in mild AD compared to age-matched control. (Reproduced with permission from Elsevier Publishers[88].)

volumes of regions of interest, tissue density, surface area, or topology. Many of these increasingly sophisticated methods provide information on differences in global or large-scale brain structure between groups of individuals or within individuals over time. These approaches include voxel-based morphometry, cortical pattern matching, hippocampal surface shape analysis, and the brain boundary shift integral (BBSI) approach[19]. While the BBSI and other heavily automated methods reduce the potential confounds that may occur when individual human operators manually delineate specific neuroanatomic structures, it is likely that some effects may be best detected by careful measurements of specific ROIs. Computational methods are advancing rapidly to enable ROI-based approaches to be performed with increasing efficiency and sophistication, including semi automated hippocampal volumetry[20], hippocampal boundary shift integral[21], and atlas-based algorithms to segment the entire brain into subcortical and cortical regions of interest[22,23].

2.2 **MR spectroscopy**

Measures of regional brain volume do not provide information about tissue composition. For example, if neuronal loss is accompanied by glial proliferation, to which T1-weighted MRI sequences are not sensitive, routine volumetric methods may not detect this aspect of pathologic change[24]. Proton magnetic resonance spectroscopic imaging (MRS) is a technique that enables the quantitation of particular neurochemical constituents of brain tissue. Metabolic components that are commonly measured include N-acetyl aspartate (NAA) and myoinositol (mI), which are thought to represent the density of living neurons and glial cells, respectively, and choline (Cho), which is a marker of cell membrane turnover. In AD patients, decreases in NAA are found in MTL, posterior cingulate, and other regions typically affected by neurofibrillary pathology early in the disease[24–26]. Levels of mI tend to be increased in AD, and Cho may be increased or unchanged. In individuals with MCI, MRS measures are different from normal ageing[26] and relate to memory performance[27]; these cross-sectional studies suggest that mI may increase prior to decreases in NAA and Cho. The combination of volumetric and spectroscopic MR measures appears to provide better diagnostic sensitivity and specificity for AD (vs. controls) than either measure alone[28]. Longitudinal MRS studies have demonstrated that changes in NAA over time relate to changes in clinical measures in AD patients[29–31]. Longitudinal changes in MRS measures have also been evaluated in AD patients during therapeutic trials with cholinergic agents[18,32,33]. Changes in both NAA and Cho correlate with changes in cognitive function. These findings indicate that AD-related changes detected by MRS may be reversible, and may reflect aspects of neuronal integrity or function. Thus, spectroscopic measures in AD may provide a bridge between traditional measures of brain structure and function.

2.3 Molecular imaging of AD pathology

Extensive efforts to develop *in vivo* methods to more directly measure AD neuropathology have begun to bear fruit. Much of this work has been directed toward the development of radiotracers that can be safely administered to humans to label proteins associated with the classic neuropathologic findings in AD. The majority of these compounds are thought to label fibrillar beta amyloid, but some reports have described labelling of tau-based proteins as well. Tracers are in development that can be detected using PET, SPECT, and even MRI. The first reports of clinical applications of these tracers have only recently appeared in the literature[34,35].

The successful visualization of markers of neuropathology in living humans is a major advance in the field and suggests that more specific *in vivo* diagnostic and monitoring capabilities may be on the horizon. In addition, these approaches may be very useful in the burgeoning efforts to improve translational research between animal models and humans. However, a number of issues will need to be addressed as part of the validation of these methods as biomarkers of AD. While visualization of a 'signal of pathology' has been demonstrated, work is still in progress to refine quantitative metrics and determine the specificity of these measures. And it has been difficult to identify clear relationships between neuropathologic (particularly amyloid burden) and clinical measures. This will likely complicate efforts to determine diagnostic sensitivity and specificity, as well as rates of change over time. Finally, it is not yet clear how early in prodromal or presymptomatic AD these pathologic imaging signals will be detectable.

3. Functional brain imaging in AD

Techniques to measure aspects of brain function *in vivo* have provided revolutionary insights into human cerebral activity at rest, during task performance, and in individuals with specific characteristics, such as the presence of clinical disease. Since functional neuroimaging tools assess inherently dynamic processes that may change over short time intervals in relation to a host of factors, these measures have unique characteristics that may offer both strengths and weaknesses as potential biomarkers for neurodegenerative disease. Functional neuroimaging measures may be affected by transient brain and body states at the time of imaging, such as arousal, attention, sleep deprivation, sensory processing of irrelevant stimuli, or the effects of substances with pharmacologic central nervous system activity. Imaging measures of brain function may also be more sensitive than structural measures to constitutional or chronic differences between individuals, such as genetics, intelligence or educational level, learning, mood, or medication use. While these may be effects of interest in certain experimental settings, they need to be controlled when the focus is on differences in disease-related changes between subject groups or within individuals over time. Functional neuroimaging data can be categorized as measures obtained 'at rest' or during task performance.

3.1 Resting blood flow and metabolism: FDG-PET and SPECT

Tomographic nuclear medicine techniques use radiolabelled compounds to detect signals related to functional properties of the brain. The two major techniques that have been applied to AD are positron emission tomography (PET) and single photon emission computed tomography (SPECT). Using PET, the regional cerebral metabolic rate of glucose can be measured (with fluorodeoxyglucose or FDG). With SPECT, regional cerebral blood flow rates (perfusion) can be measured. For over 20 years, these techniques have been applied to the study of dementia, and one of the most consistent findings in AD is a reduction, at rest, of metabolism and perfusion in posterior temporo-parietal, posterior cingulate, and frontal regions, with sparing of primary somatomotor cortices (Fig. 5.2). Animal model studies have also suggested that posterior cingulate hypometabolism may be an early feature of the disease[36] and have demonstrated that it occurs after entorhinal lesions, possibly as a result of disconnection[37].

This 'functional signature' of AD has been studied extensively as a potential marker to differentiate AD from normal ageing and other neurodegenerative diseases, and can do so in the proper clinical context with relatively high sensitivity and specificity when compared with clinical diagnoses[38]. PET or SPECT studies of AD patients followed to autopsy have demonstrated that the *in vivo* resting functional findings have relatively high sensitivity to detect *post-mortem* AD neuropathology but somewhat lower specificity[39–41]. Longitudinal studies have shown that baseline PET and SPECT measures are useful for the prediction of future cognitive decline in AD patients[42] and the early detection of disease in individuals with MCI[43]. Serial functional imaging studies have demonstrated that progressive metabolic decline correlates with cognitive decline in AD patients[44].

Tantalizing results are emerging from longitudinal studies with serial FDG-PET measures in subjects at elevated risk for clinical AD but in whom symptoms are very mild or absent. Progressive metabolic abnormalities parallel cognitive changes in both older, cognitively intact individuals[45] and subjects with mild memory impairment who carry the *ApoE* ε4 allele[46]. In individuals in their fifties, without cognitive decline, progressive metabolic alterations have been observed in ε4 carriers after two years[47].

Finally, PET and SPECT measures of resting brain function appear to be sensitive to medication effects in clinical drug trials. In AD patients given cholinesterase inhibitors, these functional brain measures relate to clinical measures in demonstrating stability or improvement in treated vs. placebo groups or in predicting response in treated patients[48,49].

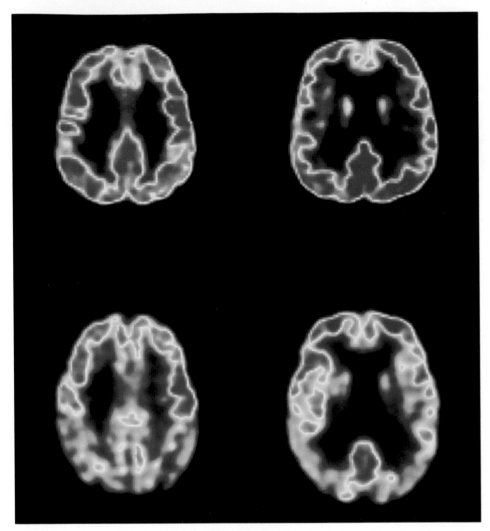

Fig. 5.2 FDG-PET data from an older control subject (top) and a patient with probable Alzheimer's disease (bottom), illustrating prominent temporoparietal hypometabolism. (Reproduced with permission from Elsevier Publishers[88].)

3.2 Task-related changes in functional imaging

A variety of functional neuroimaging techniques can be used to measure signals related to regional brain activity during the performance of cognitive tasks, including FDG PET, oxygen-15 PET, and FMRI, the focus of this chapter.

3.2.1 FMRI studies of patients with clinical AD

FMRI has been used to investigate patterns of activation during a variety of cognitive tasks in patients diagnosed with mild AD compared to older control subjects. In addition to memory, which will be discussed in detail below, aspects of language and attention have been studied. Altered patterns of frontal and temporal activation have been observed in AD patients making judgements about verbs[50]. During performance of a semantic decision-making task, AD patients with a smaller inferior frontal volume activated a relatively larger extent of this region[51]. When performing a semantic processing task (category-exemplar), AD patients activated similar frontal regions compared with controls but recruited a greater extent of these regions, as well as additional regions[52]. Similarly, although temporo-parietal activation was diminished in AD during performance of a semantic memory task, increased activation in temporal and frontal regions was also observed, suggesting possible compensatory processes[53]. During performance of a visual attention task, AD patients showed alterations in parietal activation; increased prefrontal activation was also observed compared with controls, again suggesting possible compensatory mechanisms[54].

Recent FMRI studies are beginning to reveal a link between haemodynamic changes and the well-described resting perfusion/metabolic abnormalities in AD. As discussed above, hypoperfusion/metabolism is typically seen in temporo-parietal/posterior cingulate cortical regions in AD patients during the 'resting' state. The medial parietal/posterior cingulate cortex, along with medial frontal and lateral parietal regions, appear to compose a 'default mode' network that is more active when individuals are not engaged in particular tasks, and which is thought to play a role in vigilance, readiness, or monitoring; these regions 'deactivate' (BOLD signal amplitude falls below baseline) during cognitive task performance[55]. FMRI studies of AD patients have demonstrated alterations in the deactivation and functional connectivity of these regions, suggesting that this 'default mode' network is disrupted by the disease as well[56–58].

With respect to memory, a number of FMRI studies in patients with clinically diagnosed AD, using a variety of visual stimuli, have identified decreased activation in hippocampal and parahippocampal regions compared to older control subjects during episodic encoding tasks[59–63]. Neocortical abnormalities in AD have also been demonstrated using FMRI, including decreased activation in temporal and prefrontal regions[61]. In addition to AD-related differences in task-related BOLD signal amplitude or spatial extent, the temporal dynamics of activation appear to be altered in patients with AD (see below for details)[64]. Interestingly, as has been observed in other types of tasks (mentioned above), *increased* activation in prefrontal and other regions has also been found in AD patients performing memory tasks[62,65]. Importantly, behavioural evidence that the functional alterations may serve a compensatory role was described by Grady *et al.*[65], who demonstrated that increased prefrontal recruitment in AD patients was correlated with better episodic and semantic memory performance.

Our own FMRI studies in AD have focussed on associative memory tasks — in particular, face–name association. Learning the names of new individuals we encounter can be thought of as a particularly difficult cross-modal, non-contextual, paired associate memory task. The hippocampal formation is thought to be critical in this process, acting to 'bind' together items of information into a cohesive memory[54,17] and, as above, is known to be selectively vulnerable to the early pathologic changes of AD[4].

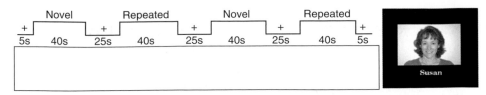

Fig. 5.3 Block design face–name associative encoding paradigm timing shown with example of face–name pair stimulus.

This aspect of cognition has been investigated using an FMRI face–name associative memory paradigm (Fig. 5.3). This 'block design paradigm' is designed to focus on the encoding of unfamiliar face–name pairs using three conditions grouped in blocks: 'novel' face–name pairs, seen only once during the scanning procedure; 'repeated' face–name pairs, shown to subjects prior to the scanning procedure and then shown repeatedly during specific blocks; and 'fixation' on a crosshair as a rest condition. The primary comparison of interest is the novel vs. repeated contrast, which holds the visual complexity of the stimuli constant and provides information about new associative learning (i.e. the encoding of novel face–name associations compared with viewing familiar face–name pairs). Subjects are instructed explicitly to try to remember the name associated with each face for later testing. All of the scanning is performed during the encoding phase and subjects are tested with a post-scan associative recognition test.

In young subjects, the encoding of novel face–name pairs reliably activates a set of brain regions, including the hippocampal formation, and fusiform and prefrontal cortices[66.] In a study of this paradigm in ageing and AD, whole-brain voxel-based methods were used to compare activation patterns in young controls (n=10), normal older controls (n=10), and patients with mild AD (n=7, mean MMSE=22.6)[62]. Young and older controls showed a similar pattern of activation to mild AD in the fusiform cortex, consistent with the relative lack of early AD pathology in these regions, and demonstrating that there is not a global decoupling of neuronal activation and haemodynamic response in normal ageing and AD subjects (Fig. 5.4a). Both young and older controls showed significant activation in the hippocampus, although the older subjects showed activation that was more limited in extent (Fig. 5.4b). The mild AD patients did not show evidence of activation within the hippocampal formation, even when the MR signal was sampled within an ROI guided by each individual subject's anatomy.

Based on a random-effects analysis, the mild AD subjects showed significantly decreased bilateral activation in the hippocampal formation compared to normal older controls. Several neocortical regions, including the precuneus, posterior cingulate, and superior frontal cortices, showed increased activation in the mild AD patients compared to older controls. These findings are consistent with other recent reports demonstrating decreased MTL activation in patients with clinical AD and suggest that additional regions, not typically activated in the task in young and older controls, may be recruited in an attempt to compensate for loss of hippocampal integrity in clinical AD.

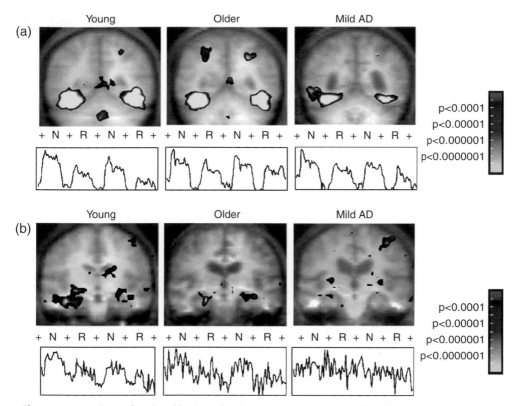

Fig. 5.4 Comparison of regional brain activation pattern as measured by BOLD FMRI during face–name pair encoding in young subjects, older control subjects, and mild AD patients, demonstrating similar pattern and degree of task-related activation in ventral temporal lobe regions (**a**) but loss of task-related pattern in medial temporal lobe regions in mild AD (**b**).

3.2.2 FMRI studies of MCI subjects

Very few FMRI studies have been published in subjects with MCI and the results, thus far, have been inconsistent. In comparison to older controls, Machulda *et al.* reported that MTL activation was decreased to a similar degree in patients with MCI and AD patients[63]. However, Small *et al.* reported heterogeneity in MTL activation in memory-impaired subjects, with some showing hypoactivation similar to that of AD patients. Other subjects showed entorhinal and hippocampal activation that was similar to controls but had decreased activation in the subiculum[59]. Recently, Johnson *et al.* used a paradigm involving the repetitive presentation of unfamiliar faces to demonstrate that MCI patients do not show the same slope of decreasing hippocampal activation with face repetition that is seen in older controls, suggesting disruption of this 'adaptive' response in the medial temporal lobe (Fig. 5.5)[67].

Focusing on separate temporal components of the BOLD signal during a face-encoding task, Rombouts *et al.*[64] found that MCI patients showed diminished early-phase activation

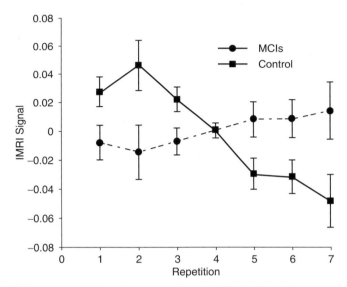

Fig. 5.5 Impaired hippocampal adaptation to repetitive stimuli in MCI. During repeated presentation of face stimuli, control subjects demonstrate a gradual decline in BOLD signal within the MTL. This 'adaptation response' is not seen in MCI patients. (Reproduced with permission from Elsevier Publishers[67].)

in occipital regions compared to older control subjects. AD patients demonstrated diminishment in this early temporal component in widespread regions compared to controls, and further diminishment in the occipital temporal component compared to MCI patients (Fig. 5.6). The three groups did not differ significantly in later phase responses, nor in mean BOLD signal when the data were modelled as a single haemodyamic response function as is often done in FMRI data analysis. These findings support the notion that FMRI is sensitive to a number of contributors to the spatiotemporal dynamics of task-related brain activity and to dynamic alterations in MCI and AD.

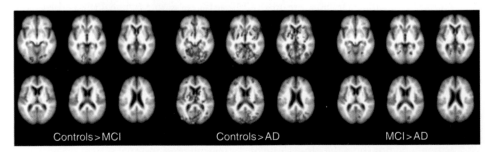

Fig. 5.6 Differences in an early temporal component of the BOLD signal during face-encoding task in older controls, MCI, and AD. Compared to controls, early BOLD response is diminished in MCI patients, specifically in the occipital lobe (left figure), but seen in widespread regions in AD patients (middle figure). Early occipital BOLD response is diminished further in AD compared to MCI (right figure). (Figure courtesy of S.A.R.B. Rombouts.)

group reported increased parietal activation in women with an *ApoE* ε4 allele[78]. Bookheimer *et al.* reported increased activation in left hippocampal, parietal, and prefrontal regions among *ApoE* ε4 carriers, compared to non-carriers, using a word–pair associative memory paradigm[79]. In addition, an increased number of activated regions in the left hemisphere at baseline was associated with a decline in memory at the two-year follow-up among the *ApoE* ε4 carriers. The authors hypothesized that this increase in activation in the *ApoE* ε4 carriers might represent the additional cognitive effort or neuronal recruitment required to adequately perform the task. Similarly increased activation in multiple brain regions was recently reported in cognitively intact older *ApoE* ε4 carriers compared to ε3 carriers, although the effect was lateralized to the right medial temporal lobe region (left hippocampal activation was greater in ε3 carriers)[80].

Our group recently identified a similar finding in the 29 older participants in the face–name associative FMRI paradigm described above. Among the entire cohort of controls, MCI subjects, and AD patients, the 13 *ApoE* ε4 carriers demonstrated greater entorhinal activation than non-carriers, in the absence of genotype-related differences in the volumes of these regions (Fig. 5.10)[69].

The data reviewed in this section indicate that FMRI can detect differences associated with genetic factors in physiologic patterns of regional brain activation during cognitive task performance in older individuals with and without cognitive impairment. These initial findings need to be investigated systematically to better elucidate their fundamental basis: for example, are genetic differences measured by FMRI related specifically to an

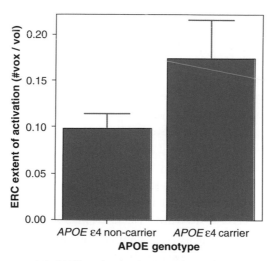

Fig. 5.10 Greater memory-related MTL activation in *ApoE* ε4 carriers. In a group of older controls, MCI subjects, and AD patients who performed a face–name associative memory task, mean spatial extent of entorhinal activation in *ApoE* ε4 carriers was greater than in ε3 carriers. Figure depicts number of voxels with task-related activation in 'novel' vs. 'repeated' contrast divided by total number of voxels in entorhinal ROI.

altered haemodynamic response or possibly to changes in resting perfusion? Are *ApoE*-related brain activation differences a lifelong characteristic of individuals with this genetic factor, or are they an indication of early AD-related neuropathology? Finally, how specific are these findings to the regional brain networks involved in the cognitive abilities investigated thus far? Answers to these questions will likely be obtained through further FMRI studies combined with other imaging modalities, and may offer novel insights into basic aspects of genetic influences on human brain function in ageing and neurodegenerative disease.

3.2.4 FMRI in differential diagnosis of dementia

The early detection and differential diagnosis of disorders causing cognitive impairment is a promising aim for further work using FMRI. Since clinical evaluation and neuropsychological testing are currently the most sensitive approaches to diagnosis, and FMRI is sensitive to both cognitive performance and clinical status, it seems reasonable to hope that the potential capability of FMRI to detect alterations in the pattern and degree of regional brain activation during task performance may provide additional useful data to accompany clinical and psychometric evaluations. However, relatively little FMRI data have been published on differential diagnosis to date.

In older individuals with cognitive symptoms, it can be difficult to distinguish a neurodegenerative process from depression — FMRI may be helpful in this setting. In a study of older individuals who had sought clinical evaluation for memory-related symptoms, Gron et al.[81] investigated the utility of FMRI to differentiate patterns of regional brain activation in those diagnosed with depression vs. AD (as well as a control group). Hippocampal activation during the memory task was decreased in AD patients compared with controls and depressed patients. In contrast, orbitofrontal and cingulate activation were greater in depressed patients than in AD subjects and controls.

Furthermore, different forms of neurodegenerative dementias may be challenging to diagnose, specifically early in their course. FMRI may provide helpful data to assist in differential diagnosis of the dementias. Rombouts et al.[82] compared regional brain activation during a working memory task in patients with fronto-temporal dementia (FTD) to that of AD patients. Although both groups activated similar fronto-parietal-thalamic regions, fronto-parietal activation was diminished in FTD patients than in AD patients.

Further insights into the utility of FMRI in assisting in differential diagnosis may potentially be gained through prospective studies of patients presenting for clinical evaluation with subtle symptoms consistent with dementia who do not yet have a clear clinical diagnosis. If such individuals are scanned using tasks they can still perform and then followed clinically, it may be possible to determine whether FMRI has predictive power in differential diagnosis.

3.2.5 FMRI and pharmacological studies

FMRI may be particularly valuable in evaluating acute and subacute effects of medications on neural activity. Alterations in memory-related activation related to the administration of pharmacological agents known to impair memory can be detected with FMRI[73,83].

The effects of cognitive-enhancing drugs on brain activation during cognitive task performance have shown that FMRI can detect changes after administration of cholinesterase inhibitors in patients with AD and MCI[84,85]. Rombouts et al.[84] found that, after receiving a single dose of galanthamine, AD patients demonstrated increased fusiform activity during a face-encoding task and increased prefrontal activity during a working memory task. Saykin et al.[85] reported that, compared to control group of healthy older individuals, MCI patients who received six weeks of donepezil showed increased prefrontal activation after this course of medication, which related to improvements in performance of a working memory task. In a recent study of galanthamine in patients with MCI, Goekoop et al.[86] found that, after patients received galanthamine for approximately one week, performance on a working memory task was improved in conjunction with increased activation in precuneus and middle frontal regions. In addition, increases in hippocampal, prefrontal, cingulate, and occipital regions were seen during an episodic encoding task, although performance did not improve on this memory task. Although these pilot studies did not include placebo-control groups to reduce potential confounding factors, such as learning effects, they indicate that FMRI is sensitive to both acute and subacute medication effects, some of which relate to behavioural change.

Although little data have been reported in MCI and AD, FMRI appears to be a promising method to investigate pharmacological effects on brain function. In particular, studies in patients with psychiatric illness suggest that FMRI may be helpful in better understanding pharmacogenetic effects that relate to response to therapy[87]. In neurodegenerative diseases, FMRI may provide an opportunity to investigate whether different drug-related changes in brain function relate to symptomatic versus disease-modifying clinical outcomes in clinical trials[88].

3.2.6 Advantages and disadvantages of FMRI in the study of cognitive impairment

FMRI has many potential advantages in studying patients with cognitive impairment, as it is a non-invasive imaging technique which does not require any injection of contrast. FMRI can be acquired on a standard clinical magnet during the same session as structural imaging. Because it is non-invasive, FMRI can be repeated many times over the course of a longitudinal study, and thus lends itself well as a measure in clinical drug trials. Perhaps the greatest potential advantage of FMRI is that we can image these patients while they are attempting to do the type of cognitive process that is causing them clinical difficulty.

There are, however, significant challenges to performing FMRI studies in cognitively impaired patients. It is likely that FMRI will not be ideal for examining patients with more severe dementia, as it is very sensitive to even small amounts of head motion. In terms of using FMRI in longitudinal or pharmacological studies, it is critical to complete further validation and reliability experiments. Although there are now a few studies of test-retest reliability in FMRI during cognitive tasks in young subjects[73,89,90], these reproducibility studies have yet to be performed in older subjects with cognitive impairment. Furthermore, additional studies are needed of the fundamental properties of the haemodynamic BOLD signal. This complex signal is generated by coupled neurovascular activity[91] and, as such, may be affected by not only altered neuronal responses but also changes in vascular reactivity. Alterations in BOLD signal-to-noise ratio and amplitude in primary sensorimotor cortices have been found in ageing and dementia[92,93], raising questions about how age- and disease-related changes in neurovascular coupling may confound group comparisons of task-related BOLD activation or deactivation.

A caveat essential to the interpretation of task-related functional neuroimaging data is that healthy individuals of any age demonstrate differences in brain activation depending on how well they are able to perform the particular task. For example, when cognitively intact individuals learn new information during FMRI scanning, the strength of this signal is related to subsequent ability to remember the information[94,95]. AD patients typically perform less well on the memory tasks, which complicates the interpretation of these data[96]. Yet MCI and AD patients may recruit additional brain tissue or regions than controls during task performance[68,97,98], as has been seen in patients with other neurological disorders[99]. The recruitment of additional brain regions during task performance by patients with neurodegenerative or other neurological disease may indicate the presence of processes attempting to compensate for damaged networks[65,68]. While the task performance factor is important to consider when designing or interpreting FMRI studies of MCI or AD, it also indicates that FMRI may be particularly sensitive to changes in cognitive function, which not only provides face validity for these measures but also supports their potential use in clinical trials of medications targeting cognition.

Since a definitive diagnosis of AD and related neurodegenerative diseases can only be made at autopsy, neuroimaging studies of these disorders face challenges related to clinicopathologic heterogeneity; this is particularly true for MCI. Although all patients with AD progress through some form of an MCI phase prior to dementia, the converse is not true. That is, some patients who fulfil MCI criteria may have non-AD disease states. Furthermore, the rate at which individuals with MCI decline within this diagnostic category and ultimately develop dementia may vary considerably. Thus, although prodromal AD may be clinically identifiable as MCI clinically[5], it is important to recognize the heterogeneity present within this clinical construct. Continued efforts to further refine clinical diagnostic[71] and staging methods[100] should help improve our understanding of the relationships between the characteristics of individuals with MCI and imaging data. Thus, while the data reviewed above indicating that FMRI is sensitive to clinical diagnosis[63,69,82] and symptom severity[68] in MCI and AD is encouraging, they also indicate that functional neuroimaging studies of these patient populations depend on rigorous clinical assessment and clear description of criteria and methodology.

4. **Conclusions**

As a variety of imaging measures of anatomy, chemistry, physiology, and pathology in AD become available, these tools may be employed in a targeted manner to advance our understanding of fundamental pathophysiological processes involved in the disease. It may also be possible to apply them to provide clinical biomarkers to improve early detection, differential diagnosis, tracking of progression, and monitoring of therapeutic response to medications. Substantial progress has already been made in validating a number of imaging biomarkers of AD against clinical and pathological data. Preliminary comparisons of imaging measures to standard cognitive or behavioural measures in clinical trials suggest that at least some types of imaging measures show changes that are expected in AD over time more consistently than behavioural measures[17].

FMRI is a particularly attractive method for studying cognitive, task-related patterns of brain activation in MCI and AD. Despite the relative infancy of the field, there have already been a number of promising FMRI studies in AD, MCI, and related disorders which highlight the potential uses of FMRI in both basic and clinical spheres of investigation. FMRI may provide novel insights into the neural correlates of memory and other cognitive abilities, and how they are altered in AD and MCI and by medications. This technique may help elucidate fundamental aspects of brain–behaviour relationships, such as the genetic influences on task-related brain physiology. Finally, FMRI measures hold promise for multiple clinical applications, including early detection and differential diagnosis, predicting future change in clinical status or cognitive performance, and as a marker of alterations in brain physiology related to potential therapeutic agents. The likely greatest potential of FMRI lies in the study of very early AD, at the point of subtle neuronal dysfunction. However, there is need for further validation studies and continued technical advances to fully realize the potential of this technology.

Acknowledgements

Supported by grants from the NIA (K23-AG22509), the NINDS (K23-NS02189), the Beeson Scholars in Aging Program (American Federation of Aging Research), and the Clinical Investigator Training Program (Harvard/MIT Health Sciences and Technology — Beth Israel Deaconess Medical Center, in collaboration with Pfizer Inc.).

References

1. Kukull, W.A., Bowen, J.D. Dementia epidemiology. *Med Clin North Am*, 2002. **86**(3): 573–90.

2. Cummings, J.L. Alzheimer's disease. *N Engl J Med*, 2004. **351**(1):56–67.

3. DeKosky, S.T., Marek, K. Looking backward to move forward: early detection of neurodegenerative disorders. *Science*, 2003. **302**(5646):830–4.

4. Petersen, R.C., *et al.* Mild cognitive impairment: clinical characterization and outcome. *Arch Neurol*, 1999. **56**(3):303–8.

5. Grundman, M., *et al.* Mild cognitive impairment can be distinguished from Alzheimer disease and normal aging for clinical trials. *Arch Neurol*, 2004. **61**(1):59–66.

6. Selkoe, D.J., *Alzheimer's disease is a synaptic failure.* Science, 2002. **298**(5594): p. 789–91.

7. Coleman, P., Federoff, H., Kurlan, R. A focus on the synapse for neuroprotection in Alzheimer disease and other dementias. *Neurology*, 2004. **63**(7):1155–62.

8. Gomez–Isla, T., *et al.* Profound loss of layer II entorhinal cortex neurons occurs in very mild Alzheimer's disease. *J Neurosci*, 1996. **16**(14):4491–500.

9. Scheltens, P., *et al.* Structural magnetic resonance imaging in the practical assessment of dementia: beyond exclusion. *Lancet Neurol*, 2002. **1**(1):13–21.

10. Killiany, R.J., *et al.* Use of structural magnetic resonance imaging to predict who will get Alzheimer's disease. *Ann Neurol*, 2000. **47**(4):430–9.

11. Dickerson, B.C., *et al.* MRI-derived entorhinal and hippocampal atrophy in incipient and very mild Alzheimer's disease. *Neurobiol Aging*, 2001. **22**(5):747–54.

12. Bobinski, M., *et al.* The histological validation of post mortem magnetic resonance imaging-determined hippocampal volume in Alzheimer's disease. *Neuroscience*, 2000. **95**(3):721–5.

13. Jack, C.R., Jr., *et al.* Antemortem MRI findings correlate with hippocampal neuropathology in typical aging and dementia. *Neurology*, 2002. **58**(5):750–7.

14. Gosche, K.M., *et al.* Hippocampal volume as an index of Alzheimer neuropathology: findings from the Nun Study. *Neurology*, 2002. **58**(10):1476–82.

15. De Leon, M.J., *et al.* Frequency of hippocampal formation atrophy in normal aging and Alzheimer's disease. *Neurobiol Aging*, 1997. **18**(1):1–11.

16. de Toledo–Morrell, L., *et al.* Hemispheric differences in hippocampal volume predict verbal and spatial memory performance in patients with Alzheimer's disease. *Hippocampus*, 2000. **10**(2):136–42.

17. Jack, C.R., Jr., *et al.* MRI as a biomarker of disease progression in a therapeutic trial of milameline for AD. *Neurology*, 2003. **60**(2):253–60.

18. Krishnan, K.R., *et al.* Randomized, placebo-controlled trial of the effects of donepezil on neuronal markers and hippocampal volumes in Alzheimer's disease. *Am J Psychiatry*, 2003. **160**(11):2003–11.

19. Fox, N.C., Schott, J.M. Imaging cerebral atrophy: normal ageing to Alzheimer's disease. *Lancet*, 2004. **363**(9406):392–4.

20. Hsu, Y.Y., *et al.* Comparison of automated and manual MRI volumetry of hippocampus in normal aging and dementia. *J Magn Reson Imaging*, 2002. **16**(3):305–10.

21. Barnes, J., *et al.* Differentiating AD from aging using semiautomated measurement of hippocampal atrophy rates. *Neuroimage*, 2004. **23**(2):574–81.

22. Fischl, B., *et al.* Whole brain segmentation: automated labeling of neuroanatomical structures in the human brain. *Neuron*, 2002. **33**(3):341–55.

23. Fischl, B., et al. *Automatically parcellating the human cerebral cortex.* Cereb Cortex, 2004. **14**(1): p. 11–22.

24. Schuff, N., *et al.* Selective reduction of N-acetylaspartate in medial temporal and parietal lobes in AD. *Neurology*, 2002. **58**(6):928–35.

25. Jessen, F., *et al.* Proton MR spectroscopy detects a relative decrease of N-acetylaspartate in the medial temporal lobe of patients with AD. *Neurology*, 2000. **55**(5):684–8.

26. Kantarci, K., *et al.* Regional metabolic patterns in mild cognitive impairment and Alzheimer's disease: a 1H MRS study. *Neurology*, 2000. **55**(2):210–7.

27. Kantarci, K., *et al.* 1H magnetic resonance spectroscopy, cognitive function, and apolipoprotein E genotype in normal aging, mild cognitive impairment and Alzheimer's disease. *J Int Neuropsychol Soc*, 2002. **8**(7):934–42.

28. Schuff, N., *et al.* Changes of hippocampal N-acetyl aspartate and volume in Alzheimer's disease. A proton MR spectroscopic imaging and MRI study. *Neurology*, 1997. **49**(6):1513–21.

29. Adalsteinsson, E., *et al.* Longitudinal decline of the neuronal marker N-acetyl aspartate in Alzheimer's disease. *Lancet*, 2000. **355**(9216):1696–7.

30. Jessen, F., *et al.* Decrease of N-acetylaspartate in the MTL correlates with cognitive decline of AD patients. *Neurology*, 2001. **57**(5):930–2.

31. Dixon, R.M., *et al.* Longitudinal quantitative proton magnetic resonance spectroscopy of the hippocampus in Alzheimer's disease. *Brain*, 2002. **125**(Pt 10):2332–41.

32. Satlin, A., *et al.* Brain proton magnetic resonance spectroscopy (1H-MRS) in Alzheimer's disease: changes after treatment with xanomeline, an M1 selective cholinergic agonist. *Am J Psychiatry*, 1997. **154**(10):1459–61.

33. Frederick, B., *et al.* Brain proton magnetic resonance spectroscopy in Alzheimer disease: changes after treatment with xanomeline. *Am J Geriatr Psychiatry*, 2002. **10**(1):81–8.

34. Shoghi–Jadid, K., *et al.* Localization of neurofibrillary tangles and beta-amyloid plaques in the brains of living patients with Alzheimer disease. *Am J Geriatr Psychiatry*, 2002. **10**(1): 24–35.

35. Klunk, W.E., *et al.* Imaging brain amyloid in Alzheimer's disease with Pittsburgh Compound-B. *Ann Neurol*, 2004. **55**(3):306–19.

36. Reiman, E.M., *et al.* Tracking Alzheimer's disease in transgenic mice using fluorodeoxyglucose autoradiography. *Neuroreport*, 2000. **11**(5):987–91.

37. Meguro, K., *et al.* Neocortical and hippocampal glucose hypometabolism following neurotoxic lesions of the entorhinal and perirhinal cortices in the non-human primate as shown by PET. Implications for Alzheimer's disease. *Brain*, 1999. **122** (Pt 8):1519–31.

38. Jagust, W.J. Neuroimaging in dementia. *Neurol Clin*, 2000. **18**(4):885–902.

39. Mega, M.S., *et al.* Mapping biochemistry to metabolism: FDG-PET and amyloid burden in Alzheimer's disease. *Neuroreport*, 1999. **10**(14):2911–7.

40. Mega, M.S., *et al.* Mapping histology to metabolism: coregistration of stained whole-brain sections to premortem PET in Alzheimer's disease. *Neuroimage*, 1997. **5**(2):147–53.

41. Bradley, K.M., *et al.* Cerebral perfusion SPET correlated with Braak pathological stage in Alzheimer's disease. *Brain*, 2002. **125**(Pt 8):1772–81.

42. Wolfe, N., *et al.* Temporal lobe perfusion on single photon emission computed tomography predicts the rate of cognitive decline in Alzheimer's disease. *Arch Neurol*, 1995. **52**(3):257–62.

43. Johnson, K.A., *et al. Preclinical prediction of Alzheimer's disease using SPECT. Neurology*, 1998. **50**(6):1563–71.

44. Jagust, W.J., *et al.* Longitudinal studies of regional cerebral metabolism in Alzheimer's disease. *Neurology*, 1988. **38**(6):909–12.

45. de Leon, M.J., *et al.* Prediction of cognitive decline in normal elderly subjects with 2-[(18)F] fluoro-2-deoxy-D-glucose/poitron-emission tomography (FDG/PET). *Proc Natl Acad Sci USA*, 2001. **98**(19):10966–71.

46. Small, G.W., *et al.* Cerebral metabolic and cognitive decline in persons at genetic risk for Alzheimer's disease. *Proc Natl Acad Sci USA*, 2000. **97**(11):6037–42.

47. Reiman, E.M., *et al.* Declining brain activity in cognitively normal apolipoprotein E epsilon 4 heterozygotes: a foundation for using positron emission tomography to efficiently test treatments to prevent Alzheimer's disease. *Proc Natl Acad Sci USA*, 2001. **98**(6): 3334–9.

48. Mega, M.S., *et al.* Cognitive and metabolic responses to metrifonate therapy in Alzheimer disease. *Neuropsychiatry Neuropsychol Behav Neurol*, 2001. **14**(1):63–8.

49. Nobili, F., *et al.* Brain perfusion follow-up in Alzheimer's patients during treatment with acetylcholinesterase inhibitors. *J Nucl Med*, 2002. **43**(8):983–90.

50. Grossman, M., *et al.* Neural basis for verb processing in Alzheimer's disease: an FMRI study. *Neuropsychology*, 2003. **17**(4):658–74.

51. Johnson, S.C., *et al.* The relationship between FMRI activation and cerebral atrophy: comparison of normal aging and alzheimer disease. *Neuroimage*, 2000. **11**(3):179–87.

52. Saykin, A.J., *et al.* Neuroanatomic substrates of semantic memory impairment in Alzheimer's disease: patterns of functional MRI activation. *J Int Neuropsychol Soc*, 1999. **5**(5):377–92.

53. Grossman, M., *et al.* Neural basis for semantic memory difficulty in Alzheimer's disease: an FMRI study. *Brain*, 2003. **126**(Pt 2):292–311.

54. Thulborn, K.R., Martin, C., Voyvodic, J.T. Functional MR imaging using a visually guided saccade paradigm for comparing activation patterns in patients with probable Alzheimer's disease and in cognitively able elderly volunteers. *AJNR Am J Neuroradiol*, 2000. **21**(3):524–31.

55. Raichle, M.E., *et al*. A default mode of brain function. *Proc Natl Acad Sci USA*, 2001. **98**(2):676–82.

56. Lustig, C., *et al*. Functional deactivations: change with age and dementia of the Alzheimer type. *Proc Natl Acad Sci USA*, 2003. **100**(24):14504–9.

57. Greicius, M.D., *et al*. Default-mode network activity distinguishes Alzheimer's disease from healthy aging: evidence from functional MRI. *Proc Natl Acad Sci USA*, 2004. **101**(13):4637–42.

58. Rombouts, S.A.R.B., *et al*. Altered resting state networks in mild cognitive impairment and mild Alzheimer's disease: an FMRI study. *Hum Brain Mapp*; 2005. **26**(4):231–9.

59. Small, S.A., *et al*. Differential regional dysfunction of the hippocampal formation among elderly with memory decline and Alzheimer's disease. *Ann Neurol*, 1999. **45**(4):466–72.

60. Rombouts, S.A., *et al*. Functional MR imaging in Alzheimer's disease during memory encoding. *AJNR Am J Neuroradiol*, 2000. **21**(10):1869–75.

61. Kato, T., Knopman, D., Liu, H. Dissociation of regional activation in mild AD during visual encoding: a functional MRI study. *Neurology*, 2001. **57**(5):812–6.

62. Sperling, R.A., *et al*. FMRI studies of associative encoding in young and elderly controls and mild Alzheimer's disease. *J Neurol Neurosurg Psychiatry*, 2003. **74**(1):44–50.

63. Machulda, M.M., *et al*. Comparison of memory FMRI response among normal, MCI, and Alzheimer's patients. *Neurology*, 2003. **61**(4):500–6.

64. Rombouts, S.A.R.B., *et al*. Delayed rather than decreased BOLD response as a marker for early Alzheimer's disease. *Neuroimage*, 2005; **26**(4):1078–85.

65. Grady, C.L., *et al*. Evidence from functional neuroimaging of a compensatory prefrontal network in Alzheimer's disease. *J Neurosci*, 2003. **23**(3):986–93.

66. Sperling, R.A., *et al*. Encoding novel face-name associations: a functional MRI study. *Hum Brain Mapp*, 2001. **14**(3):129–39.

67. Johnson, S.C., *et al*. Hippocampal adaptation to face repetition in healthy elderly and mild cognitive impairment. *Neuropsychologia*, 2004. **42**(7):980–9.

68. Dickerson, B.C., *et al*. Medial temporal lobe function and structure in mild cognitive impairment. *Ann Neurol*, 2004. **56**(1):27–35.

69. Dickerson, B.C., *et al*. Increased hippocampal activation in mild cognitive impairment compared to normal aging and AD. *Neurology* (submitted).

70. Morris, J.C., *et al*. Clinical dementia rating training and reliability in multicenter studies: the Alzheimer's Disease Cooperative Study experience. *Neurology*, 1997. **48**(6):1508–10.

71. Petersen, R.C. Mild cognitive impairment as a diagnostic entity. *J Intern Med*, 2004. **256**(3):183–94.

72. Stern, C.E., *et al*. The hippocampal formation participates in novel picture encoding: evidence from functional magnetic resonance imaging. *Proc Natl Acad Sci USA*, 1996. **93**(16):8660–5.

73. Sperling, R., *et al. Functional MRI detection of pharmacologically induced memory impairment.* *Proc Natl Acad Sci USA*, 2002. **99**(1):455–60.

74. Sperling, R., *et al*. Putting names to faces: successful encoding of associative memories activates the anterior hippocampal formation. *Neuroimage*, 2003. **20**(2):1400–10.

75. Walsh, D.M., Selkoe, D.J. Deciphering the molecular basis of memory failure in Alzheimer's disease. *Neuron*, 2004. **44**(1):181–93.

76. Saunders, A.M. Apolipoprotein E and Alzheimer disease: an update on genetic and functional analyses. *J Neuropathol Exp Neurol*, 2000. **59**(9):751–8.

77. Smith, C.D., *et al*. Altered brain activation in cognitively intact individuals at high risk for Alzheimer's disease. *Neurology*, 1999. **53**(7):1391–6.

78. Smith, C.D., *et al*. Women at risk for AD show increased parietal activation during a fluency task. *Neurology*, 2002. **58**(8):1197–202.

79. Bookheimer, S.Y., *et al.* Patterns of brain activation in people at risk for Alzheimer's disease. *N Engl J Med*, 2000. **343**(7):450–6.

80. Bondi, M.W., *et al.* FMRI evidence of compensatory mechanisms in older adults at genetic risk for Alzheimer disease. *Neurology*, 2005. **64**(3):501–8.

81. Gron, G., *et al.* Subjective memory complaints: objective neural markers in patients with Alzheimer's disease and major depressive disorder. *Ann Neurol*, 2002. **51**(4):491–8.

82. Rombouts, S.A., *et al.* Loss of frontal FMRI activation in early frontotemporal dementia compared to early AD. *Neurology*, 2003. **60**(12):1904–8.

83. Thiel, C.M., Henson, R.N., Dolan, R.J. Scopolamine but not lorazepam modulates face repetition priming: a psychopharmacological FMRI study. *Neuropsychopharmacology*, 2002. **27**(2):282–92.

84. Rombouts, S.A., *et al.* Alterations in brain activation during cholinergic enhancement with rivastigmine in Alzheimer's disease. *J Neurol Neurosurg Psychiatry*, 2002. **73**(6):665–71.

85. Saykin, A.J., *et al.* Cholinergic enhancement of frontal lobe activity in mild cognitive impairment. Brain, 2004. **127**(Pt 7):1574–83.

86. Goekoop, R., *et al.* Challenging the cholinergic system in mild cognitive impairment: a pharmacological FMRI study. *Neuroimage*, 2004. **23**(4):1450–9.

87. Bertolino, A., *et al.* Interaction of COMT (Val(108/158)Met) genotype and olanzapine treatment on prefrontal cortical function in patients with schizophrenia. *Am J Psychiatry*, 2004. **161**(10):1798–805.

88. Dickerson, B.C., Sperling, R.A. Neuroimaging biomarkers for clinical trials of disease-modifying therapies in Alzheimer's disease. *NeuroRx*, 2005. **Vol 2**: 348–60.

89. Machielsen, W.C., *et al.* FMRI of visual encoding: reproducibility of activation. *Hum Brain Mapp*, 2000. **9**(3):156–64.

90. Manoach, D.S., *et al.* Test-retest reliability of a functional MRI working memory paradigm in normal and schizophrenic subjects. *Am J Psychiatry*, 2001. **158**(6):955–8.

91. Logothetis, N.K. The underpinnings of the BOLD functional magnetic resonance imaging signal. *J Neurosci*, 2003. **23**(10):3963–71.

92. D'Esposito, M., Deouell, L.Y., Gazzaley, A. Alterations in the BOLD FMRI signal with ageing and disease: a challenge for neuroimaging. *Nat Rev Neurosci*, 2003. **4**(11):863–72.

93. Buckner, R.L., *et al.* Functional brain imaging of young, nondemented, and demented older adults. *J Cogn Neurosci*, 2000. **12 Suppl 2**:24–34.

94. Brewer, J.B., *et al.* Making memories: brain activity that predicts how well visual experience will be remembered. *Science*, 1998. **281**(5380):1185–7.

95. Wagner, A.D., *et al.* Building memories: remembering and forgetting of verbal experiences as predicted by brain activity. *Science*, 1998. **281**(5380):1188–91.

96. Price, C.J., Friston, K.J. Scanning patients with tasks they can perform. *Hum Brain Mapp*, 1999. **8**(2–3):102–8.

97. Becker, J.T., *et al.* Compensatory reallocation of brain resources supporting verbal episodic memory in Alzheimer's disease. *Neurology*, 1996. **46**(3):692–700.

98. Stern, Y., *et al.* Different brain networks mediate task performance in normal aging and AD: defining compensation. *Neurology*, 2000. **55**(9):1291–7.

99. Audoin, B., *et al.* Compensatory cortical activation observed by FMRI during a cognitive task at the earliest stage of MS. *Hum Brain Mapp*, 2003. **20**(2):51–8.

100. Daly, E., *et al.* Predicting conversion to Alzheimer disease using standardized clinical information. *Arch Neurol*, 2000. **57**(5):675–80.

6

Dementia: visualizing the metabolic changes of early Alzheimer's disease

William Wu and Scott A. Small

1. Introduction

The pathological course of Alzheimer's disease (AD) progresses slowly, taking years to cause cognitive disability, producing an often confusing array of histological and functional alterations in the brain. Despite notable inconsistencies, a consensus regarding the anatomy and physiology of AD has emerged by investigating brain tissue, both living and dead, in human patients and in mouse models of disease. Prospective neuropsychological studies have made the fundamental observation that AD begins in the hippocampal formation[1, 2]. The hippocampus itself is made up of anatomically distinct subregions, and recent microarray studies have shown that each hippocampal subregion expresses a unique molecular profile[3]. Although, over time, most subregions will manifest AD pathology, these molecular observations underlie the assumption that early on, AD selectively targets the hippocampus[4].

By investigating multiple hippocampal subregions simultaneously, a combination of in vitro[5–8] and in vivo studies[9, 10] have pinpointed the entorhinal cortex as the single hippocampal subregion most vulnerable to AD. Once germinating in the entorhinal cortex, AD progresses anatomically, spreading across multiple regions of the neocortex. Within each region, AD progresses pathophysiologically as well. Ultimately, in what can be called the 'cell-death' stage, AD is characterized by neuronal loss accompanied by amyloid plaques and neurofibrillary tangles. However, affected neurons do not die immediately, and it is now clear that there is antecedent 'cell-sickness' stage, characterized by neurons that are alive but suffer physiological and metabolic dysfunction[11]. Notably, the cell-sickness stage can occur before amyloid plaques[12] or neurofibrillary tangles[13].

The anatomy and pathophysiology of early AD informs how an imaging technique can be used as a diagnostic tool and as a tool with which to screen or validate anti-AD drugs. Currently, our greatest diagnostic challenge is reliably detecting AD in its earliest stages, when AD causes only mild forgetfulness and cognitively overlaps with normal ageing 4. In accordance with the unique molecular profiling of different hippocampal neurons, in vitro and in vivo studies have established that normal ageing spares the entorhinal cortex, targeting other hippocampal neurons, such as the granule cells of the dentate gyrus[10, 14]. Thus, a technique that can visualize cell-sickness in the entorhinal cortex should be both sensitive and specific in diagnosing AD in its earliest stages. Beyond diagnostics, the ability to accurately detect the early stage of AD is of great interest from a therapeutic point of view. For obvious reasons, drugs will more likely achieve the therapeutic goal of arresting disease progression when applied to a sick and not a dead cell. Furthermore, it is this cell-sickness stage that will be amenable to the more ambitious goal of reversing the disease process. Thus, an imaging tool that can detect cell-sickness in the entorhinal cortex can be used to screen or validate drugs that will slow, stop, or perhaps even reverse AD pathophysiology.

With these goals in mind, functional imaging techniques have received much attention. In contrast to other imaging approaches designed to visualize the later lesions of AD (cell loss or amyloid plaques), cell-sickness is fundamentally a functional defect. All functional imaging techniques are unified in their attempts to map energy metabolism and we will begin by pinning down a precise definition of 'function', establishing a clear relationship between electrophysiology, biochemistry, and energy metabolism. Metabolism is a dynamic process, constantly shifting its rates based on internal and external stimuli, and an important distinction will be made between stimuli that affect acute or basal metabolic rates. We will then review different MRI approaches designed to capture metabolic defects, which are all based on the coupling between oxygen metabolism (neurons are, of course, exclusively aerobic energy producers) and blood flow. Finally, we will conclude by comparing the different MRI approaches, highlighting the advantages and disadvantages of each for the stated clinical goals of AD.

2. **MRI correlates of metabolism**

It is important to maintain a precise definition of the 'function' in functional imaging, so as not to misinterpret its meaning or utility. Over the 50 years that the field has evolved, since the seminal work by Kety and Schmidt[15], functional brain imaging has come to imply a method that detects regional energy metabolism. Energy metabolism is best defined as the rate with which cells produce ATP, which in neurons (obligate aerobes who do not store glucose) requires the consumption of oxygen and glucose from the bloodstream. Visualizing ATP directly is challenging, but imaging techniques have been developed that can visualize correlates of oxygen and glucose consumption. With the use of radiolabelled glucose, positron emission tomography (PET) can quantify the regional rates of glucose uptake, which under certain assumptions corresponds to energy metabolism.

In contrast, MRI-based techniques have, typically, relied on the second ingredient of ATP production, oxygen consumption, with which to visualize correlates of energy metabolism. Like in any organ, an increase in oxygen consumption is accompanied by an increase in oxygen delivery (i.e. accelerated blood flow). In the brain, this relationship is governed intrinsically and with regional specificity, although the biochemical mechanisms for this regional regulation remain poorly understood. Arterial spin labelling (ASL) (a technique introduced by Detre and Alsop[16]) is the only MRI approach that can directly and absolutely quantify regional cerebral blood flow (CBF). Because post-capillary venules are low-resistant vessels, pressure shifts caused by changes in CBF lead to concomitant changes in regional cerebral blood volume (CBV). Predictably, CBV turns out to another haemodynamic variable that corresponds to oxygen consumption and that correlates with energy metabolism. In fact, metabolic-induced changes in CBV is what Roy and Sherrington measured in their historic studies over a century ago — not CBF as commonly and mistakenly thought[15]. Belliveau and Rosen introduced the first MRI-based technique, which relies on intravascular contrast agents like gadolinium to estimate regional CBV[17]. Note that in the clinical setting, this technique is often called 'perfusion' MRI, because CBV maps can be converted to CBF maps by making certain assumptions about mean transit time and arterial input functions. One limitation of this approach for the purposes of diagnostics is that it only generates a relative estimate of CBV, not an absolute quantification measured in millilitres of blood vessels per millilitres of tissue. Lin and Haake introduced a modification of this approach[18] in which a contrast agent is injected but the signal changes are measured in the steady state not the dynamic state. This approach offers the advantage of more precise quantification of CBV and greater spatial resolution[18].

Finally, deoxyhaemoglobin content is the third haemodynamic variable that correlates with oxygen consumption and energy metabolism, and which can be visualized with MRI. By having rodents breath different concentrations of oxygen, Ogawa and his colleagues were the first to show that regional differences in basal levels of deoxyhaemoglobin can visualized with MRI[19]. By using drugs to alter basal brain metabolism[20] and then by using behavioural tasks to alter metabolism more acutely[21], subsequent studies have documented that the correlation between deoxyhaemoglobin content and energy metabolism is inverted: an increase in energy metabolism will lead to a *decrease* in deoxyhaemoglobin content.

This somewhat counterintuitive inversion can be understood by examining the formulae with which deoxyhaemoglobin content is derived: deoxyhaemoglobin content = (deoxyhaemoglobin concentration x CBV). Based on Fick's principle, deoxyhaemoglobin concentration = oxygen consumption/CBF, so that deoxyhaemoglobin content = (oxygen consumption/CBF) x CBV. A range of empirical studies have established that for every unit increase in oxygen consumption, there is an approximately squared increase in CBF 22 and, thus, according to the derivations, this will lead to a decrease in deoxyhaemoglobin concentrations. Note also that because it is based on a complex and conflicting interplay between CBF and CBV, deoxyhaemoglobin content is the only MRI correlate of metabolism that is non-quantitative.

To summarize, all functional imaging is unified by attempts to visualize correlates of neuronal energy metabolism. MRI achieves this by relying on correlates of oxygen consumption — CBF, CBV, and deoxyhaemoglobin content. Among these three variables, only deoxyhaemoglobin content cannot currently be quantified absolutely.

3. **Metabolic correlates of cell sickness**

Brain metabolism is, by definition, a dynamic process, constantly shifting its rates in response to internal or external stimuli. Thus, the term 'resting' metabolism, which we and others have previously used[23], is in fact a misnomer; brain metabolism is never at rest.

More accurately, a distinction should be made between internal or external stimuli that change metabolism acutely — over milliseconds or seconds — versus stimuli that change metabolism over longer time periods, affecting basal metabolic rates. The distinction of acute vs. basal changes in metabolism lies well with the way in which investigators of metabolism have dichotomized the primary sources of neuronal energy production (Fig. 6.1). Half of neuronal ATP production is dedicated to 'bioelectric' processes[24], in particular any shift in the membrane potential. Note that a shift in post-synaptic potentials can occur with and without spike activity. The other 50% of ATP is dedicated to a long list of 'biochemical' processes, which importantly includes protein synthesis, axonal transport, and synaptogenesis[24] (Fig. 6.1).

Finally, the distinction between bioelectric and biochemical sources of energy consumption sits nicely with the two physiological mechanisms with which neurons change function' — either by changing synaptic activity or by changing synaptic strength (Fig. 6.1).

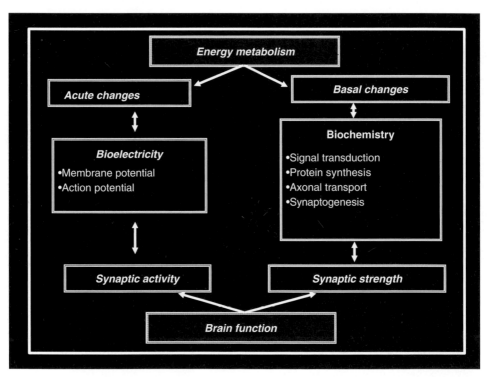

Fig. 6.1 Linking functional imaging to energy metabolism. Brain function is altered by changing either synaptic activity or by changing synaptic strength. A change in synaptic activity will shift the neuron's membrane potential, and re-normalizing the membrane potential requires energy consumption. In contrast, a change in synaptic strength, which occurs even in electrically silent neurons, is mediated by biochemical changes such as protein synthesis. These biochemical changes also require energy consumption but occur over slower time courses and affect basal metabolic rates.

Long-term increases in synaptic strength occur by increasing presynaptic neurotransmitter release, by increasing post-synaptic receptor density, or by synaptogenesis. In any case, the relatively long time courses of the biochemical mechanisms that govern these long-term effects will alter the basal metabolic rates of the neuron.

This scheme is helpful not only for understanding the different meanings of brain function vis à vis brain metabolism, but also for determining the type of function that is most informative for a particular question (Fig. 6.2). Cognitively, one can ask which brain regions change *synaptic activity* in response to a brief external stimulus (i.e. mapping sensory representation), in which case an imaging technique is required to map acute changes in energy metabolism. In contrast, asking which brain regions change *synaptic strength* in order to store the sensory representation in long-term memory is, metabolically speaking, a different question. Insofar as the biochemical mechanisms that govern synaptic strength (mechanisms that underlie long-term memory) require synaptogenesis, protein synthesis, and even axonal transport, then this change will be most evident in measures of basal metabolism (Fig. 6.2).

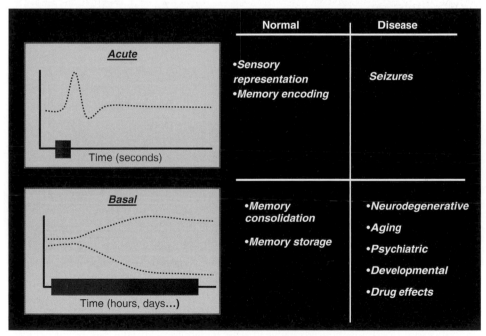

Fig. 6.2 Functional imaging can be used to map normal brain function and brain disease. **Normal brain function**: functional imaging can map changes in acute metabolism that occur during sensory representation or memory encoding, or map changes in basal metabolism that occur during memory consolidation and memory storage. **Abnormal brain function**: functional imaging can be used to map acute changes in metabolism that occur during seizure activity, or to map changes in basal metabolism that occur in most other diseases of the brain, including Alzheimer's disease.

Clinically, functional imaging is typically used to 'localize the lesion' for diagnostic purposes or for mapping the natural clinical course of disease or in response to therapeutic intervention. In the case of mapping seizures, the primary disorder is one of transient increase in synaptic activity and so a metabolic map should be sensitive to changes in bioelectricity. In contrast, the cell-sickness stage of Alzheimer's disease, or cell sickness that occurs in other physiological disorders, is characterized by a decrease in synaptic strength, not by a change in synaptic activity per se (Fig. 6.2). This has been demonstrated in humans relying on molecular markers of synaptic function[25] such as synaptophysin, and in mice relying on electrophysiological measures showing uniform deficits in basal synaptic transmission[12], or sometimes long-term potentiation. The primary change in synaptic strength accounts for why both *in vitro* and *in vivo* measures of basal metabolism uniformly detect focal deficits in these disorders, even when cell loss is not a factor.

In principle, of course, changes in basal metabolism might be difficult to detect and, in this case, using an external stimuli that acutely activates an affected brain area may further enhance lesion detection — akin to cardiac testing when a 'resting' EKG is normal or ambiguous and a stress test 'brings out the lesion'. In fact, we and others have used stimulus-induced changes in deoxyhaemoglobin content (the so-called BOLD effect) to map metabolic defects in AD (as reviewed in Chapter 5).

Nevertheless, a number of advantages are gained if a lesion can be detected in its primary basal state. Because AD does have basal metabolic defects, the BOLD response is essentially an acute-on-chronic experiment, which is prone to misinterpretation. This point can be illustrated by considering the differences in the BOLD response between primary visual cortex and motor cortex. The basal metabolic state of visual cortex is typically lower compared to the motor cortex[26], which is reflected by higher levels of basal deoxyhaemoglobin[27]. Thus, when visual cortex is stimulated, there is more deoxyhaemoglobin to be 'washed out', which will artificially amplify the BOLD response[27]. This washout effect has been invoked to account for why visual stimulation results in an artificially larger BOLD response compared to motor stimulation[27], even if the degree of neuronal stimulation is assumed equivalent. One might conclude that the motor cortex is 'dysfunctional' compared to the visual cortex, but this would obviously be a mistake, and is simply caused by differences in the basal state. Thus, differences in basal metabolic rates act as to confound when comparing the acute BOLD response between separate brain regions. A similar acute-on-chronic problem exists when comparing the same brain region between AD patients and controls, because AD reduces basal metabolic states.

A second advantage of relying on measurements of basal metabolism is the greater superior spatial resolution it affords. Higher temporal resolution is needed when setting out to measure a stimulus-induced change in acute metabolism. Like the logic of any camera, temporal resolution trades-off with spatial resolution. Although this trade-off may be irrelevant when measuring acute metabolic changes in large cortical areas, the compromise in spatial resolution makes it more difficult to reliably visualize small brain regions, such as the entorhinal cortex. Because the entorhinal cortex is only a few millimetres in dimension, MRI pulse sequences with sub-millimetre resolution have been found preferable when investigating the entorhinal cortex. When optimized, BOLD scanning has been able to visualize the entorhinal cortex. However, because the resolution is supra-millimetre, only a few pixels can be sampled from the entorhinal cortex and is, therefore, prone to error. In contrast, a sub-millimetre image — which is more easily achieved when investigating the basal metabolic state — provides dozens of entorhinal cortex pixels and, because of the high sampling, generates a more reliable metric of the entorhinal cortex.

To summarize, the cell-sickness stage of AD is characterized by a decrease in synaptic strength, reflecting chronic biochemical defects and altering basal metabolic rates. For both theoretical and practical reasons (as discussed above), an imaging technique sensitive to basal metabolism is well suited to capture cell sickness in the entorhinal cortex of early AD.

4. **MRI measures of entorhinal cortex cell sickness in AD**

Although we initially used MRI to map stimulus-induced changes in acute metabolism, because of the above considerations we have shifted our focus to explore MRI measures that capture the basal metabolic defects associated with AD.

Arterial spin labelling (ASL)[16] is a remarkable MRI technique that allows the measurement and, importantly, the absolute quantification of CBF. In our exploration of this technique, we were first interested in determining whether ASL can visualize the entorhinal cortex. We have applied this technique using different slice orientations and pixel dimensions and, consistent with other studies, we have found that an oblique coronal slice, orientated perpendicular to the hippocampal long axis, maximizes this possibility (Fig. 6.3). Unfortunately, even in this orientation, the temporal requirement of ASL, which prohibits sub-millimetre resolution, limits its ability to investigate the entorhinal cortex. First, the supra-millimetre resolution makes it difficult to reliably identify the anatomical landmarks required to distinguish the entorhinal cortex. Second, even if we convince ourselves that we can identify the entorhinal cortex, there are only a few entorhinal cortex pixels, and this low sample size is a general parametric concern (Fig. 6.3).

We have also explored whether MRI sequences sensitive to basal deoxyhaemoglobin content can be used for disease mapping. Toward this goal, we returned to Seiji Ogawa's seminal studies in which he used gradient-echo (not echo-planar) pulse sequences to show that T2*-weighted images are sensitive to basal differences in deoxyhaemoglobin content[19]. In these original studies, differences in T2*-weighted signal were detected across brain regions, according to regional differences in basal deoxyhaemoglobin content, or across time after the administration of drugs that affect basal metabolism[20].

We optimized a gradient-echo pulse sequence, maximizing the magnetic susceptibility effect so as to be most sensitive to basal deoxyhaemoglobin but, at the same time, manipulating resolution with which to best visualize the entorhinal cortex and other hippocampal subregions[23] (Fig. 6.3) As already mentioned, resolving the hippocampal subregions necessitated a pulse sequence with sub-millimetre resolution. As a proof of principle study, we used this gradient-echo pulse sequence to image patients with AD dementia compared to age-matched controls[9]. Although diminished signal was observed in all hippocampal subregions, a multivariate analysis isolated the entorhinal cortex as the primary site of signal change. Because patients already had dementia, the odds were high that the entorhinal

		Resolution	Quantification

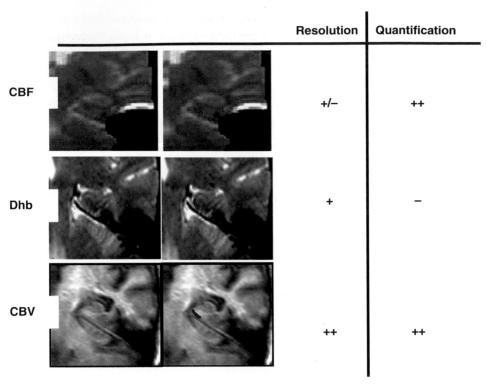

CBF — Resolution: +/−, Quantification: ++

Dhb — Resolution: +, Quantification: −

CBV — Resolution: ++, Quantification: ++

Fig. 6.3 Detecting metabolic changes in the entorhinal cortex in Alzheimer's disease. MRI can visualize three correlates of energy metabolism — cerebral blood flow (CBF), deoxyhaemoglobin content (dHB), cerebral blood volume (CBV). The MRI techniques that assess these three correlates differ along two factors — spatial resolution and degree of quantification. CBF-MRI techniques generate images that can be quantified but have relatively poor spatial resolution; dHB-MRI techniques generate images with high spatial resolution but which cannot be quantified; while CBV-MRI techniques generate images with very high spatial resolution that can be quantified. The entorhinal cortex is indicated in red in each image.

cortex of most patients had experienced cell death, not only cell sickness, and so this study did not confirm that this approach is sensitive necessarily to cell sickness.

In order to test this more clearly, we adapted our approach to be applicable to mice. We investigated a transgenic strain whose genetic manipulation led to defects in protein-synthesis dependents' long-term potentiation (i.e. a form of cell sickness) in the CA1 subregion of the hippocampus. Importantly, these mice did not develop cell loss. We observed a reliable decrease in T2*-weighted signal in the CA1 subregion of transgenic mice compared to wild-type littermates, confirming that this approach can detect cell sickness[23].

Despite these favourable findings, this approach has a number of limitations, as we point out in our paper[28]. The greatest difficulty with this approach is the fact that although T2*-weighted signal is indeed affected by basal deoxyhaemoglobin content, it is also affected by other tissue constituents. Since these other tissue constituents are not necessarily related to basal metabolism, they constitute a source of noise. Normalizing signal intensity to the whole brain or to other unaffected brain regions may correct some of these sources of noise; we cannot be sure that they correct all sources of noise. Furthermore, even if we could correct for the non-metabolic sources of noise, it is impossible to translate a difference in T2*-weighted signal into an absolute correlate of metabolism. Thus, this approach may be useful for group comparisons. However, the potentially uncorrected sources of noise and the inability to quantify a metabolic correlate are problematic for diagnostic purposes, where the precision of individual measurements is critical.

This forced us to explore the third and remaining correlate of basal metabolism, CBV. By systematically shifting the concentration of an intravascular contrast agent, the difference in MRI signal can be used to derive an estimate of CBV. Work by Belliveau and colleagues[17] introduced an approach in which rapid acquisitions are used to map how T2*-weighted signal changes over time, as gadolinium first passes through the vasculature. A relative measure of CBV can then be derived from the 'area under the curve'. Indeed, work by Gonzalez and others has shown that this MRI measure of CBV is tightly correlated with glucose uptake, as measured with PET, and can detect AD-associated metabolic deficits in the posterior parietal lobes[29]. This approach has two main limitations. First, because high temporal resolution is required to measure the rapid first pass, this approach cannot achieve the required sub-millimetre resolution. Second, as with oxygen, this approach yields only a relative, not an absolute, measure of CBV.

Most recently, we have turned to an alternative gadolinium approach developed first by Lin and Haake[18, 30]. This approach relies on T1-weighted images to measure the steady state, not dynamic, signal changes caused by the IV injection of gadolinium. We have adapted this approach in our efforts to image cell sickness in the entorhinal cortex and found that this approach provides two key advantages. First, because acquisition times can be slowed down, we can easily achieve sub-millimetre resolution, allowing us to reliably visualize the entorhinal cortex, and to do so with a relatively large pixel sampling (Fig. 6.3). Second, as argued by Lin and Haake, by normalizing the signal to an area with 100% blood, such as the sagital sinus, an absolute quantification of CBV can be generated.

To summarize, MRI can be made sensitive to three haemodynamic variables that correlate with neuronal energy metabolism, and thus all can, in principle, detect the metabolic changes associated with AD-related cell sickness. Nevertheless, important differences exist among the MRI measurements, as summarized in Fig. 6.3, with a particular emphasis placed on two factors. The first is whether the measurement can be acquired with sufficient spatial resolution with which to generate multiple sample points from the diminutive entorhinal cortex; and the second is whether the measurement generates an absolute quantification of the haemodynamic correlate, a factor critical for diagnostics. Measurements of CBF, using techniques like ASL, score high marks on quantification but, unfortunately, cannot achieve the desired sub-millimetre resolution. In direct opposition, measurements sensitive to basal deoxyhaemoglobin can be acquired with sufficient spatial resolution but, for reasons listed above, cannot be acquired quantitatively. Fortunately, measurements of CBV fulfil both requirements — sub-millimetre resolution and quantification — and, therefore, turn out to be the best MRI metric with which to visualize cell sickness in the entorhinal cortex of AD.

Indeed, based on the merits of the CBV approach, we are currently in the process of conducting two NIH-funded studies that will test its true capabilities. The first will test its diagnostic utility by measuring CBV from the entorhinal cortex and other hippocampal subregions in hundreds of healthy elders, some of whom will go on to develop AD dementia. The second will test the drug-screening utility of CBV by determining whether CBV measured in transgenic mouse models of AD can map drug efficacy.

5. Summary

During the last decade, important insights have been made into the molecular mechanisms underlying AD, and these insights have led to a justifiable optimism that we are finally on the cusp of effective treatment options. Accordingly, the ability to develop an imaging technique that can reliably detect the earliest stage of AD has become more important than ever. Not only can this technique be used to screen for efficacy among the growing number of candidate compounds designed to treat AD, but once a compound is identified, this technique can be used to determine which subjects are truly harbouring early, pre-dementia, AD.

As discussed in this chapter, we have relied on a combination of theoretical and practical considerations and series of empirical findings to home onto an MRI technique — one that measures CBV with high resolution — that we believe holds the greatest promise as a tool to detect the earliest stages of AD. Of course, theory and small-scale findings do not always predict success in clinical science. Large-scale studies are needed to confirm or refute a favoured technique and, currently, there are a number of ongoing studies that are testing basal state alterations in AD. Beyond our study measuring CBV in the entorhinal cortex and other hippocampal subregions with MRI, other studies are measuring CBF with MRI, volumetrics with MRI, glucose uptake with PET, and radiolabelling of amyloid plaques with PET. In parallel with drug development, there is justified optimism that, within the next few years, an imaging technique will be identified that can reliably detect, diagnose, and map the clinical course of the earliest stages of AD.

Acknowledgements

This work was supported in part by federal grants AG08702 and AG00949, by the Beeson Faculty Scholar Award from the American Federation of Aging, by the Institute for the Study on Aging, and the McKnight Neuroscience of Brain Disorders Award.

References

1. Jacobs, D.M., *et al.* Neuropsychological detection and characterization of preclinical Alzheimer's disease [see comments]. *Neurology*, 1995. **45**(5):957–62.
2. Masur, D.M., *et al.* Neuropsychological prediction of dementia and the absence of dementia in healthy elderly persons [see comments]. *Neurology*, 1994. **44**(8):1427–32.

3. Zhao, X., *et al.* Transcriptional profiling reveals strict boundaries between hippocampal subregions. *J Comp Neurol*, 2001. **441**(3):187–96.

4. Small, S.A. Age-related memory decline; current concepts and future directions. *Archives of Neurology*, 2001. **58**:360–4.

5. Fukutani, Y., *et al.* Neuronal loss and neurofibrillary degeneration in the hippocampal cortex in late-onset sporadic Alzheimer's disease. *Psychiatry Clin Neurosci*, 2000. **54**(5):523–9.

6. West, M.J., *et al.* The CA1 region of the human hippocampus is a hot spot in Alzheimer's disease. *Ann N Y Acad Sci*, 2000. **908**:255–9.

7. Price, J.L., *et al.* Neuron number in the entorhinal cortex and CA1 in preclinical Alzheimer disease. *Arch Neurol*, 2001. **58**(9):1395–402.

8. Schonheit, B., Zarski, R., Ohm, T.G. Spatial and temporal relationships between plaques and tangles in Alzheimer-pathology. *Neurobiol Aging*, 2004. **25**(6):697–711.

9. Small, S.A., *et al.* Evaluating the function of hippocampal subregions with high-resolution MRI in Alzheimer's disease and aging [in process citation]. *Microsc Res Tech*, 2000. **51**(1):101–8.

10. Small, S.A., *et al.* Imaging hippocampal function across the human life span: is memory decline normal or not? *Ann Neurol*, 2002. **51**(3):290–5.

11. Selkoe, D.J. Alzheimer's disease is a synaptic failure. *Science*, 2002. **298**(5594):789–91.

12. Mucke, L., *et al.* High-level neuronal expression of abeta 1–42 in wild-type human amyloid protein precursor transgenic mice: synaptotoxicity without plaque formation. *J Neurosci*, 2000. **20**(11):4050–8.

13. Oddo, S., *et al.* Amyloid deposition precedes tangle formation in a triple transgenic model of Alzheimer's disease. *Neurobiol Aging*, 2003. **24**(8):1063–70.

14. Small, S.A., *et al.* From the cover: imaging correlates of brain function in monkeys and rats isolates a hippocampal subregion differentially vulnerable to aging. *Proc Natl Acad Sci USA*, 2004. **101**(18):7181–6.

15. Small, S.A. Quantifying cerebral blood flow: regional regulation with global implications. *J Clin Invest*, 2004. **114**(8):1046–8.

16. Alsop, D.C., Detre, J.A. Reduced transit-time sensitivity in noninvasive magnetic resonance imaging of human cerebral blood flow. *J Cereb Blood Flow Metab*, 1996. **16**(6):1236–49.

17. Belliveau, J.W., *et al.* Functional cerebral imaging by susceptibility-contrast NMR. *Magn Reson Med*, 1990. **14**(3):538–46.

18. Lin, W., Celik, A., Paczynski, R.P. Regional cerebral blood volume: a comparison of the dynamic imaging and the steady state methods. *J Magn Reson Imaging*, 1999. **9**(1):44–52.

19. Ogawa, S., *et al.* Oxygenation-sensitive contrast in magnetic resonance image of rodent brain at high magnetic fields. *Magn Reson Med*, 1990. **14**(1):68–78.

20. Ogawa, S., *et al.* Brain magnetic resonance imaging with contrast dependent on blood oxygenation. *Proc Natl Acad Sci USA*, 1990. **87**(24):9868–72.

21. Ogawa, S., *et al.* Intrinsic signal changes accompanying sensory stimulation: functional brain mapping with magnetic resonance imaging. *Proc Natl Acad Sci USA*, 1992. **89**(13):5951–5.

22. van Zijl, P.C., *et al.* Quantitative assessment of blood flow, blood volume and blood oxygenation effects in functional magnetic resonance imaging. *Nat Med*, 1998. **4**(2):159–67.

23. Small, S., *et al.* Imaging physiologic dysfunction of individual hippocampal subregions in humans and genetically modified mice. *Neuron*, 2000(28):653–64.

24. Erecinska, M. Silver, I.A. ATP and brain function. *J Cereb Blood Flow Metab*, 1989. **9**(1):2–19.

25. Masliah, E., *et al.* Synaptic and neuritic alterations during the progression of Alzheimer's disease. *Neurosci Lett*, 1994. **174**(1):67–72.

26. Raichle, M.E., *et al.* A default mode of brain function. *Proc Natl Acad Sci USA*, 2001. **98**(2):676–82.

27. Davis, T.L., *et al.* Calibrated functional MRI: mapping the dynamics of oxidative metabolism. *Proc Natl Acad Sci USA*, 1998. **95**(4):1834–9.

28. Small, S.A. Measuring correlates of brain metabolism with high-resolution MRI: a promising approach for diagnosing Alzheimer disease and mapping its course. *Alzheimer Dis Assoc Disord*, 2003. **17**(3):154–61.

29. Gonzalez, R.G., *et al.* Functional MR in the evaluation of dementia: correlation of abnormal dynamic cerebral blood volume measurements with changes in cerebral metabolism on positron emission tomography with fludeoxyglucose F 18. *AJNR Am J Neuroradiol*, 1995. **16**(9):1763–70.

30. Lin, W., *et al.* Quantitative measurements of regional cerebral blood volume using MRI in rats: effects of arterial carbon dioxide tension and mannitol. *Magn Reson Med*, 1997. **38**(3):420–8.

7

Schizophrenia

Nick F. Ramsey and René S. Kahn

1. Introduction

The methodological improvements of FMRI, both in the fields of image acquisition and data analysis, call for constant re-evaluation of the type of questions that can be addressed[1]. Particularly the technological advances made in MRI technology forces the neuroimaging community to rethink the meaning of the results that are acquired in FMRI experiments and to decide on the experimental design, as technology is no longer the dominant bottleneck but the theoretical framework in which to fit the results. For instance, whereas earlier studies were mainly focussed on identifying regions that were somehow involved in performing a cognitive task, recent studies have elucidated the way in which brain regions communicate and how they function within networks[2]. It is conceivable that, in the coming decades, some of the neuronal mechanisms that form the basis of human behaviour may be captured in well-defined models, making it possible to understand pathological processes underlying mental disorders in terms of localized abnormalities of function within brain structures and of communication between structures.

This review attempts to describe what FMRI has contributed to the field of schizophrenia research. Rather than to summarize the plethora of FMRI studies on this illness, the authors have chosen to explain how FMRI has influenced ideas about the nature of brain malfunction. The most dominant subject of investigation with FMRI is undoubtedly that of information processing. This appears to be associated with two developments. Firstly, the notion that cognitive impairments are an important aspect of schizophrenia has gained significance as it has the potential to provide mechanistic explanations for a variety of seemingly unrelated clinical symptoms (e.g. see[3]). Secondly, rapid advances have been made in cognitive neuroscience — a discipline of sorts that builds on the theoretical frameworks of human cognition developed by experimental psychology and neuropsychology — providing new insights into the mechanism of normal brain function (e.g. see[4]).

In what follows, several topics of investigation in schizophrenia are reviewed briefly, with the purpose of highlighting potentially important developments in the near future. There is a focus on information processing in schizophrenia, with an attempt to explain how FMRI is changing our ideas of how the brain processes information and what the nature is of the cognitive deficits in the illness. Most of the papers referenced concern FMRI research. However, important work has been conducted using regional cerebral blood flow measurements with (PET) positron emission tomography, which is also referenced where necessary. Not all domains of impaired brain function are addressed; domains such as emotions, social cognition, and memory, although gaining interest, have, as of yet, only scarcely been investigated with FMRI. Issues like medication effects, chronicity, illness specificity (relative to other psychiatric disorders) will not be described in much detail, mainly because the diversity of the FMRI paradigms (and, consequently, the small numbers of studies that use the exact same task), precludes adequate and comprehensive assessment of these factors. However, many of the cognitive deficits persist in spite of medication, suggesting that the underlying brain dysfunctions should also be present.

Schizophrenia is a disease affecting approximately 1% of the worldwide population. It is characterized by declining social competency, negative symptoms (such as social withdrawal, affective flattening), cognitive deficits, and periodic psychotic exacerbations. The peak incidence occurs in late adolescence and early adult life and for many, but not all, individuals, it has a chronic course. Indeed, the variability in the course of illness is one of the constants over the last 100 years of research. Generally, about 25% of patients recover from their first psychosis, one third deteriorates, one third stabilizes at a lower than premorbid level, and 10–15% commit suicide. Although its aetiology is unknown, numerous findings from imaging studies strongly support the view that schizophrenia is a brain disease. Some of these brain abnormalities, such as a smaller intracranial and thalamic volume, have been associated with the genetic risk to develop schizophrenia, whereas other brain abnormalities were associated with environmental factors, including an additional reduction in whole-brain volume. Whether the reported brain abnormalities are static or increase over the course of the illness is still subject to discussion but evidence is emerging that global and focal gray matter abnormalities progress over time[5].

2. FMRI in schizophrenia

As described above, FMRI is particularly suitable for assessment of the (degree of) involvement of brain regions in particular functions. Such functions have to be invoked in a tightly controlled fashion because the time course of events is used in data analysis to search for regions where signal changes match the events associated with the task(s). For applications in schizophrenia, FMRI is mainly used to investigate cognitive processes which lend themselves to this requirement. Most FMRI studies in schizophrenia are aimed at identifying brain regions that malfunction, with the objective of associating the illness, or specific symptoms, with regionally specific neuropathology. Other studies focus more on testing a hypothesis about brain dysfunction in schizophrenia. This approach entails formulation of expectations concerning the regions that are involved and the way those regions respond to experimental manipulations incorporated in the design of task(s).

How an experiment is designed and conducted depends primarily on the type of question that one poses. For schizophrenia, these may range from relatively simple 'can we see dysfunction in the brain?' questions, to testing hypotheses about neuronal interactions. The following questions drive FMRI research in schizophrenia:

1. Are there brain regions that do not function properly? (region-specific pathology)

2. Are there abnormalities in the way brain regions communicate? (impaired networks or connectivity)

3. How does abnormal regional or network function cause symptoms of the illness? (neuronal mechanisms)

4. Are abnormalities in brain function associated with specific genes? (genetic contribution to functional deficits).

Each of these types of questions will be discussed within a specific context. FMRI studies have predominantly focussed on executive function (the main topic of this review) but also, to varying degrees, on perception and motor function, and on auditory hallucinations and language.

Studies on perceptual processes indicate that early stages of processing external information may be affected in schizophrenia[6–8], some of which (e.g. prepulse inhibition — a measure of early auditory processing) appears to be associated with a failure to engage the prefrontal cortex[8]. Functional neuroimaging studies generally find little evidence of abnormal function of primary visual cortex[9], although neuroleptic medication seems to enhance activity[11,12], supporting the notion that perceptual processes are affected through impaired top-down regulation (imposed, for instance, by focussing attention — see below) rather than through primary cortex dysfunction. Likewise, activity in the primary motor cortex appears to be normal in neuroleptic medication-free schizophrenic patients[13,14]. In most studies with patients on medication, activity in the motor system is reduced[14–16] (but see[17]), but this may be associated with confounds involving attention and rate of movements (typically finger tapping). Attention has been shown to affect the cerebral response to visual stimuli in parietal and frontal regions[18–20], as well as responses in the primary cortex to sensory[21] and auditory stimuli[22] (see Fig. 7.1 for an example of this effect), indicating that comparisons between patients and healthy subjects may be confounded by illness-related effects on top-down regulation of brain function. Such regulation most likely involves the prefrontal cortex, which is associated with executive function.

Auditory verbal hallucinations (AVH) — the most frequent type of hallucination in schizophrenia — are accompanied by activity in the perceptive language system[23–27] and in regions involved in memory and attention[26], suggesting that they can either arise from misinterpreted, normal, inner speech or from aberrant activation of the primary auditory cortex[147]. Most studies implicate the left hemisphere, where language is preferentially processed[28,29], but some investigators posit that AVH may be associated with language-related activity in the right hemisphere[30,31,148]. The latter is based, in part, on findings that patients exhibit reduced left-hemisphere dominance for language[30,31] as compared to controls who are typically strongly left-lateralized. As shown in Fig. 7.2, laterality is also reduced in healthy co-twins of schizophrenic patients[32]. The various findings indicate that cross-hemispheric communication is affected in schizophrenia[33–35], possibly by diminished suppression of spontaneous activity in the language system.

Language processing typically activates regions associated not only with language but also with executive functions (notably, working memory i.e. manipulation and brief storage of information), such as the anterior cingulate cortex and dorsolateral prefrontal cortex (DLPFC). This indicates that abnormal language function in schizophrenia[36,37] may be associated with poor executive functions. On an often used task that requires

(a) (b) (c)

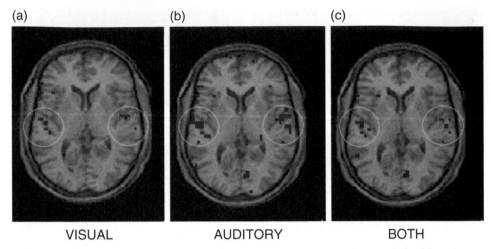

VISUAL   AUDITORY   BOTH

Fig. 7.1 Attentional modulation of primary auditory cortex activation in a single healthy subject. Subject was presented with filled circles on a screen and auditory tones simultaneously (one of each per second). Ten per cent of circles was slightly larger or smaller, and 10% of tones were slightly higher or lower in frequency. Only the instruction changed every 30 seconds: (**a**) attend to tones only and respond when a tone is deviant; (**b**) attend to circles only and respond when a circle is deviant; (**c**) attend to both modalities and respond when either is deviant. Red voxels indicate significant response to tones. Yellow circles mark primary auditory cortex. Activity to tones is enhanced when attention is directed to tones, compared to attending to circles or to both modalities, in spite of the same auditory input.

generation of words — the verbal fluency test — patients perform poorly[38,39] which, in functional neuroimaging, is often regarded as a test for frontal brain function (implicitly associated with executive function)[40–43] rather than a measure of language function per se (see Fig. 7.3). The fact that these regions play a prominent role in these studies on schizophrenia, together with the findings of normal primary cortex function, suggest that a common factor in the imaging studies may be an impairment of effective regulation and coordination of neuronal activity in multiple brain regions.

3. **Information processing**

The notion that schizophrenia is characterized by deficient executive functions (i.e. mechanisms effectuating the conscious control of cognitive processes), particularly of working memory (WM), is well established[4,36, 44–47]. Neuropsychological studies indicate that executive functions are mediated primarily by frontal brain structures, as shown in patients with frontal lobe lesions and in healthy subjects[48–50]. When *in vivo* radioactivity-based brain imaging techniques became available in the early seventies, Ingvar and Franzen[51] measured regional cerebral bloodflow in schizophrenic patients. They observed that bloodflow in the frontal cortex was reduced in comparison to healthy controls, suggesting that frontal brain function was impaired. Since then, many studies have examined frontal lobe function in schizophrenia using bloodflow (H_2–^{15}O) as well as

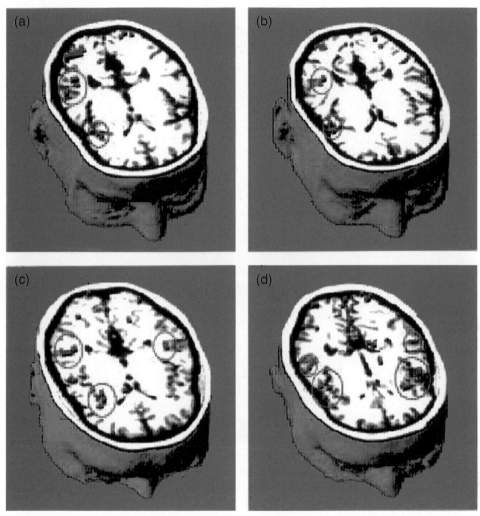

Fig. 7.2 Language activation patterns in a healthy monozygotic twin pair (**a,b**); in an unaffected co-twin (**c**); and in the twin with schizophrenia (**d**). Language-related activation is encircled (areas of Broca and Wernicke). The figure shows that both the schizophrenic patient and the unaffected co-twin exhibit more bilateral activity during language processing. (Reproduced with permission from Royal College of Psychiatrists[32].)

glucose metabolism ([18]FDG) PET measures, but the findings have not been not univocal: some found reduced activity[8,51–56]; others did not[57–59].

One of the problems associated with comparing subjects on images acquired during rest is that it is not directly relevant for brain function. Moreover, differences between groups of subjects may be a consequence of different mental processes occurring during scanning. Also, comparison of rest-state values may be confounded by non-specific effects of illness and/or medication on the cerebrovascular system or on neurophysiology. A logical next step[60] then was to assess activity during engagement in a cognitive task

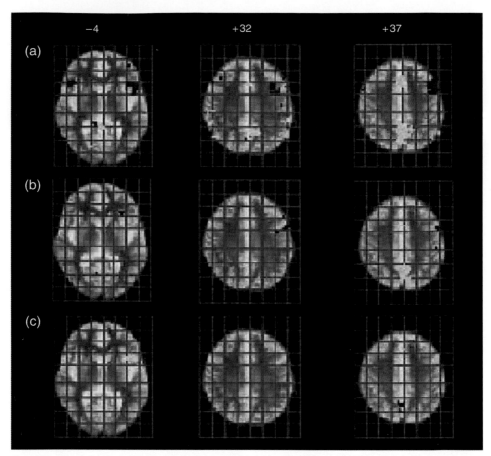

Fig. 7.3 Generic brain activation maps for FMRI data of a comparison group and a schizophrenic group and a map of significant between-group differences in power of periodic response during a verbal fluency task. Talairach z coordinates (10) are shown at the top of each column. The left side of each map represents the right side of the brain. (**a**) Generic brain activation map for comparison subjects. Red voxels are activated with maximum signal during word generation and yellow voxels are activated with maximum signal during word repetition. Voxelwise probability of type I error = 0.0002. (**b**) Generic brain activation map for schizophrenic subjects. Red voxels are activated with maximum signal during word generation and yellow voxels are activated with maximum signal during word repetition. Voxelwise probability of type I error = 0.0002. (**c**) ANCOVA map showing areas of significant between-group differences. Yellow voxels have greater power of response in comparison subjects; red voxels have greater power of response in schizophrenic subjects. Voxelwise probability of type I error = 0.01. (Reproduced with permission from American Psychiatric Association[64].)

that taxes the working memory system (i.e. to examine the brain when it is engaged in a specific mental act). For this purpose, neuropsychological tasks at which schizophrenic patients had been shown to perform poorly were modified so they could be administered while the patient was lying in the scanner. Activity measured during presentation of the task was compared to activity measured during a resting state or during another (control) task. Frontal hypofunction has since frequently been reported in patients when they were engaged in cognitive tasks that address executive function, such as the Wisconsin card sorting task (WCST)[61–63] or the verbal fluency task[40,41,64,65]. However, not all studies supported this finding[66,42,43]. Nevertheless, additional evidence was provided by studies using other tasks that were designed to address working memory function more explicitly[13,67–70]. It became widely accepted that the prefrontal cortex and, in particular, the dorsolateral prefrontal cortex, did not function properly in schizophrenic patients, and the assumption was that this was the cause of poor performance on WM tasks[4,71].

However, in the late 1990s, several studies questioned this assumption, suggesting that the concept of hypofrontality in schizophrenia is too simple, and that both the characteristics of the cognitive task used during functional imaging and performance are essential for the interpretation of functional brain imaging experiments. These studies report that under carefully controlled conditions, frontal activity is either normal[42,72] or even enhanced[73,74] in schizophrenic patients during engagement in working memory tasks, contradicting earlier reports. Authors noted that the results were associated with performance, in that equal (or enhanced) activity was observed when patients were capable of achieving a near-normal level of performance[73,42,74] (but see[13]).

3.1 More or less activity: good or bad?

Studies in healthy subjects have shown that if a WM task becomes more difficult (for instance, by increasing the amount of information that has to be processed — for an example of a parametric FMRI task, see Fig. 7.4), brain activity increases in the WM system[67,68,73,75–79]. Likewise, brain activity in the visual[80], auditory[81], and motor cortex[82,83] increases with an increasing rate of stimulus presentation or response generation. In the case of WM, activity increases until the task starts to strain the system causing an increase in errors in performance. At that point, activity declines[84,72], but performance also declines as a result of excessive demand and a concomitant failure to handle the amount of information. The decline may, therefore, reflect a decrease in the number of stimuli that are processed (i.e. skipping others) or a decrease in engagement (i.e. loss of motivation). The significance of this effect is that in healthy subjects, brain activity can rise or fall depending on the relative 'load' on the WM system[85].

For comparisons between schizophrenic patients and controls, there are two consequences to the load–response curve characteristics. Firstly, when performance is (near) optimal, brain activity is proportional to load. Consequently, reduced activity in patients at the same load and performance level as controls would indicate that patients activate as if the load is less than what it is in controls. In other words, patients would be better and physiologically more efficient than controls, which obviously is at odds with the generally accepted notion that patients are impaired. Secondly, when performance is poor, brain activity is also reduced in healthy subjects, as the result of excessive demand. Reduced activity in patients when they perform poorly is likely to result from the same mechanism. In this case, one can argue that hypoactivity in poorly performing patients is a normal phenomenon, albeit occurring at lower load than in controls. Clearly, the importance of incorporating performance in the interpretation of activity differences cannot be overemphasized[68, 86].

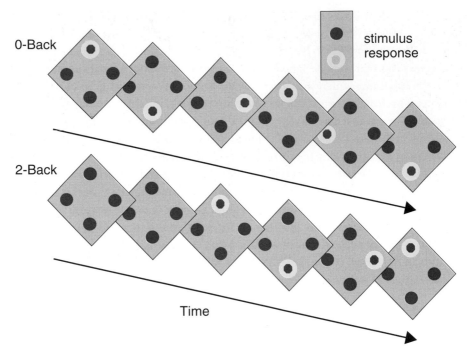

Fig. 7.4 An example is shown for a task that taxes the working memory system with different levels of difficulty (a parametric n-back task design). Two levels are shown (0-back and 2-back). The trials are presented one after the other, with a red dot as stimulus displayed on the grey diamond background, and are the same for both levels. The instruction, 0- or 2-back, indicates what the subject has to do: at 0-back he has to press the button (on a button box with the same diamond layout) corresponding to the location of the stimulus. At 2-back, the subject has to respond to the location of the stimulus that was presented two trials back. For this, the subject has to memorize the location of the current stimulus location, remember the previous one, and retrieve and respond to the stimulus presented two trials back. Correct responses are circled in yellow. The difference between 0- and 2-back is the number of items that have to be held in working memory. (Reproduced with permission from Elsevier Publishers[76].)

3.2 **DLPFC as a candidate centre of dysfunction**

Several investigators have conducted studies to take the load–response factor into account in schizophrenic patients[69,72,73,87,88]. As could be expected, activity in the WM system does increase in schizophrenic patients to normal levels, albeit at lower load levels, and it levels off or declines (depending on the brain region) at lower load levels than in controls[69,72,73]. This apparent shift in the load–response curve[85] is interpreted as reflecting a reduction of processing capacity[1,72] and of physiological efficiency[1,73,74]. An important question is whether this shift can be attributed to specific regions (notably DLPFC). In several studies, the increase in load beyond capacity resulted in a decline of activity in the DLPFC selectively, as opposed to the parietal and medial frontal cortex[13,69,72,74] (see Fig. 7.5). However, this selective decline may well be a normal response to excessive demand on WM[72], in accordance with the notion that the

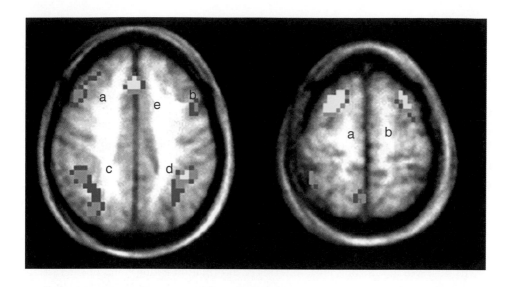

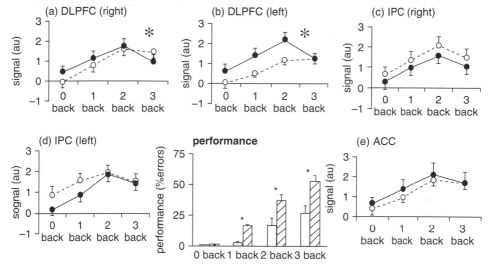

Fig. 7.5 The increase in activity that follows the increase in working memory load (task is shown in Fig. 7.2). Ten schizophrenic patients on atypical neuroleptic medication and ten healthy controls performed the task at 4 levels (0- to 3-back). The 0-back task served as the baseline for the other levels. Data from all subjects and levels were analysed together to obtain the main activity map (i.e. significant activity in both groups combined, in any of the three higher levels compared to 0-back) depicting the working memory system. Two slices of this activity map are displayed, with magnitude of activity in colour (yellow is strong activation). In each of the active regions, the FMRI signal was averaged separately for each group and each level. The graphs display the magnitude of activity for each region (DLPFC: dorsolateral prefrontal cortex; ACC: anterior cingulated cortex; IPC: inferior parietal cortex). Solid lines and striped bars represent patients. Patients exhibit a decline of activity in the DLPFC when performance approaches chance (3-back). No significant difference is seen in the other regions. (Reproduced with permission from Elsevier Publishers[72].)

load–response curve is shifted to the left[72, 85]. Nevertheless, the DLPFC remains a prominent player in the studies that support the inefficiency notion of WM in schizophrenia, given that there are multiple sources of (indirect) evidence for DLPFC dysfunction[89] (but see[90] for a critical review).

Evidence for selective DLPFC dysfunction is provided, to some degree, by other techniques. Bertolino and colleagues have shown that neuronal integrity is affected selectively in the DLPFC and hippocampus, as indicated by reduced N- acetylaspartate measures (an intraneuronal marker of neuronal functional integrity) in medication-free patients[145], and that this ratio in the DLPFC, specifically, is altered by antipsychotic medication[91] and is associated with activity in the WM network[73,92]. Laruelle and colleagues have shown that in the prefrontal cortex, sensitivity for dopaminergic neurotransmission is enhanced, both in terms of amphetamine-induced presynaptic dopamine release[93] and in terms of an up-regulation of D1 receptors[94]. Others have also attributed an important role for dopamine transmission mechanisms in the prefrontal cortex to the cognitive deficits observed in schizophrenia, in terms of information gating[95] and of interactions between dopaminergic, GABAergic, and glutamatergic neurons[96]. (For an extensive review on DLFPC function in schizophrenia see[97,89].)

The prefrontal cortex is not the only region that is under suspicion. Several studies indicate that activity in other nodes of the WM network also behave differently[64, 68,98], suggesting that the network as a whole operates inefficiently[72, 86]. Whether this is a consequence of region-selective dysfunction or of abnormal communication between regions remains to be seen. The other nodes of the WM system — the posterior parietal cortex[99] and the anterior cingulate cortex[100,101] have also been implicated in the cognitive deficits. As most of these regions are part of the same WM system(s), one of the main questions that lie ahead is how they interact in health and in schizophrenia. This interaction is not likely to be static, in the sense that it is always the same given specific circumstances. For instance, the way the brain processes information quite often depends on previous experience, adjusting processing strategies to familiarity of circumstances and using previous feedback about outcome of actions.

3.3 Functional plasticity

In functional neuroimaging, WM is generally assumed to be a static system in the sense that it responds in predictable ways to controlled settings such as WM tasks. However, it is very likely that there are multiple factors that affect how the WM system deals with demands. One is experience-induced adaptation. It is well known in neuropsychology that performance on cognitive tasks improves greatly when repeating the tests, even when the sets of stimuli are replaced with new ones to avoid recognition effects. This test–retest effect is probably due to the fact that the rules, requirements, and appearance of the tasks becomes familiar, resulting in a narrowing down of the possible stimulus features that are relevant for the task as well as the responses that are required, and, consequently, a different way of processing information.

These modulating factors pertain to a well-known dualism in human cognition — the distinction between controlled and automatic processing[102,103]. Behaviour consists of multiple components of perception, information processing, and response generation, each of which can operate in an automatic or controlled mode[104]. The distinction between these modes can best be described in terms of efficiency, in that automatic processing is effortless and relatively rigid, whereas controlled processing is effortful (claiming limited processing resources) and highly adaptive[103]. The underlying brain processes are thought to differ in that automatic processing appears to be based on long-term memory access, while controlled processing involves a conscious application of algorithms to the task[102, 103, 105, 106]. Many brain functions initially operate in controlled mode (i.e. when a task is new) and will shift into automatic mode through practice. Behaviour, including performance of FMRI tasks, is composed of multiple units, each of which may either operate in automatic mode (e.g. decode visual stimuli into letters or words, and generating the motor program to press a button) or in controlled mode (e.g. decide whether a stimulus is a target or not). Importantly, when given the chance to practise, the latter will often progress into automatic mode, resulting in faster responses and less errors[107], in which case there is a transition phase[105] from one modus to the other. Several studies have now shown that practice also leads to a reduction of brain activity[108,109].

Behavioural tests of automatization, like procedural learning tests, generally indicate that performance of schizophrenic patients improves with practice to the same degree as in normal subjects[110], although typical antipsychotic drugs may cause some disturbance[111]. The notion of inefficient processing in WM would predict that although performance improves with practice, undue claims on processing resources remain. Indeed, some behavioural studies have shown that in patients, practice of a cognitive task does not enable them to maintain good performance when a second task is added[112], as opposed to healthy subjects (e.g.[105]). A recent study reports that the reduction in brain activity following practice of a WM task[113] predicted performance in a dual task paradigm (i.e. how well performance is maintained when a second task is added) which is thought to measure processing capacity. Using the same paradigm, schizophrenic patients exhibited a normal improvement in performance, but failed to reduce activity in the WM system (Jansma *et al*, unpublished). A similar phenomenon has been reported for motor learning in schizophrenia[114]. Taken together, these studies suggest that neurophysiological inefficiency of information processing observed in schizophrenia may be associated with a failure to free processing resources that are limited by nature.

3.4 Networks and circuits

With the advent of radiological imaging techniques, the search for dysfunctional structures in schizophrenia took a flight but, at the same time, theories of dysfunctional networks gained interest, in the face of lack of convincing evidence for regional lesions. FMRI stimulated further development of network-based theories of cognition[2,115,116], providing more avenues to examine the possible mechanisms behind cognitive deficits in schizophrenia[4,117–119]. The various network approaches have, in common, that they address cognition.

To study networks, FMRI data can be used for assessment of coherence in activity between regions. Coherence is generally measured across subjects, by computing correlations between levels of activity in a predetermined set of regions (e.g. see[120]), but can also be applied to single subjects (e.g. see[121]). The analytical procedures involved are rather complex, entailing structural equation modelling and principle component analysis, but, in essence, they are aimed at explaining the variance in the data as best as possible, using a set of potential contributors (factors) including tasks, regions, and group membership. The question is, what kind of information connectivity analysis will yield[2] and whether it can provide some understanding of the neuronal mechanism underlying impaired performance in patients. Connectivity can be assessed in two ways — as correlations between brain regions ('functional connectivity'[120–122]) and as effects of one region on the activity within, or interaction between, other regions ('effective connectivity'[2,123]). Whereas functional connectivity can be performed without prior assumptions about involved regions, effective connectivity requires an explicit theoretical model stating the regions that form the network, and the expected directions of communication between each of the pairs of regions.

An interesting mechanism-oriented approach is taken by Frith, Dolan, and colleagues, who postulate that neural integration between DLPFC, superior temporal lobes, the posterior cingulate, and the medial prefrontal cortices is impaired[42,118]. They associate the degree of impairment with severity of the clinical manifestations of the disorder, and attribute an important role of both the dopamine system and DLPFC to the underlying mechanism[101,124]. Involvement of dopamine in working memory and DLPFC is indicated by non-human primate studies[125]. Dolan *et al* reported that abnormal activity in the anterior cingulate cortex (generally associated with attentional and response selection processes) and superior temporal gyrus (associated with auditory processing) in medication-free schizophrenic patients was partly normalized by the dopamine-blocking effects of apomorphine[101,124] which, the authors argue, reflects normalization of fronto-temporal interaction[124]. Connectivity between prefrontal and temporal regions is impaired[120,126,127], and this appears to be caused by impaired modulation of that connection by the anterior cingulate cortex[126]. However, others failed to replicate the fronto-temporal disconnection and reported disconnection between frontal regions (DLPFC and the anterior cingulate cortex) instead[128]. Nevertheless, the principle of viewing and approaching brain functions in terms of networks with mechanistic rules that govern interaction between regions is quite appealing and will undoubtedly be stimulated by FMRI technology. Discovering how regions communicate with each other, and how communication impairments relate to schizophrenia, will ultimately require knowledge about mechanisms underlying neuronal function and interaction. This, in turn, is most likely to be associated with intracellular processes, neurotransmitter dynamics, and, ultimately, genes and gene expression.

3.5 Genetic predisposing factors

The search for a genetic cause of schizophrenia has not been very successful, most likely due to the fact that multiple genes are involved. Twin and family studies have revealed a clear genetic contribution, but also that environmental factors determine whether or not the illness is expressed[129]. The search for specific genes has generally taken a syndrome-guided route, whereby direct links were sought between the illness and genes. A different strategy has emerged in recent years, where phenotypes are defined not on the basis of clinical symptoms but on specific traits, including cognitive functions[130], often referred to as the intermediate or endophenotype approach. Given that it is very likely that schizophrenia involves multiple genes, it is quite conceivable that the disease-promoting genotypes for each gene are present in many non-schizophrenic individuals. What distinguishes patients from healthy subjects is that patients are equipped with (one of) several sets of traits and genotypes[89] (see Fig. 7.8). One of the problems in working with behavioural phenotypes is that behaviour is, generally, an end result of multiple brain systems working in parallel and/or in synergy. When a particular system is impaired, other systems are often capable of compensating for the deficit, thereby hiding the impairment. Given that those systems must have a neuronal basis, it is likely that impaired brain function is only measurable with *in vivo* neuroimaging techniques, particularly if the impairment is mild[131,132].

For a neurobiological endophenotype approach, the choice of the phenotype is based on cognitive functions that have been shown to be disrupted in schizophrenic patients as well as in non-schizophrenic family members. From there, one searches for a gene that is associated with that function (i.e. a candidate gene)[89,130,133]. None of these impairments are selective markers for susceptibility to schizophrenia, supporting the notion that multiple impairments are required. Application of the neurophysiological measures for these impairments to the search for responsible genes requires knowledge of the brain activity pattern in healthy subjects and the abnormalities in these patterns that correspond to the behavioural deficits in schizophrenia. For several functions that meet the criteria for being potential endophenotypes, this has been assessed to varying degrees — the prefrontal cortex[73] in working memory, the prefrontal cortex[134,135] and striatum[136] in saccade inhibition, the anterior cingulate cortex[137] in attention, laterality in the language system[138] in language, and the hippocampus[139] in memory.

Weinberger and his group were one of the first to link alleles of a specific gene to brain activity and performance on the FMRI task[89,140]. The gene that encodes the enzyme catechol-o-methyl-transferase (COMT), which methylates released dopamine, is present in the general population in two types — the valine (val) and the methionine (met) allele[141] — which differ in the degree of enzyme activity. The val-val genotype exhibits a higher rate of dopamine breakdown (notably in the frontal cortex) than the met-val genotype, which in turn exhibits higher rates than met-met genotype. The COMT gene affects working memory in the sense that the met-met genotype (with more dopamine available in the synapse) is associated with better performance on an N-back WM task[140] (which is shown in Fig. 7.4) and with better efficiency of activity in the DLPFC as compared to the met-val or val-val genotype[140,142], possibly by facilitation of maintenance of information in that part of the WM system (see Fig. 7.6). The variance of WM performance that is explained by genotype appears to be small (i.e. 4%) but considering that WM is a highly complex function, involving many aspects of information handling, it is probably a realistic contribution of one gene to such a brain function[89]. Of course, this finding is a small

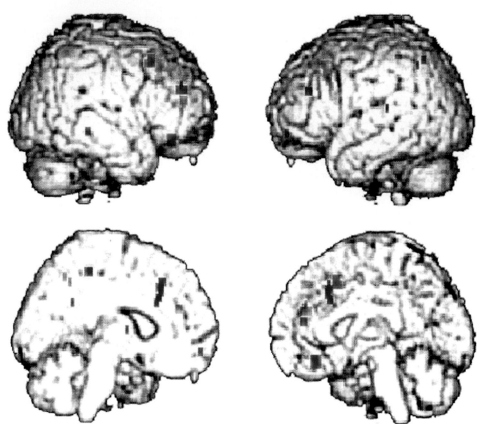

Fig. 7.6 Effect of COMT genotype on FMRI activation during the 2-back working memory task (shown in Fig. 7.4). Regions showing a significant effect of genotype on FMRI activation (voxelwise $P < 0.005$) are in red (shown clockwise from upper left in right lateral, left lateral, right medial, and left medial views, respectively). In the dorsolateral prefrontal cortex (e.g. Brodmann area 46; $x = 58$, $y = 32$, $z = 12$; cluster size = 47; $Z = 2.55$) and the anterior cingulate (e.g. Brodmann area 32; $x = 6$, $y = 60$, $z = 8$; cluster size = 77; $Z = 2.36$), val/val individuals showed a greater FMRI response (and by inference, greater inefficiency, as performance is similar) than val/met individuals, who have greater activation than met/met individuals. This shows that the met allele is associated with greater neurophysiological efficiency (i.e. less activity for same performance). (Reproduced with permission from the National Academy of Sciences[140].)

step in the process of attributing (elements of) cognitive brain functions to specific genes, but the concept is quite appealing. The various genotypes of the COMT gene are present across the human population, but as it turns out, the val allele is more frequent in patients with schizophrenia than in the general population[140].

Several other candidate genes are now being linked to brain function, such as those coding for aspects of vascular development in association with WM function[143], brain-derived neurotrophic factor (BDNF) in association with hippocampus function[146], and for the serotonin transporter in association with amygdala function[144] (see Fig. 7.7). This endophenotype approach differs from earlier approaches to identifying genes for

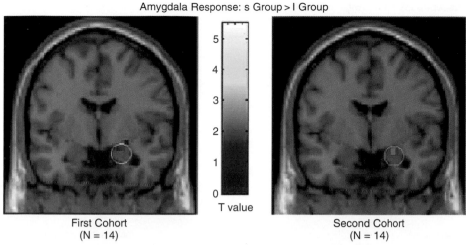

Amygdala Response: s Group > l Group

First Cohort
(N = 14)

Second Cohort
(N = 14)

Fig. 7.7 Association between BOLD response in amygdala to fearful faces and two alleles of the serotonin transporter gene 5-HTTLPR. The genotype-based parametric comparisons show significantly greater activity in the right amygdala of the short allele group (left) versus the long allele group (right), in two independent cohorts. BOLD FMRI responses in the right amygdala (white circle) are shown overlaid onto an averaged structural MRI in the coronal plane through the centre of the amygdala. Talairach coordinates and voxel level statistics ($P< 0.05$, corrected) for the maximal voxel in the right amygdala are as follows, for the first and second cohort respectively, $x = 24$ mm, $y = 8$ mm, $z = 16$ mm; cluster size = 4 voxels; voxel level corrected P value = 0.021; T score = 2.89, and $x = 28$ mm, $y = 4$ mm, $z = 16$ mm; cluster size = 2 voxels; voxel level corrected P value = 0.047; T score = 2.03. (Reproduced with permission from the American Association for the Advancement of Science[144].)

schizophrenia in that the gene need not be specific for the illness. Rather, it is viewed as one of multiple susceptibility genotypes, each of which can be found throughout the population. Only when a certain number of such genes are present within one individual, will he or she be genetically predisposed to developing the illness. Whether the person becomes schizophrenic then depends on environmental factors (see Fig. 7.8).

4. Summary

Functional neuroimaging has acquired a prominent position in schizophrenia research. Apart from being a means of describing processes in the brain and visualizing differences in brain function between patients and controls, it carries the promise of providing insight into the way cognitive functions are organized in the brain and how abnormal organization can explain cognitive deficits in schizophrenia. The imaging studies reviewed in this chapter indicate that, inasfar as there are abnormalities in function of primary cortices, they may, at least partly, be associated with impaired top-down regulation. Higher-order brain processes, such as language processing and working memory, do seem to be affected, and this may be associated with an impaired capability to exert control over regions within networks. For instance, auditory/verbal hallucinations seem

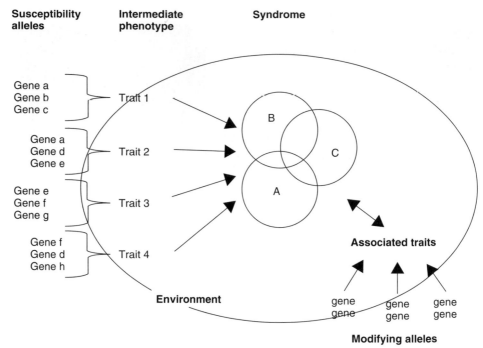

Fig. 7.8 Schematic representation of a multidimensional view of the genetic basis for schizophrenia. More than one gene can contribute to a particular trait, and multiple traits contribute to syndromes or symptoms. Traits can be used as endophenotypes associated with specific alleles. Other genes can code for traits that interact with the syndromes, such as gender and temperament. Environmental factors influence the effects of genes, traits, and syndromes on susceptibility for schizophrenia. (Reproduced with permission from Elsevier Publishers[89].)

to be associated with a reduced ability to suppress endogenous activity in the left, and possibly in the right, hemisphere language regions. WM is impaired in patients and is accompanied by hypo- or hyperactivity in the WM network, depending on the load imposed by the task, which reflects inefficiency of information processing and a resulting reduction of processing capacity.

Many of the FMRI and PET rCBF findings fit the view that schizophrenia is associated with poor attentional regulation of information processing. Although there is some indication that specific brain structures, notably the DLPFC, play a cardinal role in impaired regulation, the main emerging trend is to assess properties of communication between regions that form a network. Most advanced are theories on the dynamics of WM networks and the potential disruption that could explain cognitive deficits and, eventually, clinical symptoms. Advances in data analysis give the impression that networks can be revealed and characterized with FMRI experiments. However, this may be true for building models of brain functions, but putting models to the test in the context of psychopathology ultimately requires interventional approaches such as localized brain stimulation by means of TMS or application of psychotropic agents.

Apart from the expected developments in the design of brain activity-based models for cognitive functions and the ability to explain cognitive deficits in terms of communication within networks, the most promising approach is that of associating brain (dys)functions (i.e. endophenotypes) with genotypes. It is not clear yet whether this approach will be successful, given that brain function is governed by highly complex interactions between multiple sets of neurons, whereas genes code for the molecular make-up of cells. In other words, the gap between intra-cellular processes and brain activity patterns is still very large. Yet, this gap is much smaller than that between genes and behavioural measures. The endophenotype approach also reflects a conceptual shift in schizophrenia research towards a multidimensional view of brain dysfunction. The brain activity characteristics underlying cognitive deficits that are not necessarily specific for schizophrenia, form endophenotypes. Conforming to the notion that schizophrenia is associated with multiple genes, the multidimensional approach is based on the premise that the illness, or susceptibility for the illness, develops only when a certain number or constellation of affected genes (and associated endophenotypes) is present in an individual[89].

To summarize the functional neuroimaging studies on schizophrenia, reiterating the main questions stated earlier, there is evidence that function of the DLPFC is selectively impaired but, as of yet, there is limited evidence for significant and selective pathology in other regions. Evidence is accumulating that communication within networks that subserve WM is affected, but it is not clear yet how this translates to cognitive deficits and clinical symptoms. However, with the rapid development of mechanistic models for WM (e.g. see[4]), based on functional imaging and techniques for manipulating brain activity such as TMS, it is likely that, in the near future, theories of behavioural deficits and symptoms will incorporate specific neuronal interactions, thereby lending themselves to rigorous testing. Finally, the effort to link genes to brain activity is promising and can provide insight in the neurophysiological mechanisms underlying brain dysfunction in schizophrenia.

References

1. Ramsey, N.F., Hoogduin, H., and Jansma, J.M. 2002, Functional MRI experiments: acquisition, analysis and interpretation of data, *European Neuropsychopharmacology*, **12**:6, 517–26.

2. Friston, K. 2002, Beyond phrenology: what can neuroimaging tell us about distributed circuitry? *Ann Rev Neurosci*, **25**, 221–50.

3. Andreasen, N.C., Nopoulos, P., Oleary, D.S., Miller, D.D., Wassink, T., and Flaum, L. 1999, Defining the phenotype of schizophrenia: cognitive dysmetria and its neural mechanisms, *Biol Psychiat*, **46**:7, 908–20.

4. Cohen, J.D., Braver, T.S., and O'Reilly, R.C. 1996, A computational approach to prefrontal cortex, cognitive control and schizophrenia: recent developments and current challenges, *Philos Trans R Soc Lond B Biol Sci*, **351**:1346, 1515–27.

5. Cahn, W., Pol, H.E., Lems, E.B., van Haren, N.E., Schnack, H.G., van der Linden, J.A., *et al.* 2002, Brain volume changes in first-episode schizophrenia: a 1-year follow-up study, *Arch Gen Psychiatry*, **59**:11, 1002–10.

6. Cadenhead, K.S., Swerdlow, N.R., Shafer, K.M., Diaz, M., and Braff, D.L. 2000, Modulation of the startle response and startle laterality in relatives of schizophrenic patients and in subjects with schizotypal personality disorder: evidence of inhibitory deficits, *Am J Psychiatry*, **157**:10, 1660–8.

7. Freedman, R., Waldo, M., Bickford–Wimer, P., and Nagamoto, H. 1991, Elementary neuronal dysfunctions in schizophrenia, *Schizophr Res*, **4**:2, 233–43.

8. Hazlett, E.A., Buchsbaum, M.S., Haznedar, M.M., Singer, M.B., Germans, M.K., Schnur, D.B., *et al.* 1998, Prefrontal cortex glucose metabolism and startle eyeblink modification abnormalities in unmedicated schizophrenia patients, *Psychophysiology*, **35**:2, 186–98.

9. Braus, D.F., Weber–Fahr, W., Tost, H., Ruf, M., and Henn, F.A. 2002, Sensory information processing in neuroleptic-naive first-episode schizophrenic patients: a functional magnetic resonance imaging study, *Arch Gen Psychiatry*, **59**:8, 696–701.

10. Talairach, J., and Tournont, P., 1988, A co-planar atlas of a human brain. Theime, Stuttgart.

11. Renshaw, P.F., Yurgelun Todd, D.A., and Cohen, B.M. 1994, Greater hemodynamic response to photic stimulation in schizophrenic patients: an echo planar MRI study, *Am J Psychiatry*, **151**:10, 1493–5.

12. Taylor, S.F., Tandon, R., and Koeppe, R.A. 1997, PET study of greater visual activation in schizophrenia, *Am J Psychiatry*, **154**:9, 1296–8.

13. Barch, D.M., Carter, C.S., Braver, T.S., Sabb, F.W., MacDonald, A., III, Noll, D.C. *et al.* 2001, Selective deficits in prefrontal cortex function in medication-naive patients with schizophrenia, *Arch Gen Psychiatry*, **58**:3, 280–8.

14. Braus, D.F., Ende, G., Weber–Fahr, W., Sartorius, A., Krier, A., Hubrich–Ungureanu, P., *et al.* 1999, Antipsychotic drug effects on motor activation measured by functional magnetic resonance imaging in schizophrenic patients, *Schizophr Res*, **39**:1, 19–29.

15. Schroder, J., Wenz, F., Schad, L.R., Baudendistel, K., and Knopp, M.V. 1995, Sensorimotor cortex and supplementary motor area changes in schizophrenia. A study with functional magnetic resonance imaging, *Br J Psychiatry*, **167**:2, 197–201.

16. Schroder, J., Essig, M., Baudendistel, K., Jahn, T., Gerdsen, I., Stockert, A., *et al.* 1999, Motor dysfunction and sensorimotor cortex activation changes in schizophrenia: a study with functional magnetic resonance imaging, *Neuroimage*, **9**:1, 81–7.

17. Buckley, P.F., Friedman, L., Wu, D., Lai, S., Meltzer, H.Y., Haacke, E.M., *et al.* 1997, Functional magnetic resonance imaging in schizophrenia: initial methodology and evaluation of the motor cortex, *Psychiatry Res*, **74**:1, 13–23.

18. Corbetta, M., Akbudak, E., Conturo, T.E., Snyder, A.Z., Ollinger, J.M., Drury, H.A., *et al.* 1998, A common network of functional areas for attention and eye movements, *Neuron*, **21**:4, 761–73.

19. Courtney, S.M. and Ungerleider, L.G. 1997, What FMRI has taught us about human vision, *Curr Opin Neurobiol*, **7**:4, 554–61.

20. Culham, J.C., Brandt, S.A., Cavanagh, P., Kanwisher, N.G., Dale, A.M., and Tootell, R.B. H. 1998, Cortical FMRI activation produced by attentive tracking of moving targets, *J Neurophysiol*, **80**:5, 2657–70.

21. Johansen, B.H., Christensen, V., Woolrich, M., and Matthews, P.M. 2000, Attention to touch modulates activity in both primary and secondary somatosensory areas, *Neuroreport*, **11**:6, 1237–41.

22. Pugh, K.R., Shaywitz, B.A., Fulbright, R.K., Byrd, D., Skudlarski, P., Katz, L., *et al.* 1996, Auditory selective attention: an FMRI investigation, *Neuroimage*, **4**:3(Part 1), 159–73.

23. Bentaleb, L.A., Beauregard, M., Liddle, P., and Stip, E. 2002, Cerebral activity associated with auditory verbal hallucinations: a functional magnetic resonance imaging case study, *J Psychiatry Neurosci*, **27**:2, 110–5.

24. Dierks, T., Linden, D.E., Jandl, M., Formisano, E., Goebel, R., Lanfermann, H., *et al.* 1999, Activation of Heschl's gyrus during auditory hallucinations, *Neuron*, **22**:3, 615–21.

25. Lennox, B.R., Park, S.B., Jones, P.B., Morris, P.G., and Park, G. 1999, Spatial and temporal mapping of neural activity associated with auditory hallucinations, *Lancet*, **353**:9153, 644.

26. Shergill, S.S., Brammer, M.J., Williams, S.C., Murray, R.M., and McGuire, P.K. 2000, Mapping auditory hallucinations in schizophrenia using functional magnetic resonance imaging, *Arch Gen Psychiatry*, **57**:11, 1033–8.

27. Woodruff, P.W., Wright, I.C., Bullmore, E.T., Brammer, M., Howard, R.J., Williams, S.C., *et al.* 1997, Auditory hallucinations and the temporal cortical response to speech in schizophrenia: a functional magnetic resonance imaging study, *Am J Psychiatry*, **154**:12, 1676–82.

28. Fallgatter, A.J. and Strik, W.K. 2000, Reduced frontal functional asymmetry in schizophrenia during a cued continuous performance test assessed with near-infrared spectroscopy, *Schizophrenia Bulletin*, **26**:4, 913–9.

29. Gur, R.E. and Chin, S. 1999, Laterality in functional brain imaging studies of schizophrenia, *Schizophrenia Bull*, **25**:1, 141–56.

30. Sommer, I.E., Ramsey, N.F., Mandl, R.C., and Kahn, R.S. 2003, Language lateralization in female patients with schizophrenia: an FMRI study, *Schizophr Res*, **60**:2–3, 183–90.

31. Sommer, I.E., Ramsey, N.F., and Kahn, R.S. 2001, Language lateralization in schizophrenia, an FMRI study, *Schizophr Res*, **52**:1–2, 57–67.

32. Sommer, I.E., Ramsey, N.F., Mandl, R.C., van Oel, C.J., and Kahn, R.S. 2004, Language activation in monozygotic twins discordant for schizophrenia, *Br J Psychiatry*, **184**:2, 128–35.

33. Kircher, T.T., Liddle, P.F., Brammer, M.J., Williams, S.C., Murray, R.M., and McGuire, P.K. 2002, Reversed lateralization of temporal activation during speech production in thought disordered patients with schizophrenia, *Psychol Med*, **32**:3, 439–49.

34. Wenz, F., Schad, L.R., Knopp, M.V., Baudendistel, K.T., Flomer, F., Schroder, J., *et al.* 1994, Functional magnetic resonance imaging at 1.5 T: activation pattern in schizophrenic patients receiving neuroleptic medication, *Magn Reson Imaging*, **12**:7, 975–82.

35. Winterer, G., Egan, M.F., Radler, T., Hyde, T., Coppola, R., and Weinberger, D.R. 2001, An association between reduced interhemispheric EEG coherence in the temporal lobe and genetic risk for schizophrenia, *Schizophr Res*, **49**:1–2, 129–43.

36. Heinrichs, R.W. and Zakzanis, K.K. 1998, Neurocognitive deficit in schizophrenia: a quantitative review of the evidence, *Neuropsychology*, **12**:3, 426–45.

37. Spitzer, M., Weisker, I., Winter, M., Maier, S., Hermle, L., and Maher, B.A. 1994, Semantic and phonological priming in schizophrenia, *J Abnorm Psychol*, **103**, 485–94.

38. Bokat, C.E. and Goldberg, T.E. 2003, Letter and category fluency in schizophrenic patients: a meta-analysis, *Schizophr Res*, **64**:1, 73–8.

39. Kerns, J.G., Berenbaum, H., Barch, D.M., Banich, M.T., and Stolar, N. 1999, Word production in schizophrenia and its relationship to positive symptoms, *Psychiatry Res*, **87**:1, 29–37.

40. Bullmore, E., Brammer, M., Williams, S.C., Curtis, V., McGuire, P., Morris, R., *et al.* 1999, Functional MR imaging of confounded hypofrontality, *Hum Brain Mapp*, **8**:2–3, 86–91.

41. Curtis, V.A., Bullmore, E.T., Brammer, M.J., Wright, I.C., Williams, S.C.R., Morris, R.G., *et al.* 1998, Attenuated frontal activation during a verbal fluency task in patients with schizophrenia, *Am J Psychiatry*, **155**:8, 1056–63.

42. Frith, C.D., Friston, K.J., Herold, S., Silbersweig, D., Fletcher, P., Cahill, C., *et al.* 1995, Regional brain activity in chronic schizophrenic patients during the performance of a verbal fluency task, *Br J Psychiatry*, **167**:3, 343–9.

43. Mellers, J.D., Adachi, N., Takei, N., Cluckie, A., Toone, B.K., and Lishman, W.A. 1998, SPET study of verbal fluency in schizophrenia and epilepsy, *Br J Psychiatry*, **173**, 69–74.

44. Goldman–Rakic, P.S. 1994, Working memory dysfunction in schizophrenia, *Journal of Neuropsychiatry and Clinical Neurosciences*, **6**, 348–57.

45. Morice, R. and Delahunty, A. 1996, Frontal/executive impairments in schizophrenia, *Schizophrenia Bulletin*, **22**:1, 125–37.

46. Park, S. and Holzman, P.S. 1992, Schizophrenics show spatial working memory deficits, *Arch Gen Psychiatry*, **49**:12, 975–82.

47. Weickert, T.W., Goldberg, T.E., Gold, J.M., Bigelow, L.B., Egan, M.F., and Weinberger, D.R. 2000, Cognitive impairments in patients with schizophrenia displaying preserved and compromised intellect, *Arch Gen Psychiatry*, **57**:9, 907–13.

48. Baddeley, A. and Della, S.S. 1996, Working memory and executive control, *Philos Trans R Soc Lond B Biol Sci*, **351**:1346, 1397–403.

49. Freedman, M., Black, S., Ebert, P., and Binns, M. 1998, Orbitofrontal function, object alternation and perseveration, *Cereb Cortex*, **8**:1, 18–27.

50. Fuster, J.M. 1989, *The prefrontal cortex* Raven Press, New York.

51. Ingvar, D.H. and Franzen, G. 1974, Distribution of cerebral activity in chronic schizophrenia, *Lancet*, **2**:7895, 1484–6.

52. Alavi, A., Dann, R., Chawluk, J., Alavi, J., Kushner, M., and Reivich, M. 1986, Positron emission tomography imaging of regional cerebral glucose metabolism, *Semin Nucl Med*, **16**:1, 2–34.

53. Andreasen, N.C., O'Leary, D.S., Flaum, M., Nopoulos, P., Watkins, G.L., Boles Ponto, L. *et al.* 1997, Hypofrontality in schizophrenia: distributed dysfunctional circuits in neuroleptic-naive patients, *Lancet*, **349**:9067, 1730–4.

54. Brodie, J.D., Christman, D.R., Corona, J.F., Fowler, J.S., Gomez–Mont, F., Jaeger, J., 1984, Patterns of metabolic activity in the treatment of schizophrenia, *Ann Neurol*, **15**(Suppl), S166-9.

55. Cohen, R.M., Semple, W.E., Gross, M., Nordahl, T.E., DeLisi, L.E., Holcomb, H.H., *et al.* 1987, Dysfunction in a prefrontal substrate of sustained attention in schizophrenia, *Life Sci*, **40**:20, 2031–9.

56. Hazlett, E.A., Buchsbaum, M.S., Jeu, L.A., Nenadic, I., Fleischman, M.B., Shihabuddin, L., 2000, Hypofrontality in unmedicated schizophrenia patients studied with PET during performance of a serial verbal learning task, *Schizophrenia Research.*, **43**:1, 33–46.

57. Ebmeier, K.P., Lawrie, S.M., Blackwood, D.H., Johnstone, E.C., and Goodwin, G.M. 1995, Hypofrontality revisited: a high resolution single photon emission computed tomography study in schizophrenia, *J Neurol Neurosurg Psychiatry*, **58**:4, 452–6.

58. Jernigan, T.L., Sargent, T., III, Pfefferbaum, A., Kusubov, N., and Stahl, S.M. 1985, 18Fluorodeoxyglucose PET in schizophrenia, *Psychiatry Res*, **16**:4, 317–29.

59. Volkow, N.D., Brodie, J.D., Wolf, A.P., Angrist, B., Russell, J., and Cancro, R. 1986, Brain metabolism in patients with schizophrenia before and after acute neuroleptic administration, *J Neurol Neurosurg Psychiatry*, **49**:10, 1199–202.

60. Weinberger, D.R. and Berman, K.F. 1988, Speculation on the meaning of cerebral metabolic hypofrontality in schizophrenia, *Schizophrenia Bulletin*, **14**:2, 157–68.

61. Berman, K.F., Zec, R.F., and Weinberger, D.R. 1986, Physiologic dysfunction of dorsolateral pre-frontal cortex in schizophrenia. II. Role of neuroleptic treatment, attention, and mental effort, *Arch Gen Psychiatry*, **43**, 126–35.

62. Milner, B. 1964, Some effects of frontal lobectomy in man, in *The granular cortex and behavior* (eds. J. M. Warren and K. Akert), McGraw–Hill, New York, pp. 313–34.

63. Weinberger, D.R., Berman, K.F., and Zec, R.F. 1986, Physiological dysfunction of dorsolateral prefrontal cortex in schizophrenia 1: regional cerebral bloodflow (rCBF) evidence, *Arch Gen Psychiatry*, **43**, 114–25.

64. Curtis, V.A., Bullmore, E.T., Morris, R.G., Brammer, M.J., Williams, S.C., Simmons, A., *et al.* 1999, Attenuated frontal activation in schizophrenia may be task dependent, *Schizophr Res*, **37**:1, 35–44.

65. Yurgelun–Todd, D.A., Waternaux, C.M., Cohen, B.M., Gruber, S.A., English, C.D., and Renshaw, P.F. 1996, Functional magnetic resonance imaging of schizophrenic patients and comparison subjects during word production, *Am J Psychiatry*, **153**:2, 200–5.

66. Dye, S.M., Spence, S.A., Bench, C.J., Hirsch, S.R., Stefan, M.D., Sharma, T., *et al.* 1999, No evidence for left superior temporal dysfunction in asymptomatic schizophrenia and bipolar disorder — PET study of verbal fluency, *Brit J Psychiat*, **175**, 367–374.

67. Callicott, J.H., Ramsey, N.F., Tallent, K., Bertolino, A., Knable, M.B., Coppola, R., *et al.* 1998, Functional magnetic resonance imaging brain mapping in psychiatry: methodological issues illustrated in a study of working memory in schizophrenia, *Neuropsychopharmacology*, **18**: 3, 186–96.

68. Fletcher, P.C., McKenna, P.J., Frith, C.D., Grasby, P.M., Friston, K.J., and Dolan, R.J. 1998, Brain activations in schizophrenia during a graded memory task studied with functional neuroimaging, *Arch Gen Psychiatry*, **55**:11, 1001–8.

69. Perlstein, W.M., Carter, C.S., Noll, D.C., and Cohen, J.D. 2001, Relation of prefrontal cortex dysfunction to working memory and symptoms in schizophrenia, *Am J Psychiatry*, **158**:7, 1105–13.

70. Stevens, A.A., Goldman–Rakic, P.S., Gore, J.C., Fulbright, R.K., and Wexler, B.E. 1998, Cortical dysfunction in schizophrenia during auditory word and tone working memory demonstrated by functional magnetic resonance imaging, *Arch Gen Psychiat*, **55**:12, 1097–103.

71. Weinberger, D.R. and Berman, K.F. 1996, Prefrontal function in schizophrenia: confounds and controversies, *Philos Trans R Soc Lond B Biol Sci*, **351**:1346, 1495–503.

72. Jansma, J.M., Ramsey, N.F., van der Wee, N.J., and Kahn, R.S. 2004, Working memory capacity in schizophrenia: a parametric FMRI study, *Schizophr Res*, **68**:2–3, 159–71.

73. Callicott, J.H., Bertolino, A., Mattay, V.S., Langheim, F.J., Duyn, J., Coppola, R., *et al*. 2000, Physiological dysfunction of the dorsolateral prefrontal cortex in schizophrenia revisited, *Cereb Cortex*, **10**:11, 1078–92.

74. Manoach, D.S., Press, D.Z., Thangaraj, V., Searl, M.M., Goff, D.C., Halpern, E., *et al*. 1999, Schizophrenic subjects activate dorsolateral prefrontal cortex during a working memory task, as measured by FMRI, *Biol Psychiatry*, **45**:9, 1128–37.

75. Braver, T.S., Cohen, J.D., Nystrom, L.E., Jonides, J., Smith, E.E., and Noll, D.C. 1997, A parametric study of prefrontal cortex involvement in human working memory, *NeuroImage*, **5**:1, 49–62.

76. Jansma, J.M., Ramsey, N.F., Coppola, R., and Kahn, R.S. 2000, Specific versus nonspecific brain activity in a parametric n-back task, *NeuroImage*, **12**:6, 688–97.

77. Klingberg, T., Osullivan, B.T., and Roland, P.E. 1997, Bilateral activation of fronto-parietal networks by incrementing demand in a working memory task, *Cerebral Cortex*, **7**:5, 465–71.

78. Manoach, D.S., Schlaug, G., Siewert, B., Darby, D.G., Bly, B.M., Benfield, A., *et al*. 1997, Prefrontal cortex FMRI signal changes are correlated with working memory load, *Neuroreport*, **8**:2, 545–9.

79. Rypma, B., Prabhakaran, V., Desmond, J.E., Glover, G.H., and Gabrieli, J.D.E. 1999, Load-dependent roles of frontal brain regions in the maintenance of working memory, *Neuroimage*, **9**:2, 216–26.

80. Vafaee, M.S., Meyer, E., Marrett, S., Paus, T., Evans, A.C., and Gjedde, A. 1999, Frequency-dependent changes in cerebral metabolic rate of oxygen during activation of human visual cortex, *J Cerebr Blood Flow Metabol*, **19**:3, 272–7.

81. Dhankhar, A., Wexler, B.E., Fulbright, R.K., Halwes, T., Blamire, A.M., and Shulman, R.G. 1997, Functional magnetic resonance imaging assessment of the human brain auditory cortex response to increasing word presentation rates, *J Neurophysiol*, **77**:1, 476–83.

82. Ramsey, N.F., Van den Brink, J.S., van Muiswinkel, A.M., Folkers, P.J., Moonen, C.T., Jansma, J.M., *et al*. 1998, Phase navigator correction in 3D FMRI improves detection of brain activation: quantitative assessment with a graded motor activation procedure, *Neuroimage*, **8**:3, 240–8.

83. Sadato, N., Ibanez, V., Deiber, M.P., Campbell, G., Leonardo, M., and Hallett, M. 1996, Frequency-dependent changes of regional cerebral blood flow during finger movements, *J Cerebr Blood Flow Metab*, **16**:1, 23–33.

84. Callicott, J.H., Mattay, V.S., Bertolino, A., Finn, K., Coppola, R., Frank, J.A., *et al*. 1999, Physiological characteristics of capacity constraints in working memory as revealed by functional MRI, *Cerebral Cortex*, **9**:1, 20–6.

85. Manoach, D.S. 2003, Prefrontal cortex dysfunction during working memory performance in schizophrenia: reconciling discrepant findings, *Schizophr Res*, **60**:2–3, 285–98.

86. Ramsey, N.F., Koning, H.A., Welles, P., Cahn, W., van der Linden, J.A., and Kahn, R.S. 2002, Excessive recruitment of neural systems subserving logical reasoning in schizophrenia, *Brain*, **125**:8, 1793–807.

87. Carter, C.S., Perlstein, W., Ganguli, R., Brar, J., Mintun, M., and Cohen, J.D. 1998, Functional hypofrontality and working memory dysfunction in schizophrenia, *Am J Psychiatry*, **155**:9, 1285–7.

88. Manoach, D.S., Gollub, R.L., Benson, E.S., Searl, M.M., Goff, D.C., Halpern, E., *et al.* 2000, Schizophrenic subjects show aberrant FMRI activation of dorsolateral prefrontal cortex and basal ganglia during working memory performance, *Biol Psychiatry,* **48**: 2, 99–109.

89. Weinberger, D.R., Egan, M.F., Bertolino, A., Callicott, J.H., Mattay, V.S., Lipska, B.K., *et al.* 2001, Prefrontal neurons and the genetics of schizophrenia, *Biol Psychiatry,* **50**:11, 825–44.

90. Zakzanis, K.K. and Heinrichs, R.W. 1999, Schizophrenia and the frontal brain: a quantitative review, *J Intern Neuropsychological Soc,* **5**:6, 556–66.

91. Bertolino, A., Callicott, J.H., Mattay, V.S., Weidenhammer, K.M., Rakow, R., Egan, M.F., *et al.* 2001, The effect of treatment with antipsychotic drugs on brain N- acetylaspartate measures in patients with schizophrenia, *Biol Psychiatry,* **49**:1, 39–46.

92. Bertolino, A., Esposito, G., Callicott, J.H., Mattay, V.S., Van Horn, J.D., Frank, J.A., *et al.* 2000, Specific relationship between prefrontal neuronal N-acetylaspartate and activation of the working memory cortical network in schizophrenia, *Am J Psychiatry,* **157**:1, 26–33.

93. Laruelle, M. 2000, The role of endogenous sensitization in the pathophysiology of schizophrenia: implications from recent brain imaging studies, *Brain Res Brain Res Rev,* **31**:2–3, 371–84.

94. Abi–Dargham, A., Mawlawi, O., Lombardo, I., Gil, R., Martinez, D., Huang, Y., *et al.* 2002, Prefrontal dopamine D1 receptors and working memory in schizophrenia, *J Neurosci,* **22**:9, 3708–19.

95. Braver, T.S., Barch, D.M., and Cohen, J.D. 1999, Cognition and control in schizophrenia: a computational model of dopamine and prefrontal function, *Biol Psychiat,* **46**:3, 312–28.

96. Goldman–Rakic, P.S. and Selemon, L.D. 1997, Functional and anatomical aspects of prefrontal pathology in schizophrenia [see comments], *Schizophrenia Bulletin,* **23**:3, 437–58.

97. Bunney, W.E. and Bunney, B.G. 2000, Evidence for a compromised dorsolateral prefrontal cortical parallel circuit in schizophrenia, *Brain Res Brain Res Rev,* **31**:2–3, 138–46

98. Honey, G.D., Bullmore, E.T., and Sharma, T. 2002, De-coupling of cognitive performance and cerebral functional response during working memory in schizophrenia, *Schizophr Res,* **53**:1–2, 45–56.

99. Quintana, J., Wong, T., Ortiz–Portillo, E., Kovalik, E., Davidson, T., Marder, S.R., *et al.* 2003, Prefrontal-posterior parietal networks in schizophrenia: primary dysfunctions and secondary compensations, *Biol Psychiatry,* **53**:1, 12–24.

100. Carter, C.S., MacDonald, A.W., III, Ross, L.L., and Stenger, V.A. 2001, Anterior cingulate cortex activity and impaired self-monitoring of performance in patients with schizophrenia: an event-related FMRI study, *Am J Psychiatry,* **158**:9, 1423–8.

101. Dolan, R.J., Fletcher, P., Frith, C.D., Friston, K.J., Frackowiak, R.S., and Grasby, P.M. 1995, Dopaminergic modulation of impaired cognitive activation in the anterior cingulate cortex in schizophrenia, *Nature,* **378**:6553, 180–2.

102. Logan, G.D. 1988, Toward an instance theory of automatization, *Psychological Review,* **95**: 492–527.

103. Shiffrin, R. M. and Schneider, W. 1977, Controlled and automatic human information processing: II. Perceptual learning, automatic attending and a general theory, *Psychological Review,* **84**, 127–90.

104. Gilbert, C.D., Sigman, M., and Crist, R.E. 2001, The neural basis of perceptual learning, *Neuron,* **31**:5, 681–97.

105. Strayer, D.L. and Kramer, A.F. 1990, An analysis of memory-based theories of automaticity, *J Exp Psychol Learn Mem Cogn,* **16**:2, 291–304.

106. LaBerge, D. and Samuels, S.J. 1974, Towards a theory of automatic information processing in reading, *Cognitive Psychology,* **11**, 1–12.

107. Schneider, W. and Shiffrin, R.M. 1977, Controlled and automatic human information processing: I. Detection, search and attention, *Psychological Review,* **84**, 1–66.

108. Buchel, C., Coull, J.T., and Friston, K.J. 1999, The predictive value of changes in effective connectivity for human learning, *Science,* **283**:5407, 1538–41.

109. Jansma, J.M., Ramsey, N.F., Slagter, H.A., and Kahn, R.S. 2001, Functional anatomical correlates of controlled and automatic processing, *J Cogn Neurosci*, **13**:6, 730–43.

110. Schmand, B., Brand, N., and Kuipers, T. 1992, Procedural learning of cognitive and motor skills in psychotic patients, *Schizophr Res*, **8**:2, 157–70.

111. Kumari, V., Gray, J.A., Honey, G.D., Soni, W., Bullmore, E.T., Williams, S.C., *et al.* 2002, Procedural learning in schizophrenia: a functional magnetic resonance imaging investigation, *Schizophr Res*, **57**:1, 97–107.

112. Granholm, E. and Asarnow, R.F. 1996, Dual-task performance operating characteristics, resource limitations and automatic processing in schizophrenia, *Neuropsychology*, **10**, 11–21.

113. Ramsey, N.F., Jansma, J.M., Jager, G., Van Raalten, T.R., and Kahn, R.S. 2004, Neurophysiological factors in human information processing capacity, *Brain*, **127**, 517–25.

114. Kodama, S., Fukuzako, H., Fukuzako, T., Kiura, T., Nozoe, S., Hashiguchi, T., *et al.* 2001, Aberrant brain activation following motor skill learning in schizophrenic patients as shown by functional magnetic resonance imaging, *Psychol Med*, **31**:6, 1079–88.

115. Horwitz, B., Friston, K.J., and Taylor, J.G. 2000, Neural modeling and functional brain imaging: an overview, *Neural Netw*, **13**:8–9, 829–46.

116. Mcintosh, A.R. 2000, Towards a network theory of cognition, *Neural Netw*, **13**:8–9, 861–70.

117. Braver, T.S. and Cohen, J.D. 1999, Dopamine, cognitive control, and schizophrenia: the gating model, *Prog Brain Res*, **121**, 327–49.

118. Dolan, R.J., Fletcher, P.C., Mckenna, P., Friston, K.J., and Frith, C.D. 1999, Abnormal neural integration related to cognition in schizophrenia, *Acta Psychiat Scand*, **99**(Suppl. 395), 58–67.

119. Weinberger, D.R. 1993, A connectionist approach to the prefrontal cortex, *J Neuropsychi Clin Neurosci*, **5**, 241–253.

120. Friston, K.J., Frith, C.D., Fletcher, P., Liddle, P.F., and Frackowiak, R.S. 1996, Functional topography: multidimensional scaling and functional connectivity in the brain, *Cerebral Cortex*, **6**:2, 156–64.

121. Bullmore, E.T., Rabehesketh, S., Morris, R.G., Williams, S.C.R., Gregory, L., Gray, J.A., *et al.* 1996, Functional magnetic resonance image analysis of a large scale neurocognitive network, *Neuroimage*, **4**, 16–33.

122. Mcintosh, A.R. 1999, Mapping cognition to the brain through neural interactions, *Memory*, **7**:5–6, 523–48.

123. Buchel, C. and Friston, K. 2000, Assessing interactions among neuronal systems using functional neuroimaging, *Neural Netw*, **13**:8–9, 871–82.

124. Fletcher, P.C., Frith, C.D., Grasby, P.M., Friston, K.J., and Dolan, R.J. 1996, Local and distributed effects of apomorphine on fronto-temporal function in acute unmedicated schizophrenia, *J Neurosci*, **16**:21, 7055–62.

125. Sawaguchi, T. and Goldman–Rakic, P.S. 1991, D1 dopamine receptors in prefrontal cortex: involvement in working memory, *Science*, **251**:4996, 947–50.

126. Fletcher, P., McKenna, P.J., Friston, K.J., Frith, C.D., and Dolan, R.J. 1999, Abnormal cingulate modulation of fronto-temporal connectivity in schizophrenia, *Neuroimage*, **9**:3, 337–42.

127. Lawrie, S.M., Buechel, C., Whalley, H.C., Frith, C.D., Friston, K.J., and Johnstone, E.C. 2002, Reduced frontotemporal functional connectivity in schizophrenia associated with auditory hallucinations, *Biol Psychiatry*, **51**:12, 1008–11.

128. Spence, S.A., Liddle, P.F., Stefan, M.D., Hellewell, J.S., Sharma, T., Friston, K.J., *et al.* 2000, Functional anatomy of verbal fluency in people with schizophrenia and those at genetic risk. Focal dysfunction and distributed disconnectivity reappraised, *Br J Psychiatry*, **176**, 52–60.

129. Tsuang, M. 2000, Schizophrenia: genes and environment, *Biol Psychiatry*, **47**:3, 210–20.

130. Gottesman, I.I. and Gould, T.D. 2003, The endophenotype concept in psychiatry: etymology and strategic intentions, *Am J Psychiatry*, **160**:4, 636–45.

131. Callicott, J.H. 2003, An expanded role for functional neuroimaging in schizophrenia, *Curr Opin Neurobiol*, **13**:2, 256–60.

132. Hariri, A.R. and Weinberger, D.R. 2003, Imaging genomics, *Br Med Bull*, **65**, 259–270.

133. Freedman, R., Adams, C.E., Adler, L.E., Bickford, P.C., Gault, J., Harris, J.G., *et al.* 2000, Inhibitory neurophysiological deficit as a phenotype for genetic investigation of schizophrenia, *Am J Med Genetics*, **97**:1, 58–64.

134. McDowell, J.E. and Clementz, B.A. 2001, Behavioral and brain imaging studies of saccadic performance in schizophrenia, *Biol.Psychol*, **57**:1–3, 5–22.

135. Muri, R.M., Heid, O., Nirkko, A.C., Ozdoba, C., Felblinger, J., Schroth, G., *et al.* 1998, Functional organisation of saccades and antisaccades in the frontal lobe in humans: a study with echo planar functional magnetic resonance imaging, *J Neurol Neurosurg Psychiatry*, **65**:3, 374–77.

136. Raemaekers, M., Jansma, J.M., Cahn, W., Van Der Geest, J.N., Der Linden, J.A., Kahn, R.S., *et al.* 2002, Neuronal substrate of the saccadic inhibition deficit in schizophrenia investigated with 3-dimensional event-related functional magnetic resonance imaging, *Arch Gen Psychiatry*, **59**:4, 313–20.

137. Carter, C.S., Mintun, M., Nichols, T., and Cohen, J.D. 1997, Anterior cingulate gyrus dysfunction and selective attention deficits in schizophrenia: [15O]H2O PET study during single-trial Stroop task performance, *Am J Psychiatry*, **154**:12, 1670–5.

138. Sommer, I.E., Ramsey, N.F., Mandl, R.C., and Kahn, R.S. 2002, Language lateralization in monozygotic twin pairs concordant and discordant for handedness, *Brain*, **125**:12, 2710–18.

139. Heckers, S., Rauch, S.L., Goff, D., Savage, C.R., Schacter, D.L., Fischman, A.J., *et al.* 1998, Impaired recruitment of the hippocampus during conscious recollection in schizophrenia, *Nat Neurosci*, **1**:4, 318–23.

140. Egan, M.F., Goldberg, T.E., Kolachana, B.S., Callicott, J.H., Mazzanti, C.M., Straub, R.E., *et al.* 2001, Effect of COMT Val108/158 met genotype on frontal lobe function and risk for schizophrenia, *Proc Natl Acad Sci USA*, **98**:12, 6917–22.

141. Lachman, H.M., Papolos, D.F., Saito, T., Yu, Y.M., Szumlanski, C.L., and Weinshilboum, R.M. 1996, Human catechol-O-methyltransferase pharmacogenetics: description of a functional polymorphism and its potential application to neuropsychiatric disorders, *Pharmacogenetics*, **6**:3, 243–50.

142. Mattay, V.S., Goldberg, T.E., Fera, F., Hariri, A.R., Tessitore, A., Egan, M.F., *et al.* 2003, Catechol O-methyltransferase val158-met genotype and individual variation in the brain response to amphetamine, *Proc Natl Acad Sci USA*, **100**:10, 6186–91.

143. Wassink, T.H., Nopoulos, P., Pietila, J., Crowe, R.R., and Andreasen, N.C. 2003, NOTCH4 and the frontal lobe in schizophrenia, *Am J Med Genet*, **118B**:1, 1–7.

144. Hariri, A.R., Mattay, V.S., Tessitore, A., Kolachana, B., Fera, F., Goldman, D. 2002, Serotonin transporter genetic variation and the response of the human amygdala, *Science*, **297**:5580, 400–3.

145. Bertolino, A. Callicott, J.H., Elman, I., Mattay, V.S., Tedeschi, G., Frank, J.A., *et al.* 1998, Regionally specific neuronal pathology in untreated patients with schizophrenia: a proton magnetic resonance spectroscopic imaging study, *Biol Psychiatry*, **43**:9, 641–8.

146. Honey, G.D., Bullmore, E.T., Soni, W., Varatheesan, M., Williams, S.C., and Sharma, T. 1999, Differences in frontal cortical activation by a working memory task after substitution of risperidone for typical antipsychotic drugs in patients with schizophrenia, *Proc Natl Acad Sci USA*, **96**:23, 13432–7.

147. Stephane, M., Barton, S., and Boutros, N.N. 2001, Auditory verbal hallucinations and dysfunction of the neural substrates of speech, *Schizophr Res*, **50**:1–2, 61–78.

148. Leonhard, D. and Brugger, P. 1998, Creative, paranormal, and delusional thought: a consequence of right hemisphere semantic activation?, *Neuropsychiatry Neuropsychol Behav Neurol*, **11**:4, 177–83.

8

Depression and anxiety disorders

Dick J. Veltman

1. Introduction

Depression and anxiety disorders are, by far, the most common psychiatric disorders, with a lifetime prevalence estimated as high as 16% for major depressive disorder alone[1]. Similar figures have been reported for anxiety disorders[2]. In the widely used *Diagnostic and Statistical Manual of Mental Disorders*[3], major depressive disorder (MDD; also termed unipolar depression) has been brought under the heading of 'mood disorders', together with dysthymia (i.e. chronic mild depression), various types of bipolar disorder (or manic depressive disorder), and some additional, sometimes provisional, diagnoses. Similarly, since the 1980s, anxiety disorders have been grouped together in the *DSM*. This category includes 'pure' (non-phobic) anxiety disorders, in which patients may experience anxiety symptoms without clearly identifiable external cues, and phobic disorders, the symptoms of which are triggered by specific objects or situations. Non-phobic anxiety disorders are panic disorder (PD) and generalized anxiety disorder (GAD), both formerly lumped together under the name of anxiety neurosis. Phobic disorders include agoraphobia (which usually occurs in the context of panic disorder), social phobia, and the so-called specific phobias, e.g. for animals (snakes, spiders) or specific situations (elevators, airplanes). Finally, obsessive compulsive disorder (OCD) and post-traumatic stress disorder (PTSD) have been classified as anxiety disorders, again with a few residual categories for completeness' sake.

Comorbidity among anxiety disorders is high, not only for PD and agoraphobia, but also for PD and GAD, and for PD and social phobia. In addition, depressive episodes are common in anxiety disorders, and panic attacks frequently co-occur in MDD. Although this would suggest a shared predisposition and/or pathogenetic mechanism between depression and anxiety disorders, their aetiology is still insufficiently clear, with the exception of PTSD.

Over the last two decades, neuroimaging research has added considerably to our understanding of neurobiological mechanisms in psychiatric disorders. Apart from schizophrenia (see Chapter 7), most work has been done for major depressive disorder and obsessive compulsive disorder, followed by panic disorder, PTSD, and phobic disorders. In the present chapter, we will review imaging studies focussing on these disorders and MRI studies in particular. To this end, we will briefly discuss clinical features for each disorder, followed by an overview of imaging research performed to date. Given the scope of the field, we will not attempt to provide an exhaustive review, but rather discuss key findings and common methodological themes across diagnostic categories.

2. Neuroimaging in psychiatry: methodology

2.1 Technical aspects

Neuroimaging modalities used in psychiatry research encompass both structural (morphological) and functional techniques. With regard to neuroanatomical imaging, computerized (axial) tomography (CT) has been rendered obsolete due to its inherently poor contrast between white and gray matter, and structural MRI (sMRI) is now the method of choice. Functional imaging includes, primarily, techniques to assess neural activity, either directly, as in electroencephalography (EEG) and magnetoencephalography (MEG), or indirectly, as in PET/SPECT and FMRI. Tracers commonly used for functional studies in PET (positron emission tomography) are ^{15}O-labelled water and ^{18}F-labelled glucose (^{18}F-deoxyfluoroglucose, FDG): regional differences in tracer uptake reflect changes in perfusion and glucose metabolism, respectively. For SPECT (single photon emission computed tomography), most flow studies have been performed using ^{99}Tc-HMPAO (hexamethylenepropylamine oxime) or ^{133}Xenon. Due to the long half-life of naturally occurring isotopes as used in SPECT, and of ^{18}F (109 minutes) in PET, temporal resolution is low, so that only a single scan can be acquired during each session. In contrast, the half-life of ^{15}O is circa 2 minutes, so that ^{15}O-PET scans can be repeated after 10 minutes, permitting up to 12 scans per session. Before the advent of functional MRI, ^{15}O-PET was widely used for imaging studies involving task vs. baseline comparisons. However, over the last decade, FMRI has gradually taken over because of its advantages of greater spatial and especially temporal resolution, and absence of radiation exposure. The temporal resolution of EEG and MEG is superior to FMRI (in the millisecond range), but spatial resolution is generally limited, so that MEG is still infrequently used in psychiatry research.

In this chapter, we will therefore discuss mostly (F)MRI and PET/SPECT studies. Both MRI and PET/SPECT can also be used for biochemical imaging. For MR spectroscopy, this can be achieved by imaging ^{1}H in molecules containing, for example, CH_3, NH_2, or OH groups, or isotopes such as ^{7}Li, ^{13}C, ^{19}F, and ^{31}P (e.g. adenosine triphosphate — ATP). Molecules whose relative concentrations can be assessed using MRS are choline, lactate, glutamatergic compounds (Glx), and N-acetyl aspartate (NAA, a marker of neuronal viability). In PET/SPECT, tracers can be synthesized designed to bind specifically to various types of neuroreceptors; at present, successful ligands have been developed for dopaminergic, serotonergic (Fig. 8.1), and GABA-ergic receptors, among others. PET has advantages over SPECT (better spatial resolution and data quantification), but is also much more expensive, because an on-site cyclotron is needed to produce PET-isotopes.

2.2 Study design

Whereas technical issues regarding data acquisition and post-processing of volumetric MR and ligand PET/SPECT studies are often highly complex, the overall design is not. Basically, for a group of patients, a single scan is made for each subject, which are compared

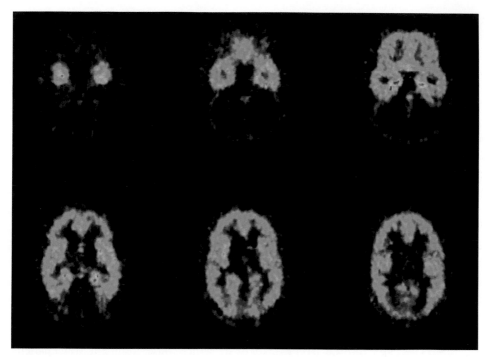

Fig. 8.1 PET image showing binding of [11C]WAY-100635 to 5HT1a receptors.

to those of one or more control groups. For volumetric MRI, this may entail the acquisition of several scans of different modalities (e.g. T_1 and T_2 weighted), to improve segmentation into white matter, gray matter, and cerebrospinal fluid (CSF). Similarly, PET images are usually coregistered to anatomical MR scans to facilitate manual drawing of regions of interest (ROIs). Equally straightforward (compared with these cross-sectional, between-group designs) are longitudinal (within-subject) designs, in which patients are rescanned, for example, after therapy. To exclude non-specific changes, more sophisticated factorial (mixed) designs are necessary, in which a group of healthy control subjects and/or a placebo group is also scanned twice. Similar considerations apply for functional studies in which only a single scan can be acquired, as in HMPAO-SPECT and FDG-PET. A major disadvantage of the latter type of investigation (so-called resting-state studies) is that there is little control over subjects' mental activity; in other words, experimental conditions are difficult to constrain. As a result, differences between patients and healthy controls may present interpretation problems (for example, due to increased anticipation anxiety in the patient group). For this reason, researchers have switched to multi-scan techniques (^{15}O-PET and FMRI) which permit within-session comparisons between two or more conditions, usually 'task vs. baseline'.

In psychiatry research, investigators have used symptom provocation (or symptom capture) designs, alternating 'symptom' and 'baseline' conditions, and cognitive paradigms with both neutral and emotional stimuli. These latter paradigms are generally based on previous neuropsychological findings of cognitive dysfunctions in psychiatric patients (e.g. impaired working memory in schizophrenia). Therefore, functional imaging during performance of such tasks aims at identifying the neural substrate of specific cognitive abnormalities in various psychiatric disorders. Although this approach has clear methodological advantages over the single-scan, resting-state measurements described previously, it should be noted that ^{15}O-PET and FMRI generally provide only relative measurements. Absolute quantification of BOLD-FMRI data is physiologically meaningless; consequently, FMRI is blind to baseline differences, which may therefore act as a confounder.

3. Mood disorders: major depression

3.1 Clinical aspects

As noted earlier, major depressive disorder (MDD) is the single most common psychiatric disorder, as well as one of the most common medical conditions. MDD is characterized by single or recurrent episodes of depressed mood, or loss of interest or pleasure in nearly all activities, lasting at least two weeks. Additional symptoms include changes in appetite, body weight, and sleeping behaviour, loss of energy, and concentration problems. Feelings of guilt or hopelessness are common, and may be associated with a preoccupation with death or suicidal ideation. MDD is often complicated by panic attacks, which may meet the criteria for panic disorder, and alcohol or substance abuse. Although MDD patients may have EEG abnormalities as well as alterations in hypothalamic-pituitary-adrenal (HPA) axis functioning, the diagnosis of MDD is primarily made based on a clinical interview. However, additional laboratory tests may be used to rule out depression due to a general medical condition (neurological or endocrine).

The aetiology of MDD is still insufficiently known, as both constitutional and environmental factors (e.g. adverse life events) have been implicated. In addition, twin and family studies have shown a strong genetic component. Treatment strategies proven effective in MDD include interpersonal and cognitive psychotherapy, the use of antidepressant drugs, and electroconvulsive therapy (ECT). Although ECT is presumably more effective than either psychotherapy or pharmacotherapy, its use is still limited, due to serious side-effects. However, over the last few years, promising results have been obtained using repetitive transcranial magnetic stimulation (rTMS), which is (far) less invasive (for an overview see[4]). Most antidepressant drugs are neurotransmitter transport blockers, usually of serotonin, and to a lesser extent of noradrenalin and dopamine. Newer antidepressants are more selective at blocking serotonin reuptake compared with older compounds, which may also possess antihistaminergic, anticholinergic, and antiadrenergic properties. Therefore, selective serotonin reuptake inhibitors (SSRIs) usually produce fewer side-effects, although their clinical efficacy also tends to be smaller[5].

A major problem when treating MDD is that conventional therapeutic strategies are only effective in about 50% of all patients, whereas the remainder shows no or only a partial response to treatment[6]. Furthermore, about half of MDD patients will suffer from another episode within the first year after discontinuation of antidepressant medication; moreover, identification of relapse predictors has been problematic[7].

3.2 Neuroanatomical studies in MDD

Neuroanatomical studies in MDD have indicated structural abnormalities in various brain structures in MDD, including the prefrontal and anterior cingulate cortex[8], the orbitofrontal cortex[9], the basal ganglia, and the medial temporal lobe[10] (for an overview). Most recent studies have focussed on hippocampal atrophy, which has been linked to HPA axis hyperactivity in MDD[11]. Elevated glucocorticoid levels may ultimately lead to loss of glucocorticoid receptor (GR) containing cells in the hippocampus that mediate suppression of corticotropin-releasing hormone (CRH) from the paraventricular nucleus (PVN) of the hypothalamus, thereby establishing a positive feedback loop. It has been hypothesized that defective regulation of corticosteroid receptor gene expression may contribute to altered HPA axis function in MDD. In rodents, an increase in GR and miner-alocorticoid receptor density in the hippocampus and hypothalamus has been shown after 2–5 weeks of antidepressant therapy, suggesting a possible mechanism for the normalization of HPA axis hyperactivity observed in MDD patients[12].

With regard to hippocampal volume loss, about half of the MRI studies published until now have indicated decreased hippocampal volume in MDD, either left-sided, right-sided, or bilateral ([13]; cf. Fig. 8.2), whereas in the other studies, no significant differences were found compared with healthy control subjects. These inconsistencies may have been

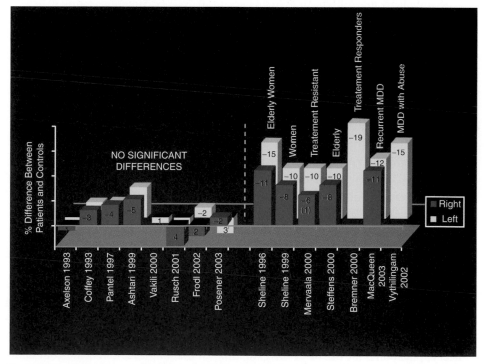

Fig. 8.2 Overview of structural MR studies in depressive disorder showing decreased hippocampal volume. (Reproduced with permission from Elsevier Publishers[20].)

partly due to the inclusion of the amygdala with the hippocampus in some studies, as hippocampal atrophy has been observed primarily when the hippocampus was considered as a discrete structure[14]. Indeed, amygdala volume was found to be increased in MDD, at least in first-episode patients[15]. Hippocampal atrophy was found to be associated with illness duration[16], in particular duration of untreated episodes[17] and poor clinical outcome[18]. Moreover, it has been demonstrated that the hippocampi in currently depressed patients were smaller than in remitted MDD patients[19]. Another recent study found that successful antidepressant therapy was associated with improved mnemonic abilities in MDD patients, but failed to show an increase in hippocampal volume[20]. Thus, current evidence supports the notion of hippocampal atrophy in MDD.

3.3 Biochemical studies in MDD

PET and SPECT ligand studies in MDD have focussed on serotonergic transmission, targeting $5HT1_a$ and $5HT2_a$ receptors as well as 5HT transporter sites. Studies using $5HT2_a$ ligands have produced mixed results, showing decreased, increased, and unchanged binding in MDD patients relative to healthy controls as well as pre/post therapy ([21] for an overview). With regard to cortical $5HT1_a$ receptors, in several studies a decreased PET-ligand binding in MDD patients, relative to controls, has consistently been observed[22,23]. This reduction persisted after successful antidepressant therapy, indicating that lowered $5HT1_a$ binding availability is a trait feature of MDD[24]. Results for serotonin transporter receptor ligands have been similarly inconsistent, as both increased and decreased binding relative to healthy controls has been observed in MDD. 5HT transporter ligands have also been used for monitoring drug therapy, to assess changes in receptor binding whilst subjects were taking standard dosages of paroxetine or citalopram[25]. Finally, serotonergic transmission in MDD has been investigated with the aid of alpha-[(11)C]methyl-l-tryptophan[26]. Compared with age- and sex-matched controls, in MDD patients, regional uptake of labelled tryptophan was significantly decreased in several (para)limbic cortical regions, such as the anterior cingulate cortex and mesial temporal cortex. Thus, most of the available evidence is compatible with the hypothesis of lowered serotonergic transmission in MDD.

Other transmitter systems have received less attention in MDD. Striatal dopaminergic reactivity in MDD during amphetamine challenge was found to be normal[27]; also, a SPECT study using the benzodiazepine receptor ligand [(123)I]iomazenil found no evidence of altered gamma amino butyric acid (GABA)-ergic binding in MDD[28].

Magnetic resonance spectroscopy (MRS) studies in MDD have been rare until now. In a preliminary study, a decreased GABA to choline ratio in the occipital cortex was observed in MDD[29]. Other studies have reported decreased glutamate/glutamine (Glx) concentrations in the dorsolateral prefrontal cortex in MDD, normalizing after electroconvulsive therapy[30], and decreased NAA/creatine ratios in the caudate nucleus together with increased choline/ creatine ratios in the putamen, suggesting subcortical metabolic abnormalities in MDD[31]. Although interesting, these isolated findings clearly need replication. A potential clinical application is the use of ^{19}F-MRS to monitor brain uptake of fluorine-containing antidepressant drugs, such as fluvoxamine or fluoxetine[32].

3.4 Resting-state studies in MDD

Since the 1980s, a considerable number of resting-state studies in MDD have been performed, using either HMPAO-SPECT or FDG-PET. Overall, these studies have provided evidence for decreased dorsal prefrontal perfusion and glucose uptake in MDD, together with increased perfusion and metabolism in ventral prefrontal and other limbic regions[10]. Consistently reported are frontal and cingulate changes. While less common, other limbic and subcortical regions including the hippocampus, amygdala, posterior cingulate, striatum, and thalamus have also been implicated[33]. These abnormalities have been found in both primary (idiopathic) and secondary MDD. Moreover, functional alterations were found to be associated with illness severity and tended to be more pronounced in familial MDD. Successful therapy is associated with changes in regional metabolism, although the direction of these changes is not uniform across treatment modalities[34].

Interestingly, changes in regional glucose uptake in MDD patients after successful therapy (limbic decreases and neocortical increases) were in the opposite direction compared to changes in regional cerebral blood flow in healthy volunteers during induced sadness[35]. In particular, dorsolateral prefrontal activity was inversely correlated to ventral (subgenual) cingulate activity in both groups. Transient sadness paradigms have been employed in healthy volunteers to mimic depressed states, whereas in recovered MDD patients, tryptophan depletion (TD) has been used to induce temporary relapses by lowering serotonergic transmission. Induced sadness has been found to increase limbic, paralimbic, and subcortical perfusion (e.g. [36]). In remitted MDD patients, but not in control subjects, TD compared with sham depletion resulted in increased glucose uptake in the orbitofrontal cortex, anterior and posterior cingulate cortex, and ventral striatum[37]. These changes were found both in patients experiencing a relapse during TD and those who did not, indicating that increased metabolism in these regions, which have been associated with affective stimulus evaluation and generating behavioural responses, is a trait abnormality in MDD.

3.5 Activation studies

3.5.1 Affective paradigms

A disadvantage of tryptophan depletion, as discussed in the previous paragraph, is that it takes several hours before the effects wear off, so that TD and sham depletion sessions need to be conducted on different testing days. Therefore, the sensitivity of such a design is likely to be reduced due to session-to-session variability. To circumvent this problem, researchers have used within-session psychological mood induction paradigms in MDD, for example, by presenting subjects with scripts of sad autobiographical memories[38]. In depressed patients, induced sadness vs. neutral state was associated with CBF changes in various cortical and subcortical regions, including the cingulate cortex and medial orbitofrontal cortex. These changes, however, were in the opposite direction compared with the TD results of Neumeister et al.[37], which may have been due to differences in medication status.

The use of idiosyncratic stimuli, such as autobiographical scripts, provides a powerful tool for *in vivo* investigation of the neural substrate of psychiatric symptoms, but has several methodological drawbacks. First, compared with standardized stimuli, a design employing individually tailored stimuli entails a loss of homogeneity, and comparability between groups and/or subjects is reduced. Second, intensity and duration of induced symptoms are often difficult to control. For example, in the Liotti *et al.* study[38], a flexible ^{15}O-PET scanning protocol was necessary, so that each scan was acquired only when subjects had reached the desired emotional state or had returned to baseline. Such prolonged rests, however, reduce design efficiency and may introduce confounders such as excessive subject movement[39]. Third, induction of full-blown symptom states may lead not only to changes in regional CBF but also in global CBF, due to increased arousal and/or hyperventilation.

A more controlled way to investigate the neural substrate of affective symptoms is to present subjects with standardized emotional vs. neutral stimuli, such as pictures from the International Affective Picture System (IAPS)[40] (Fig. 8.3) or pictures of faces with various emotional expressions, for example, the Ekman set[41] (Fig. 8.4). Using the latter paradigm, Thomas *et al.*[42] found increased amygdala responses to emotional vs. neutral faces in anxious but not in normal children, whereas in depressed children, amygdala responses were blunted. The decreased left amygdala response in depressed children was interpreted as evidence for diminished approach behaviour, whereas increased right amygdala responsiveness in anxious children was thought to reflect increased avoidance behaviour[42].

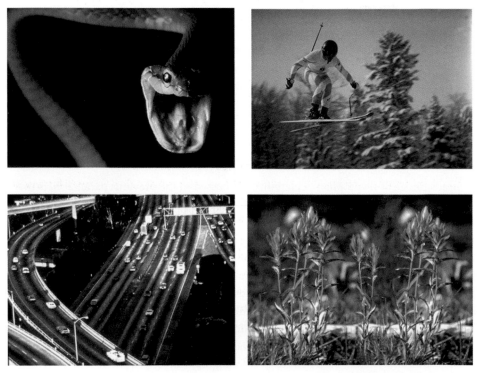

Fig. 8.3 Example pictures from the International Affective Picture System (IAPS). (Reproduced with permission from Blackwell Publishing[40].)

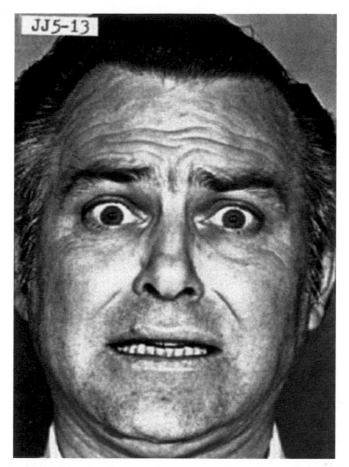

Fig. 8.4 Example picture from the Ekman and Friesen picture set of emotional faces.

A blunted response in the amygdala to anxious faces has also been found in adults with MDD[43]. In contrast, Sheline et al.[44] found increased left amygdala responses for masked fearful and happy faces masked with neutral faces in MDD patients compared with healthy controls, resolving after antidepressant therapy. In agreement with these latter findings, increased left amygdala responses to overtly presented sad faces in MDD was reported by Fu et al.[45]. However, these results with regard to amygdala hyperactivity in MDD were only partially confirmed by other investigators[46,47]. Davidson et al.[46] used IAPS pictures to investigate responses to emotional pictures in MDD patients before and after treatment with venlafaxine — a mixed serotonin-noradrenalin reuptake inhibitor. Before treatment, increased activity in the visual cortex was observed in MDD patients relative to control subjects, as well as decreased insular and anterior cingulate activity, the latter normalizing after two and eight weeks of drug treatment, respectively. The authors concluded that decreased insular and anterior cingulate cortex activity reflected blunted emotional responding in MDD patients. However, in the Davidson et al. study, amygdala activity in MDD patients did not differ from controls. In the Surguladze study[47], a parametric design was employed. Healthy individuals were found to have linear increases in response in the bilateral fusiform gyri and right putamen to expressions of increasing happiness, whereas in MDD subjects, linear increases in response in the left putamen, left parahippocampal gyrus/amygdala, and right fusiform gyrus to expressions of increasing sadness were observed. Differential effects of positively and negatively valenced stimuli in MDD relative to healthy controls were also observed, albeit not in the amygdala, in a study employing a picture-caption paradigm[48] and by Lawrence et al.[49] who used pictures of sad and happy faces.

Increased activity in visual processing pathways during presentation of negative stimuli, as found in several of the above-reviewed studies, has been explained as resulting from upstream modulating activity from the amygdala[50]. On the other hand, the evidence for abnormal amygdala activation in MDD during presentation of emotional pictures, and faces in particular, appears to be mixed. Whether these inconsistencies are due to methodological issues (e.g. medication use) or differences in state anxiety, is insufficiently clear, as most studies did not provide anxiety ratings. In the Sheline et al. study[44], amygdala signal in MDD patients was not correlated with severity of depression or anxiety ratings. However, as the authors pointed out, these negative results may have been caused by low statistical power due to their small sample size and suboptimal assessment of state anxiety.

Studies employing verbal stimuli — single words rather than scripts — to provoke limbic activity in MDD patients have been sparse. An exception is the study by Siegle et al.[51] in which prolonged amygdala responses to negative words compared with healthy controls was found; amygdala activity in patients continued even when subjects switched to a non-emotional working memory task designed to provoke cortical activity elsewhere in the brain, thereby shutting off the amygdala. In MDD patients, amygdala activity was related to self-reported rumination measures, suggesting that these processes are clinically relevant.

3.5.2 Cognitive paradigms

In imaging research, study designs comparing emotional vs. neutral words have mainly been used to highlight increased response bias while performing a cognitive task in MDD, for example, facilitation or interference during a 'go/no go' task[52]. Neuropsychological studies have identified a number of cognitive deficits in MDD which have been associated with dysfunction of medial temporal lobe structures, which are critically involved in episodic memory[53], and of various prefrontal regions[54]. Of these, the dorsolateral prefrontal cortex is primarily involved in executive functions, including working memory and planning. The anterior cingulate cortex has been associated with attentional processes, including error monitoring and response selection. Finally, the orbitofrontal cortex is involved in emotional decision making, for example, by assessing the significance of positive or negative feedback[55].

Although neuropsychological findings have not been wholly consistent, a number of studies have shown that MDD patients perform worse during tasks tapping DLPFC function, such as verbal fluency, working memory, set shifting, and planning[56]. Verbal fluency can be measured by asking the subject to provide, within a short time, from a given category, as many examples as possible (e.g. towns whose name begins with a B). Thus, verbal fluency tasks assess both semantic retrieval and working memory. Working memory (WM) has been defined as the capacity to keep information on-line for immediate use[57]. Two types of WM tasks can be discriminated — maintenance (usually delayed match to sample) and manipulation tasks. During a maintenance task, subjects are presented with a number of letters or objects (encoding phase); after a few seconds, the set disappears (retention phase) and a cue stimulus is presented, to which the subject has to respond whether it was in the set or not (responding phase). Manipulation WM tasks are similar to maintenance tasks but require additional changing or updating of each memory set (e.g. the n-back task) (Fig. 8.5). Imaging research in healthy subjects has shown that the ventrolateral prefrontal cortex (VLPFC) is primarily involved during maintenance tasks, whereas DLPFC activity is increased while performing manipulation WM tasks. At higher loads, DLPFC is likely to be also recruited during maintenance tasks[58]. A widely used set-shifting task is the Wisconsin card sorting task (WCST), in which the subject is required to sort the cards according to shape, colour, or number of the symbols shown on the cards. After some time, the sorting rule is changed unbeknownst to the subject who has to discover the new rule and change his/her strategy accordingly. Finally, a classic planning task is the Tower of London (ToL) task[59], in which subjects are shown a starting and a target configuration and have to work out the minimum number of steps in between (Fig. 8.6).

With regard to anterior cingulate function, investigators have used selective attention paradigms such as the Stroop colour–word task and, in particular, so-called modified or

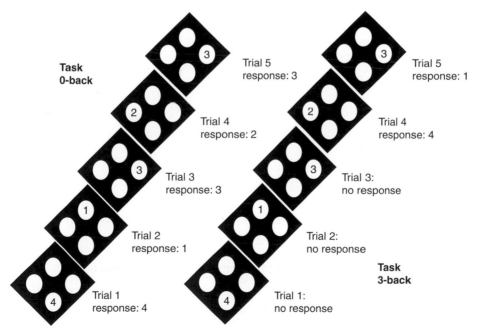

Fig. 8.5 Schematic representation of a spatial n-back working memory task. (Reproduced with permission from Elsevier Publishers[173].)

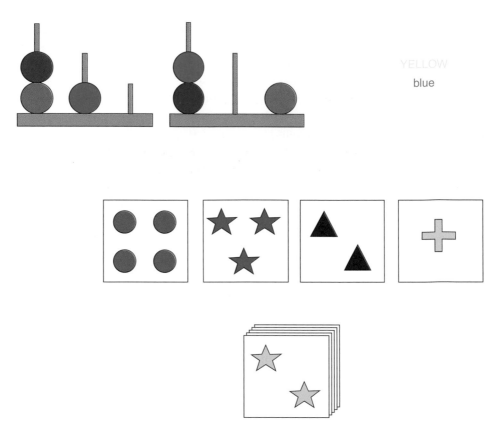

Fig. 8.6 Examples of neuropsychological tasks adapted for FMRI: (top left) Tower of London task; (top right) Stroop colour word naming task; (middle and lower) Wisconsin Card Sorting Task.

emotional versions of the task. In the standard version, subjects are requested to name the colour of the letters (e.g. yellow) while ignoring the colour word (e.g. red; see Fig. 8.6). In the modified version, congruent and incongruent colour words are substituted by neutral (e.g. table) or emotionally negative (e.g. cancer) words. Orbitofrontal function has been probed with the aid of gambling tasks, for example, the Bechara task[55]. In this task, the subject has to draw cards from one of four decks, each card being followed by feedback (i.e. gaining or losing points or money). Two decks are associated with high rewards but even greater losses, whereas the other two provide smaller rewards but also smaller losses, and the subject has to learn that the latter decks are more advantageous in the long run.

Imaging studies in MDD using cognitive paradigms have been relatively sparse. In an early PET study, Smith *et al.*[60] compared eight recovered MDD patients following trypto-phan depletion vs. sham depletion, observing diminished anterior cingulate activity during performance of a verbal fluency task. Videbech *et al.*[61] also employed a verbal fluency para-digm during PET to investigate prefrontal function in 41 MDD patients and 46 controls. As expected, MDD patients performed worse than control subjects; however, prefrontal activation patterns in both groups were similar. In contrast, in the only FMRI study published to date, Okada *et al.*[62] found attenuated activity in the anterior cingulate cortex and left DLPFC in their sample of ten MDD patients, compared with ten healthy controls. Thus, the relationship between impaired verbal fluency and prefrontal hypofunction in MDD is not yet clear.

Barch *et al.*[63] also used FMRI to investigate prefrontal function in 14 MDD patients, compared with 38 schizophrenia patients and 49 healthy controls, during performance of a verbal (letters) and a non-verbal (non-famous faces) 2-back task. Schizophrenia patients were found to perform worse during both versions of the task, but MDD patients did not differ significantly from control subjects. Imaging data revealed decreased DLPFC activation in schizophrenia patients but not in depressed patients, relative to healthy controls. While these findings indicate that DLPFC dysfunction is more pervasive in schizophrenia compared with MDD, it should be noted that Barch *et al.* did not use a parametric n-back task[58,64], so that WM deficits at a higher task load may have been missed[65].

Imaging studies using planning or selective attention tasks in MDD have been rare. George *et al.*[66] performed a PET study using a Stroop paradigm containing both standard and emotional stimuli in a group of 11 patients with either unipolar or bipolar depression, and reported decreased anterior cingulate activity in patients compared with controls. Similar findings were reported by Elliott *et al.*[67], who used a Tower of London task in a PET study in six MDD patients and six healthy control subjects. However, in neither study performance ratings of MDD patients were below those of control subjects. In a follow-up study, Elliott *et al.*[52] employed an emotional 'go/no go' paradigm during functional MR imaging in ten MDD patients and 11 control subjects. In this study, subjects were requested to respond (go) to, for example, happy words (targets) while ignoring (no go) sad or neutral words (distracters), and vice versa. Although behavioural results were similar in both groups, in MDD patients a blunted response to emotional stimuli, in particular happy items, was found in the ventral anterior cingulate cortex. In addition, an increased dorsal medial prefrontal response was observed in MDD patients for sad words but, in healthy controls, for happy words, indicating a group-specific, mood-congruent response bias.

Finally, in a recent FMRI study, Steele *et al.*[68] used a gambling task to investigate differences in error signal (defined as the difference between the predicted and observed monetary gains) between MDD patients and control subjects. MDD patients were found to display greater rostral anterior cingulate and posterior parahippocampal activity relative to controls, explained as reflecting emotional-motivational processing and dysfunctional associative learning, respectively. Unfortunately, differences in orbitofrontal activity could not be assessed due to susceptibility artefact[68].

In summary, imaging studies employing prefrontal tasks have provided mixed results in MDD. Task-related DLPFC activity in MDD is generally not abnormal, with the possible exception of verbal fluency paradigms. In contrast, blunted anterior cingulate cortex activation, both of its rostral and dorsal subdivisions, has been consistently observed in MDD. Thus, whereas resting-state studies have shown hypofunction of both the DLPFC and dorsal cingulate cortex in MDD, the above-reviewed studies provide support only for the involvement of the ACC in cognitive deficits in MDD. Moreover, most task paradigms failed to elicit differences in performance between patients and control groups, again with the possible exception of verbal fluency. Because verbal fluency is likely to rely on intact medial temporal lobe as well as dorsolateral prefrontal function, such deficits may reflect medial temporal abnormalities as well[69,54]. As noted earlier, a number of neuropsychological studies have reported deficits in declarative memory in MDD[70], which has been associated with hippocampal volume loss due to neurotoxic effects of high levels of endogenous glucocorticoids[11]. As was also discussed earlier, hippocampal volume is inversely correlated with illness duration, in particular length of untreated episodes; moreover, memory deficits were found to be worse in recurrent vs. first-episode MDD[71]. Moreover, MDD patients perform better during long-term memory tasks after successful antidepressant treatment[20]. It has been shown that in patients with Cushing's syndrome, which is characterized by extremely high endogenous corticosteroid levels due to an adrenal tumour, episodic memory is also compromised. After surgical removal of the tumour, not only memory function was found to be improved, but hippocampal volume was also increased[72].

Bremner *et al.*[73] investigated episodic encoding in 18 unmedicated MDD patients and nine controls. In the control condition, subjects were read a list of word pairs and asked to count the number of Ds (shallow encoding), whereas in the task condition, a paragraph was read while subjects were instructed to remember it and imagine the scene during the following PET scan (deep encoding). Although memory performance for both shallow and deep encoding was similar for both groups, control subjects displayed increased hippocampal and anterior cingulate activity compared with MDD patients. Inferior prefrontal activity was higher in MDD patients, explained as increased effort[73].

4. Anxiety disorders: obsessive compulsive disorder

4.1 Clinical aspects

Obsessive compulsive disorder (OCD) is a neuropsychiatric disorder characterized by intrusive thoughts (obsessions) and repetitive, ritualized behaviour (compulsions). Common themes for these obsessions are contamination, aggression, and sexuality; compulsive behaviours are typically checking, washing/cleaning, arranging (so-called symmetry behaviour), and hoarding. Although OCD was formerly believed to occur infrequently, recent epidemiological data have indicated that OCD is a fairly common disorder, with lifetime prevalence figures ranging between 1% and 3% (e.g. [74]).

Treatment modalities for OCD are only moderately successful and include cognitive behavioural therapy and antidepressant drug treatment. Both the tricyclic antidepressant, clomipramine, and selective serotonin reuptake inhibitors have proven efficacy in OCD, whereas noradrenergic antidepressants are not effective. However, a considerable number of patients do not show significant improvement in response to SSRIs alone, implying that a solitary disturbance in 5-HT transmission cannot fully account for the pathophysiology of OCD[75]. Clinical research has indicated that a considerable number of these SSRI-refractory cases may benefit from antipsychotic drugs in addition to SSRIs[76]. If untreated, OCD tends to have a chronic-relapsing course, with often considerable morbidity due to time-consuming ritualistic behaviours necessary to alleviate anxiety-provoking obsessions.

Since the third edition of the *Diagnostic and Statistical Manual*[77], OCD has been classified as an anxiety disorder. Comorbidity occurs frequently in OCD, in particular, major depressive disorder, phobic disorders, and Tourette's syndrome (TS). In addition, patients with OCD often present soft neurological signs; moreover, obsessive compulsive symptoms have been observed as part of neurological disorders such as Huntington's disease and Sydenham's chorea, and in patients with lesions of the striatum (caudate nucleus and putamen), globus pallidus, and prefrontal cortex[78]. These clinical findings point to the involvement of prefrontal-striatal circuits in the aetiology of OCD, which has been further underlined by neurosurgical results in intractable OCD, since all proposed methods directly or indirectly disconnect these loops[79].

Since the 1980s, neuroimaging tools have been employed to investigate the pathogenesis and aetiology of OCD. As in MDD, these include volumetric, resting-state, and activation studies; biochemical studies, however, have been rare, with the exception of MRS in childhood OCD.

4.2 Neuroanatomical studies in OCD

To date, over 20 volumetric imaging studies in OCD have been published, the majority being MRI studies. Early studies have focussed on striatal abnormalities, with most studies reporting normal volumes[80,81], although both decreased[82] and enlarged[83] striatal volumes have also been found. Similarly, conflicting findings have been reported for the ventral prefrontal cortex, including the anterior cingulate cortex and the medial temporal cortex[84,85]. These inconsistencies may be due to several methodological issues, for example, scanning details (imaging modality, scanner type, sequences), subject inclusion criteria (comorbidity, medication status), and analysis methods (e.g. neuroanatomical definitions of ROIs). In addition, in most studies, sample sizes were only modest. An exception is a recent study by Pujol *et al.*[86], which included 72 OCD patients and 72 age- and sex-matched control subjects. In this study, voxel-based morphometry (VBM) was used instead of ROIs. In VBM, all structural images are warped to a template, as is necessary for group voxel-by-voxel comparisons. This can be either a standard or a study-specific template (i.e. created from all individual images); the latter being preferable when studying, for example, children or elderly subjects. Although global brain shape variability disappears during this transformation, voxel values are adjusted for volume changes: greater voxel values (higher density) indicate a larger volume at that location[87].

VBM has several advantages over ROI-based methods, as it avoids time-consuming manual segmentation of anatomical structures, with its often low interrater reliability. On the other hand, VBM is sensitive to, for example, differences in subject positioning and movement, and group differences, overall, contrast between WM and GM. Moreover, the smoothing step during image preprocessing may obscure differences in small structures. In the Pujol *et al.* study, reduced gray matter density in OCD relative to control subjects was found in the medial frontal gyrus, medial orbitofrontal cortex, and left anterior insula. A relative increase was observed in the bilateral ventral putamen and anterior

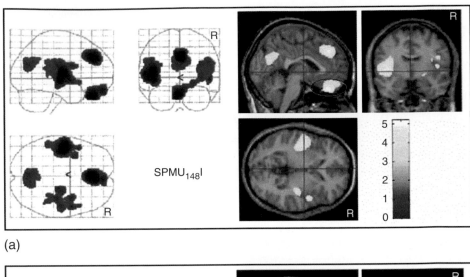

(a)

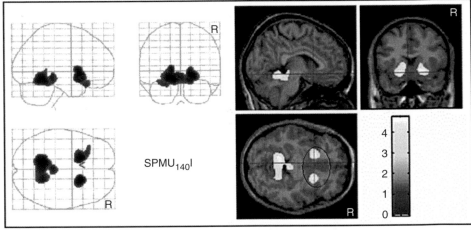

(b)

Fig. 8.7 Statistical parametric map showing voxels with significantly (**a**) reduced and (**b**) increased gray matter density in obsessive-compulsive disorder. (Reproduced with permission from the American Medical Association[86].)

cerebellum (Fig. 8.7). In both groups, gray matter volume was inversely correlated with age, with the exception of the ventral striatum in OCD patients. Structural abnormalities in OCD were not correlated to age of onset, disease severity, comorbid anxiety and/or depression, and treatment history. A lack of normal age-related GM decline was also observed in the dorsolateral prefrontal cortex in juvenile OCD[88]; in an earlier study, these authors had reported increased thalamic volumes in juvenile OCD, normalizing after SSRI treatment[89]. These latter findings are compatible with the hypothesis of OCD as a neurodevelopmental disorder, in which normal pruning is defective[90].

4.3 Biochemical studies in OCD

To date, PET/SPECT ligand studies in OCD have been rare, and have mainly focussed on dopaminergic transmission. Iodine-labelled [^{123}I]-2β-carbomethoxy-3β-(4-iodophenyl)-tropane ([^{123}I] β-CIT) is a SPECT radiotracer with high affinity to monoamine transporters[91] and, thus, can be used to visualize the human central dopamine (DAT) and serotonin transporters (SERT) *in vivo*[92]. Although β-CIT lacks specificity within the monoamine transporter family, distinct brain regions have been found to be related to DA and 5-HT binding; whereas striatal β-CIT uptake mainly reflects binding to DAT. In other subcortical regions, including the hypothalamus, thalamus, midbrain, and pons, β-CIT uptake has been predominantly associated with SERT availability[93]. Alternative radiotracers used to visualize DAT and SERT are the SPECT-ligand iodine-labelled N-(3-iodopropen-2-yl)-2β-carbomethoxy-3β-(4-chlorophenyl)tropane ([^{123}I] IPT) and the PET-ligand C-11 labelled trans-1,2,3,5,6,10 β-hexahydro-6-[4–9methylthio)phenyl]-pyrrolo-[2,1-a]-isoquinoline ([^{11}C] McN 5652), respectively.

So far, ligand studies focussing on SERT and DAT in OCD have shown conflicting results. Pogarell *et al.*[94] found increased β-CIT binding in the midbrain and pons of medication-naive OCD patients, reflecting increased SERT availability. Midbrain β-CIT binding was highest in patients with childhood or adolescence symptom onset, suggesting a more pronounced serotonergic dysfunction in early- compared to late-onset OCD. In contrast, other studies have reported unchanged[95] or reduced[96] SERT availability, using [^{11}C] McN5652 PET and [^{123}I] β-CIT SPECT, respectively.

Recently, Denys *et al.*[97] performed a radiolabelled iodobenzamide ([^{123}I] IBZM) SPECT study, investigating D_2 receptor binding in ten OCD patients and ten healthy control subjects. Decreased D_2 receptor binding in the left caudate nucleus and a reduced left compared to right caudate volume was found in OCD. The authors suggested that the decreased [^{123}I] IBZM binding reflects postsynaptic dopamine D_2 receptor down-regulation by competition with high concentrations of endogenous dopamine. This explanation is in accordance with the hypothesis of an imbalance between direct and indirect pathways of the frontal-striatal circuits in OCD, due to increased inhibition of the indirect pathway by D_2 neurons[98]. Increased synaptic concentrations of endogenous dopamine may result from decreased serotonergic inhibition of dopamine transmission.

In support of the results of Denys *et al.*, Kim *et al.*[99], using [^{123}I] IPT SPECT, found increased DAT binding in the right basal ganglia and a tendency toward an increased DAT binding in the left basal ganglia. In contrast, Pogarell *et al.*[94] reported normal striatal β-CIT binding in a smaller sample of mostly medication-naive OCD patients. Inconsistencies between these studies may be explained by various methodological issues, such as differences in age, gender, medication history, comorbidity, and/or genetic predisposition. Moreover, most studies did not include medication-naive patients, which is important since SSRI treatment may lead to a long-term decrease in SERT availability.

Compared with PET/SPECT, magnetic resonance spectroscopy (MRS) is less invasive, as possible risks when using ionizing radiation are avoided. Thus, MRS is particularly useful for child/adolescent psychiatric research, and for longitudinal studies involving repeated measurements. Most MRS studies in OCD have been performed by Rosenberg and coworkers, investigating early-onset OCD in children and adolescents[100]. An important methodological limitation of MRS is that data acquisition is usually restricted to a single voxel or small volume in the striatum, thalamus, or prefrontal cortex, so that studies are difficult to compare. Decreased NAA signal in the left[101] and right striatum[102] has been found in adult OCD, whereas striatal volumes were unchanged, suggesting that MRS enables early detection of decreasing cell density. In contrast to these studies, Ohara et al.[103] found normal viability of neuronal cells in the putamen and pallidum in medicated OCD patients. The caudate nucleus, however, was not included.

Differences in medication status cannot explain this inconsistency since Rosenberg et al. also found normal thalamic[104] and striatal NAA signal[105] in their medication-naive paediatric OCD patients. In addition, NAA concentrations have also been found to be increased in the DLPFC[106] of children with OCD. Moreover, it has been suggested that the reported reductions in right and left medial thalamic NAA/(Cho+Cr) and NAA/Cho ratios in paediatric OCD[107] actually reflected an increase in Cho levels rather than a decrease in NAA[104]. Therefore, the possible role of cholinergic dysfunction in the pathophysiology of OCD warrants further investigation.

Dysfunctional glutamatergic neurotransmission and/or altered serotonergic modulation of glutamatergic transmission at the level of the caudate nucleus may also be involved in the pathogenesis and maintenance of OCD symptoms[108]. Glutamate is the primary excitatory neurotransmitter in the CNS, and increased glutamatergic neurotransmission in specific frontal-striatal regions may contribute to obsessive compulsive symptoms. Glutamate receptor antagonists have been shown to reduce OCD-like behaviour in mice[109]. Moreover, in a family-based association study, variants of the glutamate sub-unit receptor gene were associated with the susceptibility to develop OCD[110]. MRS results have provided additional evidence for dysfunctional glutamatergic neurotransmission in OCD. Comparing 11 medication-naive paediatric OCD patients to 11 healthy control children, Rosenberg et al.[105] reported increased left caudate Glx concentrations in OCD. After 12 weeks of paroxetine treatment, Glx levels had normalized. Interestingly, successful cognitive behavioural therapy did not induce a reduction in striatal Glx[111]. However, the disease specificity of glutamatergic dysfunction in OCD still has to be addressed, since altered Glx concentrations in the ACC have been found in OCD as well as in MDD[112].

4.4 Resting-state studies in OCD

Compared with healthy controls, resting-state studies (mostly HMPAO-SPECT or FDG-PET) have frequently shown increased metabolism or rCBF for OCD patients in the OFC (either bilaterally[113–115], left-lateralized[116,117], or right-lateralized[118,119]) and in the bilateral[120,121] or left [117] ACC, the left frontotemporal cortex[115], the left insula[118], and the right dorsal parietal cortex[114]. Also, elevated metabolism and rCBF have often been found in subcortical structures, such as the bilateral[122,123] or right[115,117] thalamus, the bilateral[116] or right[123] head of caudate nucleus, and the bilateral putamen/pallidum[124]. These findings point toward hyperactive (orbito)frontal-striatal circuitry in mediating OCD symptoms. This hypothesis receives further support from frequently observed positive correlations between these metabolic alterations and symptom severity in OCD patients[125]; moreover, functional correlations between these areas tend to diminish after successful treatment, as has been repeatedly demonstrated[126–128].

Conflicting findings have also been reported: *decreased* metabolism and rCBF have been found in the above-mentioned structures as well, for the right OFC[125,129], left ACC[125], left lateral temporal cortex[129], left parietal cortex[118,129], bilateral[114] or right[129,130,131] caudate nucleus, bilateral putamen[130], and right[129] thalamus. Some of these opposing functional abnormalities were also correlated with clinical OCD rating scores[125,129]. However, metabolism and rCBF have been consistently found to be decreased in the bilateral dorsolateral/superior prefrontal cortex[129,131,132].

Differences between these studies with respect to the identified structures and to the direction of aberrant activity in OCD subjects may be due to several methodological issues, concerning both patient characteristics and technical (imaging) aspects. The latter may include differences in reporting of absolute versus relative metabolic or rCBF rates, the use of ROIs versus voxel-by-voxel analyses, and the criteria adopted for delineating the applied ROIs. With regard to the former, the inclusion in some studies of OCD patients who used anti-obsessional medication may have presented a confound[116,129,132], since the use of medication may induce brain metabolic alterations over time[133]. Another confounder in differentiating OCD and healthy subjects may have been the use of patient samples with concurrent major depression[125]. A final factor with regard to patient characteristics that may have skewed findings between patients and controls across resting-state studies is the inclusion of OCD groups with different symptom profiles, because these clinical subdimensions are likely to be associated with distinct neurophysiological correlates[123,134].

Apart from cross-sectional designs, resting-state studies have been conducted longitudinally in OCD patients (i.e. at baseline and following treatment either with antidepressant medication or cognitive behavioural therapy (CBT)). These studies point towards a decrease in baseline-elevated metabolism or rCBF in the OFC[135–137], ACC[138,139], caudate nuclei[124,126–128,133,135,137,140], putamen[133,140], and thalamus[133]. These changes were found both after medication and CBT. Importantly, these neurophysiological changes at follow-up were significantly greater in responders compared to non-responders[133,137,139] and/or were associated with decreases in OCD symptom severity[121,126–128,135,136,138] or in general functioning[124]. However, discrepant findings with regard to post-treatment metabolic rates in OCD patients have also been reported, such as a further increase in pre-treatment elevated right caudate metabolism after trazodone[116], an increase in right putamen metabolism[135], and a decrease in bilateral caudate glucose uptake[128] both before and after clomipramine treatment.

Despite these few discordant findings, the overall impression is that improvement of OCD symptoms is accompanied by a normalization of frontal-striatal circuit activity. However, in most studies, the control group was not rescanned, so that treatment effects were potentially confounded with time (order) effects. Moreover, in some studies, pre/post treatment changes may have been due to medication use[128,140] or improvement in comorbid depression.

Finally, resting-state studies have been used to predict treatment response. Swedo et al.[136] found that lower pre-treatment metabolism in the right OFC and right ACC predicted better short-term (two months) outcome after clomipramine treatment, whereas lower left caudate activity predicted better long-term (one year) response. Based on analyses from previously published data[126,127], Brody et al.[141] demonstrated that higher pre-treatment activity in the left OFC was associated with greater improvement in the CBT group, yet less improvement in the fluoxetine-treated group. Similarly, Saxena et al.[137] found bilateral lower OFC pre-treatment metabolism to be a good predictor for paroxetine response. Thus, decreased activity in OCD-associated brain regions at baseline is related to better outcome after medication treatment, whereas the opposite (i.e. increased activity at baseline) may be true for CBT. However, in the study of Hoehn–Saric et al.[139], higher pre-treatment rCBF in the OFC, basal ganglia, and cingulate areas was associated with better clinical outcome after medication. This discrepant finding may have been due to the inclusion of an OCD patient sample with comorbid depression.

In summary, resting-state studies have indicated that OCD pathophysiology is mediated by hyperactivity in frontal-striatal circuits, involving the OFC, caudate nucleus, putamen, and thalamus. A recent quantitative meta-analysis showed that significant hyperactivity in OCD across resting-state studies was actually limited to the orbital gyrus and the head of the caudate nucleus[142]. These functional abnormalities appear to be state-related, as brain activity in these structures tends to normalize upon successful treatment with antidepressants or CBT.

4.5 Activation studies

4.5.1 Affective paradigms

Another strategy to differentiate between state and trait aspects of OCD is represented by symptom provocation designs. By alternating rest and symptom states within a session, the role of time (order) effects, as discussed in the previous section, can be ruled out. Overall, the most consistent finding is provocation-induced activation of various frontal-striatal regions, such as the OFC 143,[144–150], ACC[144,147], striatum[78,144,146,149,150], and thalamus[78,149,150]. In contrast to the *increased* activation in *ventral* prefrontal regions, OCD patients showed *decreased dorsal* prefrontal activation during the symptomatic state[78,151]. In some, but not all studies, activation of the middle temporal lobe structures, such as the amygdala, was also observed[78,146,147,151]. Moreover, OCD patients with predominant contamination fear showed increased activity in the insular cortex, implicated in disgust perception[143,146,148].

Inconsistencies across studies are again likely due to methodological issues, with regard to technical aspects of imaging (e.g. imaging modality, ROIs vs. whole-brain data acquisition and analyses, correction for motion artefacts), patient selection (e.g. medication status, comorbidity, symptom heterogeneity, sample size), and stimulus paradigms (e.g. randomized vs. off-on designs, tactile vs. visual, idiosyncratic vs. standardized stimuli). Many provocation studies used tactile stimuli ('dirty' vs. 'clean'), which necessitated ritualistic behaviour (e.g. hand washing), interrupting the scanning session, so that a balanced order paradigm was precluded[144–147,152].

Whereas most OCD symptom provocation studies investigated contamination fear in 'washers', Cottraux and colleagues[153] included OCD patients with prominent *checking* rituals. OCD patients, as well as controls, showed increased orbitofrontal perfusion during the provoked compared to the neutral state. In addition, provocation-induced rCBF in the basal ganglia was higher in controls compared to OCD patients. In a recent PET study in 11 medication-free OCD patients and ten healthy control subjects, decreased caudate activation in OCD patients compared to controls during provocation of contamination fear was also observed[151]. Since most studies which report increased provocation-induced caudate activation lack a healthy control group[78,144,150], it cannot be excluded that basal ganglia activity reflects processing of emotional information, also present in healthy volunteers. Moreover, in OCD patients, recruitment of frontal-striatal circuitry may be decreased, rather than increased, compared to controls[151,153]. Therefore, it seems likely that the failure of the frontal-striatal circuit in OCD patients to control the processing of negative disease-related stimuli results in an inadequate fear response, as shown by increased amygdala activation in patients relative to controls. However, as noted earlier, amygdala activation has not been consistently found in previous studies, but mostly in small subgroups and/or at lower statistical thresholds[146,147], or not at all[143,144,148–150,153]. This inconsistency may be explained partly by the use of ROIs excluding the amygdala[150,153], small sample size[144,146], use of medication[143,149], and differences in stimulus paradigm. Although the amygdala receives multimodal sensory information, projections from visual processing areas are particularly prominent[154]. Therefore, salient visual stimuli may give rise to amygdala activation more easily than tactile or auditory stimuli. Amygdala involvement in OCD during symptom states is in agreement with studies using fear paradigms in healthy subjects[155–159], supporting the role of the amygdala as a key structure in evaluating the behavioural significance of external stimuli and fear responses[160].

OCD is a clinically heterogeneous disorder. Factor-analytic studies have consistently identified at least four stable symptom dimensions: contamination/washing, aggressive/checking, hoarding, and symmetry/ordering[161,291]. As stated earlier, different neuronal mechanisms may underlie the heterogeneous symptoms of the various OCD dimensions. In two-symptom provocation studies, differentiation between OCD subcategories has been investigated[143,149]. Phillips and colleagues compared 'checkers' and 'washers' using standardized visual stimuli. Similar to the results of Cottraux et al., 'checkers', as well as normal control subjects, showed increased activation of frontal-striatal regions, whereas insular activity was observed in 'washers'. A methodological drawback of this study is that only washing-relevant, not checking-relevant, stimuli were presented. The latter approach was adopted by Mataix–Cols et al.[149], who used general aversive, washing-related, checking-related, hoarding-related, and neutral visual stimuli in a heterogeneous group of OCD patients. Whereas ventral regions of the frontal-striatal circuits were activated during washing-related provocation, checking-related stimuli induced recruitment of dorsal regions of these circuits. Unfortunately, no symptom subtype by stimulus subtype interaction analyses were reported. In future research, it would be interesting to combine the two strategies, thus comparing both patient symptom dimensions and stimulus sub-type within the same study design.

Two studies have been performed to investigate the correlation between pre-treatment response during symptom provocation and the efficacy of treatment with selective sero-tonin reuptake inhibitors (SSRIs). Rauch and colleagues[145], in a small sample of OCD patients with contamination fear, found lower bilateral orbitofrontal and higher bilateral posterior cingulate activation to be predictive of a better response to the SSRI, fluvoxamine. Hendler *et al.*[162], using SPECT, investigated a large group of OCD patients with mixed symptoms. Before treatment, responders showed less provocation-induced activity in the dorsal ACC than non-responders — although these results might have been biased by differences in comorbid depressive symptoms. An additional post-hoc ROI analysis showed that prospective responders also had significantly more pre-treatment provocation-induced activity in the right caudate nucleus than non-responders. Following six months of SSRI (sertraline) treatment, symptom provocation led to increased activation in the left anterior temporal cortex in responders, but not in non-responders. Whether these results reflect biological subtypes of the disorder with differential sensitivity to SSRIs, or merely differences in pre-treatment symptom severity, or comorbid depressive sympto-matology, awaits further investigation.

4.5.2 Cognitive paradigms

Similar to major depressive disorder, OCD is associated with a number of cognitive deficits, as indicated by neuropsychological research. Although results of these studies have not been wholly consistent, impairments appear to stand out in the field of executive function-ing and (non-verbal) memory, especially in application of organizational strategies to effectively complete such tasks[163,164].

So far, cognitive paradigms during functional neuroimaging in OCD have been relatively sparse and have been used to investigate different, often unrelated, cognitive domains. In one of the first of such designs, Rauch and colleagues[165], using $H_2^{15}O$ PET, showed a lack of bilateral striatal activation during successful *implicit* learning in OCD patients, in con-trast to healthy subjects. Instead, patients recruited (para)hippocampal regions that nor-mally serve the processing of *explicit* learning and memory. This finding was replicated in a small (N = 6) OCD sample during FMRI instead of PET scanning[166]. The authors argued that (para)hippocampal brain areas are engaged during task performance in OCD to compensate for frontal-striatal dysfunction. This hypothesis received support from a neuropsychological study that showed a failure of implicit learning in OCD when subjects had to simultaneously perform an explicit memory task[167]. Employing a verbal fluency paradigm during FMRI, Pujol *et al.*[168] found increased left DLPFC activation for OCD subjects while performing the task, as well as elevated residual activation during a subsequent resting period. According to the authors, these functional alterations indi-cated enhanced DLPFC responsiveness to cognitive challenges, and diminished ability to suppress activation during rest in the same area.

Differential activations in the DLPFC between OCD and healthy controls were also found in a recent study on planning capacity using the Tower of London task. In this study, it was found that dorsal frontal-striatal regions were recruited to a lesser extent in OCD patients compared with control subjects[169] (Fig. 8.8). Instead, ACC, VLPFC, parahippocampal gyrus, and dorsal brain stem activity was found in patients. The hypothesis of compensatory activity in posterior brain regions in OCD patients has received additional support from another recent study using a (modified) Stroop task[170]. During performance of a standard stroop task, posterior regions (the fusiform area, parahippocampal gyrus, insula, brain stem, precuneus, and parietal cortex) were activated in OCD patients but not in controls during cognitive interference (i.e. incongruent vs. congruent colour naming). Moreover, in an emotional analogue of this task, processing of OCD-related vs. neutral words during colour naming was associated with enhanced activation of the VLPFC, dorsal ACC, putamen, and amygdala in OCD compared to controls (Fig. 8.9). OCD subjects showed greater responses during emotional interference (i.e. emotional vs. neutral words) only for OCD-related words, but hypochondriasis and PD patients reacted for both OCD- and panic-related words. Also, patients with OCD recruited a predominantly *ventral* system for processing this disease-specific emotional material, as opposed to the other patient groups in which a *dorsal* system for processing emotional cues was additionally observed. These two activation pathways correspond to the ventral and dorsal system involved in generating and controlling emotional responses, respectively, proposed by Phillips *et al.*[171,172] (Fig. 8.10).

In a spatial n-back paradigm (see Fig. 8.5), also using FMRI, van der Wee *et al.*[173] found diminished performance at the highest task load level in OCD subjects, although activity in regions normally found in spatial working memory (e.g. the bilateral DLPFC and parietal cortex) was similar to control subjects. However, in OCD subjects, the ACC was engaged to a greater extent at all load levels. The authors concluded that spatial

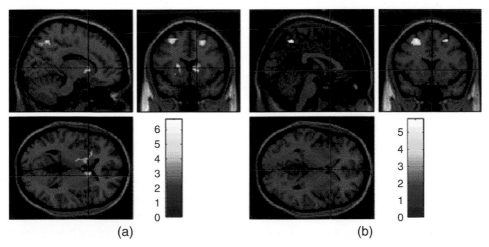

(a)   (b)

Fig. 8.8 SPM showing voxels with significantly increased activity during performance of a parametric Tower of London task vs. baseline, in healthy controls (**a**) and OCD patients (**b**). (Reproduced with permission from the American Medical Association[169].)

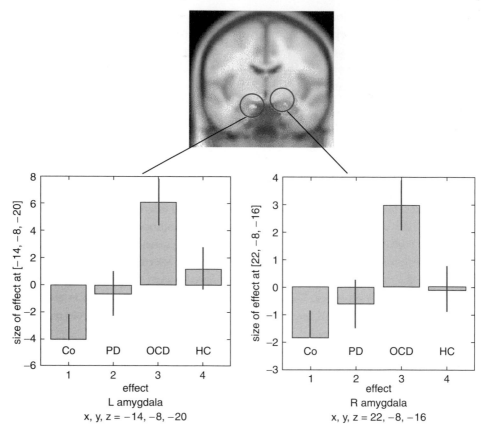

Fig. 8.9 Effect sizes (FMRI) in bilateral amygdala during performance of an emotional Stroop task (OCD-related words vs. neutral words) in healthy control subjects (Co) and patients with panic disorder (PD), obsessive compulsive disorder (OCD), and hypochondriasis (HC). (Reproduced with permission from the American Medical Assocation[170].)

working memory capacity is normal in OCD, but performance is impaired at the highest load level due to ACC interference. Increased ACC activity unrelated to performance is in line with data from Ursu et al.[174], who used a response-conflict (continuous perform-ance) task in OCD and normal subjects during FMRI. They found increased ACC activity both during errors and during correct trials encompassing high-conflict situations. Previously, increased *error-related* ACC activity had been found as heightened and pro-longed error-negativity responses during false trials in an ERP paradigm, using a variant of the Stroop task[175]. However, the results of van der Wee et al.[173] and Ursu et al.[174] extend these findings by showing that increased ACC activity is also present during correct responses, across task paradigms. This may reflect an enhanced and dysfunctional action monitoring in OCD subjects, regardless of actual task performance. It may represent the neuronal substrate of the subjective feelings of doubt, despite correct task performance, characteristic of this disorder.

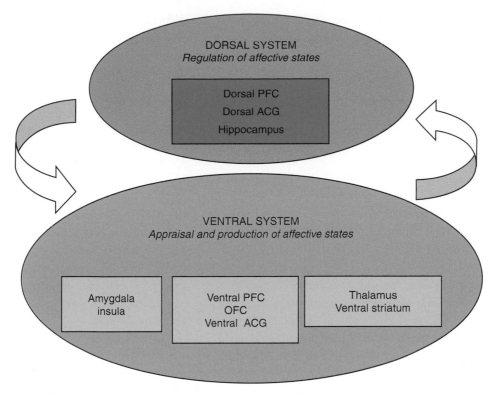

Fig. 8.10 Schematic representation of dorsal and ventral CNS systems involved in generating and controlling affective responses. PFC = prefrontal cortex; ACG = anterior cingulate gyrus; OFC = orbitofrontal cortex. (Reproduced with permission from Elsevier Publishers[172].)

5. Post-traumatic stress disorder

5.1 Clinical aspects

Post-traumatic stress disorder (PTSD) is unique among anxiety disorders as it has a clearly defined aetiology: after exposure to an extreme stressor, individuals experience intense fear and/or helplessness, followed by persistent re-experiencing of the event (flashbacks or nightmares), avoidance of stimuli associated with the event, numbness of general responsiveness, and increased arousal. Such traumatic events may include military combat, physical or sexual assault, and natural or manmade disasters. Apart from these core symptoms, PTSD patients may have impaired affect modulation, various somatic symptoms, and impulse control problems, the latter particularly as a consequence of childhood trauma. PTSD is a frequently occurring disorder and comorbidity with major depressive disorder and other anxiety disorders is high. About half of PTSD cases resolve after several months, whereas in others, symptoms may last longer than a year, with (partial) remissions and relapses[3]. Although the onset of PTSD is, by definition, associated with life events (i.e. trauma), vulnerability to develop PTSD may be determined, in part, by genetic factors. Effective treatment options for PTSD are exposure-based — either cognitive behavioural therapy (psycho-education/cognitive restructuring, exposure, and anxiety management)[176] or eye movement desensitization and reprocessing (for an overview, see[7]). In addition, SSRIs may prove effective[178].

5.2 Neuroanatomical and biochemical studies in PTSD

Structural imaging studies in PTSD have focussed on hippocampal volume loss, although abnormalities in other brain regions, such as the corpus callosum, parietal cortex, and anterior cingulate cortex[179] have also been reported. As in major depressive disorder, hippocampal damage in PTSD has been associated with high levels of circulating gluco-corticoids[11]. In several early volumetric MRI studies, decreased hippocampal volume in PTSD patients has been reported[180–182], although in other studies, no significant differences have been found[183,184]. Since PTSD patients generally have lower cortisol levels compared with healthy controls (e.g. Yehuda *et al.* 2004), this would predict that hippocampal volume loss occurs early during the course of PTSD. However, Bonne *et al.*[185] were unable to detect hippocampal changes in their sample of 37 traumatized subjects, scanned one week and six months after the traumatic event. Also, hippocampal volume was similar in subjects who developed PTSD (10) and those who did not.

In contrast, Wignall *et al.*[186] found decreased hippocampal volume early (mean, five months) after the traumatic event in 15 PTSD patients compared with 11 control subjects, and Lindauer *et al.*[187] reported decreased hippocampal volume in 14 traumatized police officers with PTSD compared to 14 who were traumatized without developing PTSD. Moreover, Lindauer *et al.* were able to rule out comorbid depression and substance abuse (in particular, alcohol) as potential confounders. A similar study in women with early childhood sexual abuse revealed that traumatized women with PTSD had a smaller hippocampal size compared to both traumatized women without PTSD and healthy control subjects[188]. Whereas these latter findings support the hypothesis that PTSD, not trauma, is associated with hippocampal atrophy, Winter and Irle[189] found that adult burn victims, both with and without PTSD, had smaller hippocampi compared with controls. Another unresolved issue is the role of genetic factors, as it has been shown that both Vietnam veterans with PTSD and their co-twins without combat experience had smaller hippocampi compared to control subjects[190].

In summary, although most studies have indicated an association between PTSD and decreased hippocampal size, it is insufficiently clear whether this represents a vulnerability factor, a result of trauma, or of PTSD. Additional support for the latter view has been provided by Vermetten *et al.*[191], who demonstrated that antidepressant treatment in PTSD resulted in improved episodic memory function as well as increased hippocampal volume (Fig. 8.11).

With regard to biochemical studies, ^{1}H-MRS in PTSD has revealed decreased NAA concentrations in the hippocampus[192,193], the anterior cingulate cortex[183], but not the occipital cortex, arguing against generalized NAA changes in PTSD[192]. Ligand studies in PTSD have focussed on GABA-ergic and serotonergic transmission. Bremner *et al.*[194] found decreased prefrontal [(123)I]iomazenil binding in 13 Vietnam veterans with PTSD

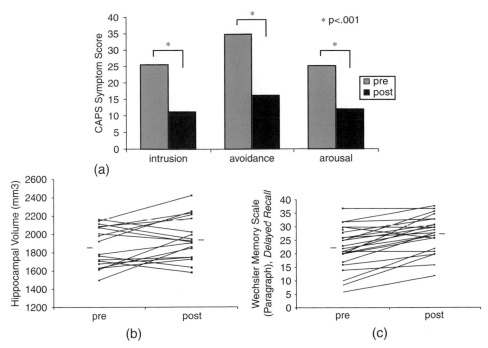

Fig. 8.11 Symptom reduction (**a**), increased hippocampal volume (**b**), and improved memory function (**c**) in PTSD patients before and after antidepressant therapy. (Reproduced with permission from Elsevier Publishers[191].)

compared with 13 controls. However, Fujita et al.[195] were unable to replicate this finding in their sample of 19 Gulf War veterans vs. 19 controls, which may have been due to differences in illness duration and/or severity. In the only published 5HT ligand study to date, Bonne et al.[196] likewise failed to detect differences in 5HT1a binding in 12 medication-free PTSD patients relative to 11 control subjects. Thus, whereas lowered NAA concentrations in PTSD are compatible with decreased hippocampal and cingulate neuronal integrity, abnormalities in neurotransmitter systems have not been clearly demonstrated.

5.3 Resting-state and activation studies in PTSD

Functional imaging studies in PTSD have sought to demonstrate changes in resting-state activity between patients and controls, or before and after treatment, whereas activation studies have mainly used symptom provocation designs. In addition, a few studies have aimed at investigating hippocampal function using memory tasks.

Resting-state studies have provided some evidence for increased perfusion of the (medial) prefrontal cortex and basal ganglia compared with healthy controls[131,197] as well as in cerebellum and temporal regions[197,198]. Medial prefrontal perfusion was found to decrease after SSRI treatment, regardless of clinical response[199].

Several investigators have used HMPAO-SPECT to perform symptom vs. rest comparisons in PTSD. Liberzon *et al.*[200] compared rCBF changes while their subjects listened to either white noise (baseline) or combat sounds on two different testing days. In all subjects (14 PTSD, 11 with combat experience but without PTSD, 14 healthy controls), Liberzon *et al* observed increased anterior cingulated/medial prefrontal perfusion, but only PTSD subjects showed additional increased perfusion of the medial temporal lobe. Lindauer *et al.*[187] investigated 30 traumatized police officers with and without PTSD, and found decreased medial prefrontal and increased right cuneus perfusion in PTSD subjects during listening to trauma scripts relative to neutral scripts. Similar paradigms have been used in single-session activation studies (i.e. PET and FMRI). Pissiota *et al.*[201] used a combat vs. neutral sounds paradigm during PET, observing increased perfusion in sensorimotor, midbrain, and amygdaloid regions in their sample of PTSD war veterans. However, no control group was included in their study.

Trauma vs. neutral scripts were employed in several PET and FMRI studies in PTSD. Bremner *et al.*[202] used PET to investigate 22 women with childhood sexual abuse with and without PTSD. Listening to trauma vs. neutral scripts was associated with increased activity in the posterior cingulate, anterior lateral PFC, and motor cortex. PTSD patients showed less activation in the anterior cingulate cortex and ventromedial prefrontal cortex, as well as deactivations in visual processing areas and the hippocampus. Using a similar design, Shin *et al.*[203] found greater rCBF increases in the orbitofrontal cortex and anterior temporal pole in eight traumatized women with PTSD but smaller increases in the anterior cingulate cortex compared with eight traumatized women without PTSD.

Lanius *et al.*[204] used functional MR imaging to compare nine traumatized subjects with and nine without PTSD and observed less activation in the thalamus, anterior cingulate, and medial prefrontal cortex in PTSD subjects during trauma vs. neutral scripts. In a follow-up study[205], these authors compared ten traumatized subjects with and ten without PTSD during three script-induced emotional states, and found decreased thalamic and rostral anterior cingulate activation in PTSD subjects during all emotional states. Thus, most provocation studies indicate decreased responsiveness of the medial prefrontal and anterior cingulate cortex in PTSD. To investigate this issue further, Shin *et al.*[206] conducted a functional MR study in 16 Vietnam veterans, eight of whom had PTSD. Subjects were asked to perform a modified Stroop task, consisting of neutral, generally negative, and combat-related words. PTSD subjects were found to perform slower and committed more errors than non-PTSD subjects across conditions. During combat-related vs. generally negative words, non-PTSD subjects showed increased rostral anterior cingulate activity, whereas PTSD subjects did not. The authors concluded that their data, as well as those of earlier studies, were compatible with a neuroanatomical model of PTSD that posits a failure of the medial prefrontal cortex to inhibit a hyperresponsive amygdala[206]. However, in most of the studies reviewed so far, no increased amygdala activity in PTSD subjects was found, which may have been due to the use of word stimuli[206]. Indeed, in two studies employing either combat-related pictures or fearful faces, increased amygdala activity in PTSD groups was observed[207,208].

6. **Panic disorder**

6.1 **Clinical aspects**

The hallmark of panic disorder (PD) is the occurrence of panic attacks, defined as sudden urges in anxiety or distress, accompanied by physical symptoms such as palpitations, shortness of breath, paresthesias, and sweating, and cognitions such as fear of fainting or having a heart attack. During the early stages of the disorder, these attacks tend to occur unexpectedly, 'out of the blue', but may become associated with particular situations, such as being in a crowd or on public transport. Patients with PD are likely to develop anticipatory anxiety (i.e. for the next attack to occur) and may avoid situations in which they have experienced previous attacks, resulting in secondary agoraphobia. Substance abuse, in particular alcohol abuse, is another complication of PD; in addition, comorbidity of MDD, hypochondriasis, and other anxiety disorders is high. Although the aetiology of PD is unknown, both genetic and environmental factors are presumed to contribute to its onset.

As noted earlier, PD is a relatively 'new' syndrome, being introduced in the *DSM* in 1980. The dissection of the former anxiety neurosis into panic disorder (of which spontaneous panic attacks are the key symptom) and generalized anxiety disorder (characterized by chronic apprehension and worry) was based on observations that panic attacks respond to antidepressant treatment whereas chronic anxiety can be alleviated by benzodiazepine use. In addition, panic attacks can be experimentally provoked by a number of chemical substances, including lactate infusions, carbon dioxide inhalation, and various sympathicomimetic drugs, suggesting a neurobiological aetiology. A variety of pathogenetic models for PD have been proposed, including effort (lactate) intolerance, carbon dioxide hypersensitivity[209], dysregulation of various neurotransmitter systems, and psychophysiological mechanisms (e.g. interpreting palpitations as a symptom of a heart attack will lead to increased arousal, and so on)[210]. In these neurobiological models, an attempt has been made to associate the various symptoms of PD to a specific neuroanatomical substrate. For example, panic attacks have been postulated to originate in (dysfunctional) brain stem foci, whereas anticipatory anxiety and maladaptive cognitions were linked to limbic structures and the prefrontal cortex, respectively[211]. With the advent of neuroimaging techniques, neurobiological research into the pathophysiology of PD has received new impetus.

6.2 **Neuroanatomical studies in PD**

Early qualitative MRI studies investigating neuroanatomical changes in lactate-sensitive PD patients reported increased focal abnormalities in the medial temporal cortex, mainly involving the right hemisphere[212]. Later studies, using quantitative volumetric MRI methods, have revealed decreased volumes of left and right temporal lobes in PD patients compared to healthy control subjects[213], in particular, the amygdala[214,215], hippocampus[214], and parahippocampal gyrus[216]. Whether volume reduction of the amygdala predisposes to PD or rather reflects a neurodegenerative process secondary to the disorder is not yet clear.

However, no significant correlation was found between volumetric changes of the amygdala on the one hand and duration of the symptoms, number of panic attacks, and demographic variables on the other hand, suggesting a primary rather than a secondary process[215].

6.3 Biochemical studies in PD

Biochemical studies in PD have focussed on the GABA-benzodiazepine receptor complex, based on the anxiolytic effects of benzodiazepines. Conventional benzodiazepines act as receptor agonists and facilitate the inhibitory effects of GABA, resulting in their sedative, anxiolytic, and anticonvulsant effects. Inverse agonists, such as FG7142, in contrast, were found to produce opposite effects (i.e. increased anxiety and arousal)[217]. Flumazenil and its synthetic analogue, iomazenil, are antagonists, blocking the effects of both agonists and inverse agonists, but having few intrinsic effects themselves[218]. Although this spectrum of agonist activities at the benzodiazepine receptor may explain pharmacological effects in human anxiety, aberrant patterns have been found in PD. Panic disorder patients, compared to healthy controls, were found to be less sensitive to the conventional benzodiazepine, diazepam, using saccadic eye movement velocity as a dependent measure, suggesting decreased sensitivity of the GABA-benzodiazepine complex in brainstem regions controlling saccadic eye movements[219]. In addition, whereas conventional benzodiazepines are effective in reducing anticipatory anxiety in PD patients, high-potency benzodiazepines are usually necessary to abort a panic attack.

Abnormal benzodiazepine receptor functioning in PD may be explained by several mechanisms[220]. First, PD patients may have an overproduction of an endogenous inverse agonist and/or a deficiency in an endogenous full agonist. Another hypothesis posits a shift in benzodiazepine receptor 'set-point' towards the inverse agonist direction. This hypothesis would predict reduced efficacy of benzodiazepines agonists, increased efficacy of inverse agonists, and the emergence of partial inverse agonist actions for antagonists, such as flumazenil. Indeed, administration of flumazenil to PD patients resulted in an increase of panic attacks and subjective anxiety in comparison to controls[220,221]. Moreover, this anxiogenic effect of flumazenil argues against the presence of endogenous anxiogenic (inverse agonist) ligands.

Several studies have investigated benzodiazepine receptor function in PD using ^{123}I-iomazenil SPECT[222,223] or ^{11}C-flumazenil PET[224,225]. Early SPECT studies were limited by non-quantitative analysis methods, the presence of comorbid diagnoses, use of antidepressants, and the inclusion of diseased control subjects. Moreover, BZR availability may change over time: whereas most studies reported baseline differences, Bremner et al.[223] were able to compare PD patients who panicked during the scan with PD patients who did not. Compared to the non-panickers, panickers showed decreased benzodiazepine receptor binding in the prefrontal cortex. Baseline differences in benzodiazepine receptor binding have been reported for several brain regions, mainly the prefrontal and temporal cortices, although the direction of these changes was not uniform[222–224]. In contrast, no differences were found by Abadie et al.[225], which may be explained by the inclusion of patients with other anxiety disorders instead of only PD. In addition, Malizia et al.[224] reported a global reduction in benzodiazepine receptor binding, with the greatest differences in the right orbitofrontal cortex and insula, but no whole-brain differences were found by Bremner *et al.*[223].

Whereas most findings indicate decreased binding (global as well as regional) compared to control subjects, the underlying mechanism is not yet clear. Malizia *et al.*[224] suggested that modification of GABA$_A$-subunit composition (for instance, by increased expression of α_6 subunits to which flumazenil does not bind) may be the result of genetic polymorphisms or environmentally induced modification of receptor configuration. Also, increased concentration of brain GABA may induce down-regulation of the GABA-benzodiazepine receptor complex[226]. However, Goddard *et al.*[227], using MRS, found a 20% decrease, not an increase, in occipital cortex GABA levels in PD patients compared to controls. Finally, structural brain abnormalities, such as temporal lobe atrophy, may contribute to decreased flumazenil binding.

So far, most ligand studies in PD have focussed on the GABA-ergic system. Recently, Neumeister *et al.*[228] reported the results of the first serotonergic ligand study in PD. In a PET study in 16 unmedicated PD patients and 15 healthy volunteers, 5-HT$_{1A}$ receptor binding was assessed using ^{18}F-trans-4-fluoro-N-2-[4-(2-methoxyphenyl)piperazin-1-yl]ethyl]-N-(2-pyridyl)cyclohexanecarboxamide (FCWAY). PD patients, compared to controls, showed lower 5-HT$_{1A}$-receptor binding in the anterior and posterior cingulate cortex and in the raphe nuclei. No significant differences were found between PD patients with or without a comorbid depressive disorder.

6.4 Resting-state studies in PD

Early resting-state studies reported abnormally low ratios of left-to-right parahippocampal blood flow and increased whole-brain perfusion in PD patients who subsequently panicked during lactate infusion, compared to PD patients who were non-responders and healthy controls[229,230]. However, in a later report, it was shown that these differences were due, at least in part, to vascular or muscular changes caused by teeth clenching[231]. Nordahl and colleagues[232,233] investigated cerebral glucose metabolism using ^{18}FDG-PET in unmedicated PD patients during an auditory discrimination task. Although their results did not confirm increased whole-brain metabolism as reported by Reiman *et al.*[230], metabolic asymmetry in the (para)hippocampal region was replicated. This left-to-right asymmetry persisted following imipramine treatment[233]. In addition, PD patients showed decreased metabolism in the left inferior parietal and anterior cingulate cortices, and increased metabolism in the medial orbitofrontal cortex compared to healthy controls[232]. Post-treatment metabolic measurements showed a decrease in the posterior orbitofrontal cortex in treated PD patients compared to untreated patients[233]. In another FDG-PET study, Bisaga *et al.*[234] reported increased left-sided hippocampal and parahippocampal metabolic rates in PD patients compared to normal subjects in six female, lactate-sensitive, medication-free PD patients and six female, healthy control subjects. In addition, relatively decreased metabolism was reported for the right inferior parietal and superior temporal cortices.

Using ^{Tc99m}HMPAO SPECT, De Christofaro *et al.*[235] found significantly greater left-to-right asymmetry in the bilateral inferior prefrontal cortex in seven lactate-sensitive, drug-naive

PD patients compared with five normal subjects, explained as increased right-sided cerebral blood flow. In contrast to previous findings, hypoperfusion was found bilaterally in the hippocampal region in the PD group. Also using SPECT, but without lactate provocation prior to scanning, Eren et al.[236] found a significant decrease in perfusion bilaterally in the inferior frontal cortex in their PD patients. In contrast, Lucey et al.[131,237] did not find any difference between PD patients and controls, but instead reported reduced metabolism in the caudate nucleus and the prefrontal cortex in OCD and PTSD patients compared to controls and PD patients.

In summary, resting-state measurements in PD have shown involvement of the (para)hippocampal and medial prefrontal regions, although lateralization and direction of these effects have been inconsistent, which may reflect prolonged effects of pre-test lactate challenge, vascular and muscular artefacts, as well as differences in anticipatory anxiety.

6.5 Activation studies in PD

As discussed earlier, symptom provocation studies in PD have been extensively performed using various pharmacological probes, and these paradigms have also been employed during functional imaging studies. Of these, carbon dioxide inhalation is likely to induce an increase in global CBF which may confound panic-associated rCBF changes. Moreover, CO_2 challenge is anxiogenic not only in PD patients but also in patients with specific phobias, and even healthy controls, limiting its use as a research tool. Lactate infusion, on the other hand, has long been considered a possible biological marker for PD, although its mechanism of action is still insufficiently known. Stewart et al.[238] used Xenon-133 SPECT to measure regional CBF changes in ten medication-free PD patients and five healthy control subjects before and during lactate challenge. Six out of ten PD patients and none of the control subjects experienced a panic attack during the infusion. Whereas whole-brain perfusion showed a marked increase in controls and non-panicking PD patients, in responders, only a small increase or even decrease in CBF was found, presumably due to vasoconstriction secondary to hyperventilation. In their $H_2^{15}O$ PET study, Reiman et al.[239] found increased perfusion in several brain regions, mainly in the bilateral temporal cortex, during lactate-induced panic attacks, but not in non-panicking PD patients and controls. However, activation of these temporal regions was also observed during anticipatory anxiety in healthy volunteers[240].

As an alternative to carbon dioxide and lactate, researchers have used compounds of which the pharmacological properties are more clearly defined. Cholecystokinin (CCK_4), as well as its analogue, pentagastrin, has a high affinity for CCK_B-receptors. This subtype of CCK receptors is especially abundant in several brain regions implicated in fear responses, such as the rostral brainstem, hippocampus, and amygdala, as well as several parts of the cerebral cortex[241–243]. A close functional relationship between the GABA-ergic system and CCK has been found in rats/rodents; benzodiazepines have been shown to antagonize CCK-induced activation of hippocampal neurons[244] and CCK significantly enhanced GABA release in the striatum, frontal cortex, and hippocampus[245]. CCK_B-receptor agonists have been found to induce severe anxiety, in a dose-dependent manner, in PD patients but, to a lesser extent, in healthy controls also[246,247]. CCK_4-induced anxiety could be antagonized in PD patients using the CCK_B-antagonist L-365,260[248]. In addition, pretreatment with the serotonin-noradrenalin reuptake inhibitor, imipramine, or the selective serotonin reuptake inhibitor, fluvoxamine, decreased the vulnerability for CCK_B-agonists in PD patients[249,250]. Using PET, Benkelfat et al.[251] reported increased regional CBF in the claustrum-insular-amygdalar region, the anterior cingulate cortex, and the cerebellar vermis after CCK administration in healthy volunteers. Javanmard et al.[252] extended these findings by showing that CCK-induced rCBF changes may vary over time. Early CCK-induced rCBF increases were observed in the hypothalamic region, whereas subsequent measurements showed increased regional CBF in the claustrum-insular region. In addition, decreased regional CBF was found in the medial frontal cortex.

Until now, only one imaging study in PD has been performed using pentagastrin as panicogenic agent. Boshuisen et al.[253] compared brain perfusion before pentagastrin challenge ('anticipatory anxiety') and after challenge-induced panic symptoms had subsided ('rest') in 17 PD patients and 21 healthy volunteers. Before and after pentagastrin challenge, differences between PD patients and healthy control subjects were found in similar limbic and paralimbic regions, although these activation patterns differed in intensity. Thus, increased activity in PD patients relative to control subjects was found in the parahippocampal gyrus, superior temporal cortex, hypothalamus, anterior cingulate cortex, and midbrain; decreased activation was reported for the precentral gyrus, inferior frontal cortex, right amygdala, and anterior insular cortex. The occurrence of panic in PD patients, as well as increased anxious arousal in controls, was correlated with increased regional CBF in the parahippocampal gyrus, basal ganglia, and parts of the prefrontal cortex, and decreased perfusion in the precentral gyrus, thalamus, and other parts of the prefrontal cortex. Paradoxically, activation of the hypothalamus and bilateral amygdala was found during pentagastrin-induced anxiety in controls but not in PD patients[254]. In addition, partial normalization of the regional CBF patterns was found after successful pharmacological treatment[254]. Thus, the results of Boshuisen et al. failed to demonstrate a clear-cut neuroanatomical differentiation between anticipatory anxiety and panic, as proposed by the model of Gorman et al.[211].

Yohimbine, an α_2-adrenergic receptor antagonist, enhances synaptic availability of noradrenalin (NA) and increases sympathetic activity by blocking pre-synaptic α_2-autoreceptors. The locus coeruleus (LC) has a key role in noradrenergic mediation of physiological arousal. A drawback of yohimbine is that its anxiogenic effects are not specific for PD, but have been found in PTSD as well[255]. Compared to control subjects, PD patients show more yohimbine-induced subjective anxiety and increased cardiovascular biochemical responses, despite similar increases in NA levels[256,257]. Also, levels of 3-methoxy-4-hydroxyphenylglycol (MHPG), the peripheral marker of central NA turnover, are increased in PD patients following administration of yohimbine[256].

Drugs that reduce locus coeruleus firing rate, such as the α_2-adrenergic agonist, clonidine, have been shown to possess antipanic properties[258]. Acute clonidine administration also produced a greater decrease in anxiety and plasma MHPG levels of PD patients compared to normal volunteers, supporting the hypothesis of noradrenergic dysregulation in PD[259,260].

Moreover, treatment with the serotonin reuptake inhibitor, fluvoxamine, reduced yohimbine-induced anxiety in PD patients[261], illustrating the interaction between noradrenergic and serotonergic systems. In healthy volunteers, yohimbine produced a significant decrease in global perfusion and increased regional CBF in medial frontal and insular cortices, as well as the thalamus and cerebellum[262]. Since all subjects hyperventilated after yohimbine challenge, decreased global perfusion may at least partly be explained by hyperventilation-induced hypocapnia. An early, and so far the only, imaging study with yohimbine-challenge in PD patients was performed by Woods *et al.*[263]. Using ^{99m}TcHMPAO SPECT, regional CBF changes were measured after a bolus injection of yohimbine in six medication-free PD patients and six healthy control subjects. All PD patients and only one control subject experienced higher anxiety levels in response to yohimbine. Yohimbine decreased frontal cortical flow in PD patients, but not in controls.

Finally, serotonergic agonists have been used in PD research. Whereas long-term (2–4 weeks) use of SSRIs in PD is associated with increased serotonergic transmission and clinical improvement, patients may at first experience an exacerbation of their symptoms. Moreover, acute administration of 5HT may induce fear-like behaviour in animals. Panic-reducing effects of chronic SSRI treatment may result from several projections of the 5HT raphe nuclei, in particular modification of unconditioned fear responses by inhibition of locus coeruleus and periaquaeductal gray (PAG) activity, and inhibition of hypothalamic release of corticotropin-releasing hormone. In addition, it has been hypothesized that 5-HT facilitates conditioned fear responses (e.g. generalized and anticipatory anxiety) via activation of the limbic structures such as the amygdala and hippocampus. So far, only one imaging study using fenfluramine challenge in PD has been published[264]. To compare regional CBF before and after fenfluramine challenge, $H_2{}^{15}O$ PET was used in nine PD patients and 18 healthy volunteers. The study design lacked a placebo control condition. At baseline, PD patients showed decreased regional CBF in the left posterior parietal-superior temporal cortex compared to controls. Following fenfluramine challenge, a greater increase in perfusion in the same region was found in PD patients compared to control subjects. However, since fenfluramine-induced panic attacks, if present, subsided within 5 minutes of fenfluramine administration and the post-fenfluramine PET scans were acquired at 20 and 35 minutes after challenge, these rCBF changes are unlikely to reflect the actual panic attack.

In addition to these PET/SPECT pharmacological challenge designs, a small number of studies in PD have been published in which functional MRI was employed. Bystritsky *et al.*[265] used an imaginary exposure paradigm in six PD patients and six healthy control subjects, who performed directed imagery of neutral, moderate, and high anxiety-related situations based on an individually determined behavioural hierarchy. Increased activation during high anxiety blocks compared to neutral blocks was found in the right inferior frontal cortex, right hippocampus, bilateral anterior cingulate cortex extending into the anterior prefrontal gyrus, and posterior cingulate cortex extending into the precuneus. Although anxiety ratings were significantly higher in PD patients compared to controls, no panic attacks occurred during the experiment. Increased activation in the amygdala could not be visualized, due to local signal drop out.

Maddock *et al.*[266] compared six PD patients with eight control subjects while making valence judgments of threat-related and neutral words using functional MRI. Compared to healthy volunteers, PD patients showed increased activation of the left posterior cingulate and dorsolateral prefrontal cortex in response to threat-related words. In addition, PD patients had significantly greater right-to-left asymmetry in the parahippocampal region. Although PD patients reported more anxiety during the test than did control subjects, no amygdala response was observed. Van den Heuvel *et al.*[170], in a study in PD, OCD, and hypochondriasis referred to earlier, investigated the disease specificity and neuroanatomical correlates of cognitive and emotional Stroop interference effects. PD patients showed minimal interference on colour naming of incongruent colour words (i.e. the cognitive variant of the task). However, in contrast to the results of Maddock *et al.*[266], increased right-sided amygdala and hippocampal activation was found in PD patients in response to panic-related threat words, associated with increased response latency. Although PD patients did not panic during the experiment, they also showed increased activation of the rostral brainstem during colour naming of panic-related threat words. Hypochondriasis patients showed a similar activation pattern as PD patients, but without the amygdala response.

7. Phobic disorders

7.1 Clinical aspects

Apart from agoraphobia, which is usually diagnosed in the context of Panic disorder, the *DSM* recognizes social phobia and various specific phobias. Social phobia, or social anxiety disorder (SAD), is characterized by fear of social situations, in particular during public performance. In specific phobias, excessive fear can be triggered when patients are exposed to specific objects or situations (e.g. animals such as spiders and snakes, seeing blood or receiving an injection, flying, heights). Therefore, a shared aspect of phobic disorders is that threat appraisal of specific cues or situations possessing ethological significance is dysfunctional. Both social phobia and specific phobias are common, and usually start in early adolescence or mid-teens. Phobias tend to have a strong familiar component and, as is the case with all anxiety disorders, comorbidity is high. Treatment of choice for specific phobias is (cognitive) behavioural therapy, as medication has been found ineffective; in SAD, antidepressant drug therapy (SSRIs) may provide additional benefit.

7.2 Neuroanatomical and biochemical studies in social and specific phobias

To date, MR volumetric and PET/SPECT biochemical studies in social phobia and specific phobias have been rare. In an early study, Potts *et al.*[267] failed to detect differences in total cortical volume and basal ganglia volume between their sample of 22 SAD patients and 22 controls. In the only morphometric MR study in animal phobia published until now, Rauch *et al.*[268] found increased cortical thickness in various paralimbic as well as visual cortical regions in 10 animal phobia patients compared with 20 healthy controls.

The authors speculated that this abnormality was due to defective pruning, although the alternative explanation (increased cortical thickness due to 'overuse' of emotional and visual processing circuitry) could not be ruled out.

In SAD, a small number of biochemical imaging studies have been performed. Tiihonen et al.[269] compared striatal dopamine transporter binding using β-CIT SPECT in 11 SAD patients and 11 matched control subjects. DAT-binding was significantly lower in SAD patients, suggesting that drugs possessing dopamine reuptake inhibiting properties, such as monoamine oxidase inhibitors, may be useful when treating SAD. Evidence for lowered dopaminergic transmission in SAD was also reported by Schneier et al.[270], who found decreased IBZM-binding in ten SAD patients compared with ten control subjects. Recently, Phan et al.[271] found increased Glx concentrations in the anterior cingulate but not in the occipital cortex in ten SAD patients compared with ten control subjects; moreover, Glx concentrations were correlated with symptom severity. Both findings are in need of replication, however.

7.3 Resting-state and activation studies in social and specific phobias

Resting-state studies in SAD and specific phobias have mostly been performed using HMPAO-SPECT. Baseline perfusion was investigated by Stein and Leslie[272] who did not find differences between 11 patients with generalized SAD and 11 control subjects. In contrast, van der Linden et al.[273] and Carey et al.[274] demonstrated decreased temporal and medial prefrontal perfusion after antidepressant treatment in SAD and other anxiety disorders. Most perfusion studies, however, have used symptom provocation paradigms. In SAD, it has been found that perfusion of the amygdala region increases during public speaking[275] and its anticipation[276], although these findings were not corroborated in another recent PET study[277]. Using FMRI, Birbauer et al.[278] found increased amygdala responses to faces in SAD in a small study. Similar findings were reported by Schneider et al.[279] in an aversive conditioning paradigm in 12 SAD patients and 12 controls, and Stein et al.[280], who compared responses to angry/contemptuous and happy faces in 15 SAD patients and 15 controls. Thus, most studies point to increased amygdala responsiveness to disease-specific cues in SAD.

In specific phobias, older PET/SPECT symptom provocation studies failed to show amygdala activity during symptom vs. baseline conditions, which has been explained as a result of rapid habituation[281]. Paquette et al.[282] were similarly unable to demonstrate amygdala activity during presentation of spider pictures, which may also have been due to habituation during each stimulus block[283]. In their event-related FMRI study, Dilger et al. found increased amygdala activity in nine spider-phobia subjects vs. nine control subjects during presentation of spider pictures, but not snakes or mushrooms. In a recent PET study, Veltman et al.[284] also found increased activity in visual processing areas and medial temporal regions, including the right amygdala, during spider vs. butterfly pictures in 11 spider-phobia patients. In addition, prolonged exposure to spider pictures was associated with a significant decrease in anxiety ratings as well as a significant linear decrease

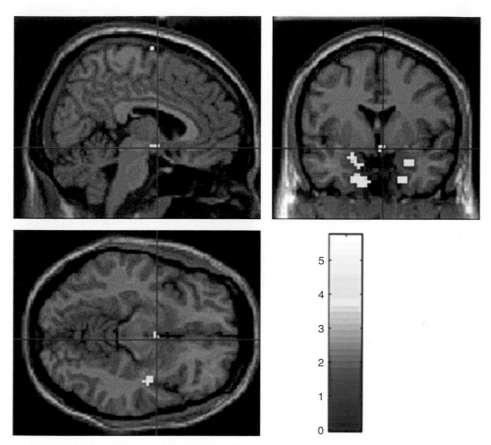

Fig. 8.12 Habituation (decreased perfusion) in the bilateral anterior MTL in spider-phobia patients during continuous viewing of spider pictures. (Reproduced with permission from Elsevier Publishers[284].)

in bilateral anterior MTL activity, supporting the hypothesis of amygdala involvement in habituation to phobic stimuli (Fig. 8.12). In contrast, amygdala responses to fearful vs. neutral faces in specific phobia were similar to those of healthy controls[285], suggesting that amygdala hyperresponsivity in small animal phobia may be restricted to disease-specific stimuli.

Functional imaging studies using cognitive paradigms have been rare. Response bias to disease-relevant words vs. neutral words in spider-phobia patients was investigated by Straube *et al.*[286] who found increased task-related activity in the prefrontal cortex, the insula, and the posterior cingulate cortex in patients but not in controls, implicating these regions in processing disease-specific verbal stimuli. In contrast, Martis *et al.*[287] found normal striatal recruitment during performance of a serial response task in ten phobia subjects compared with ten normal control subjects, implying a different pathophysiological mechanism compared with OCD[165,166].

8. Concluding remarks

Although neuroimaging research in psychiatry is still a new field, a considerable amount of data has been collected over the last two decades with regard to depressive disorder and various anxiety disorders. However, drawing general conclusions is somewhat problematic since studies directly comparing two (or more) psychiatric groups have been rare. Moreover, there is considerable heterogeneity across studies with regard to methodological issues, both at the hardware level (imaging modality, differences in tracers (PET/SPECT) and scanning sequences (MRI)), with regard to experimental design (e.g. stimulus paradigms), and subject inclusion criteria. Nevertheless, at this juncture, several convergent lines of evidence can be discerned.

With regard to volumetric studies, the majority of structural MRI data have indicated hippocampal volume loss in both major depressive disorder and post-traumatic stress disorder, whereas preliminary data have indicated medial temporal atrophy in panic disorder as well. In OCD, hippocampal atrophy has not been observed, whereas in simple phobia, if anything, medial temporal gray matter volume is increased. In MDD, hippocampal volume loss has been observed bilaterally, with a small preponderance of left-sided abnormalities, whereas in PTSD, lateralization differences have not been clearly established. In MDD and PTSD, but not PD, neuropsychological data have shown episodic memory dysfunction, resolving after successful therapy. In PTSD, successful SSRI treatment may even lead to normalization of hippocampal volume, similar to patients with Cushing's syndrome after adrenalectomy. Therefore, it has been hypothesized that hippocampal volume loss in PTSD and Cushing's syndrome results from regression of dendritic processes, whereas in MDD, loss of neurons and/or glia may occur[11].

Whereas the weight of the evidence points to the role of glucocorticoid involvement in HC atrophy, other mechanisms, such as failure of adult hippocampal neurogenesis have also been postulated. In addition, the pathogenetic mechanism of focal prefrontal volume loss in MDD is not yet clear. However, since subgenual volume loss was found to be similar in adolescent and middle-aged MDD patients, this may reflect a genetically determined vulnerability to mood disorders[8]. A neurodevelopmental mechanism (defective pruning) may also underlie morphological abnormalities in OCD. With regard to biochemical studies in MDD and anxiety disorders, the picture is less clear, with the possible exception of decreased serotonergic transmission in MDD. This finding, however, may not be specific for MDD. Other findings, for example the involvement of dopamineric and glutamatergic pathways in OCD, and GABA-ergic transmission in panic disorder, although promising, are in clear need of replication. Considerable evidence has been presented through resting-state studies showing decreased dorsal prefrontal perfusion and metabolism in MDD. Increased activity during rest has been observed, albeit less consistently, in ventral prefrontal and other limbic areas. In PTSD, panic disorder, and SAD, increased activity in limbic regions during neutral states has also been observed. In OCD, there is abundant evidence for striatal-ventral prefrontal hyperactivity as well as decreased dorsal prefrontal metabolism, whereas data for medial temporal metabolism have been negative.

A disturbed balance between hyperactive limbic regions involved in stimulus evaluation and generating an emotional response, and dorsal regions controlling this response, has been postulated as a central mechanism in MDD by Phillips *et al.*[171,172]. In their model, the amygdala has a key role in appraisal and identification of emotional significance of a stimulus, whereas the insula is implicated in disgust. These structures are also assumed to be involved in generating emotional responses, together with the orbitofrontal cortex, ventral anterior cingulate cortex, and ventral striatum (nucleus accumbens). In contrast, the dorsal prefrontal and anterior cingulate cortex and the hippocampus are likely to be involved in response control. Whereas resting-state studies in MDD generally are in accordance with this model, studies using emotional stimuli, including symptom provocation paradigms, have produced mixed results, which may have been due to differences in state anxiety. Moreover, imaging studies using cognitive paradigms have not yet yielded convincing evidence with regard to dorsal prefrontal dysfunction in MDD. Although Phillips *et al.*[172] did not extend their model to anxiety disorders, it may provide a framework for conceptualizing prefrontal dysfunction in OCD[288]. In contrast, current pathogenetic models for PD[289], phobic disorders, and PTSD are all 'amygdalocentric'[290].

In PTSD and agoraphobia, abnormalities in stimulus appraisal have been linked to fear-conditioning models, whereas constitutional factors are presumably more relevant in specific phobias. Most functional imaging studies in PTSD have indicated decreased reactivity of medial prefrontal and hippocampal regions, whereas increased amygdala activity has proved to be difficult to demonstrate, not only in PTSD but also in PD and specific phobias. However, studies designed to circumvent prefrontal influence[290], for example by manipulating attentional processes or by presenting masked stimuli, have provided evidence that stimulus appraisal in MDD and several anxiety disorders is primarily defective. Until now, few studies have included different patient groups, so that the specificity of positive findings remains to be addressed. It has been hypothesized that a similar fear network is involved in PD, PTSD, SAD, and major depression[289]. In this view, these disorders share a common genetic vulnerability and which syndrome becomes manifest, and to what degree, is determined primarily by environmental factors. Such a model might explain not only the high comorbidity between depression and various anxiety disorders, but also the effectiveness of serotonergic antidepressants in these disorders. Future research will need to address these issues by comparing various anxiety disorders and depression, and to address state-trait issues in longitudinal studies as well as twin designs. Finally, future research will benefit from multimodal designs which may yield converging data and system approaches focussing on dysfunctional neural networks rather than isolated cortical regions.

References

1. Kessler RC, Berglund P, Demler O, Jin R, Koretz D, Merikangas KR, *et al*. National Comorbidity Survey Replication. The epidemiology of major depressive disorder: results from the National Comorbidity Survey Replication (NCS-R). *JAMA*, 2003, **289**(23):3095–105.
2. Alonso J, Angermeyer MC, Bernert S, Bruffaerts R, Brugha TS, Bryson H, *et al*. Prevalence of mental disorders in Europe: results from the European Study of the Epidemiology of Mental Disorders (ESEMeD) project. *Acta Psychiatr Scand Suppl*. 2004, **420**:21–7.

3. American Psyciatric Association. *Diagnostic and Statistical Manual of Mental Disorders, 4th revised edition*. APA, 2000.

4. Gershon AA, Dannon PN, Grunhaus L. Transcranial magnetic stimulation in the treatment of depression. *Am J Psychiatry*, 2003, **160**(5):835–45.

5. Richelson E. Interactions of antidepressants with neurotransmitter transporters and receptors and their clinical relevance. *J Clin Psychiatry*, 2003, **64** (Suppl 13):5–12.

6. Fava M. The role of the serotonergic and noradrenergic neurotransmitter systems in the treatment of psychological and physical symptoms of depression. *J Clin Psychiatry*, 2003, **64** (Suppl 13):26–9.

7. Kennedy N, Abbott R, Paykel ES. Remission and recurrence of depression in the maintenance era: long-term outcome in a Cambridge cohort. *Psychol Med*, 2003, 33(5):827–38. [Comment in: *Evid Based Ment Health*, 2004, 7(1):6. Psychol Med, 2003, **33**(5):769–74.]

8. Botteron KN, Raichle ME, Drevets WC, Heath AC, Todd RD. Volumetric reduction in left subgenual prefrontal cortex in early onset depression. *Biol Psychiatry*, 2002, **51**(4):342–4.

9. Bremner JD, Vythilingam M, Vermetten E, Nazeer A, Adil J, Khan S, *et al*. Reduced volume of orbitofrontal cortex in major depression. *Biol Psychiatry*, 2002, **51**(4):273–9.

10. Drevets WC. Neuroimaging studies of mood disorders. *Biol Psychiatry*, 2000, **48**(8):813–29.

11. Sapolsky RM. Glucocorticoids and hippocampal atrophy in neuropsychiatric disorders. *Arch Gen Psychiatry*, 2000, **57**(10):925–35.

12. Barden N. Implication of the hypothalamic-pituitary-adrenal axis in the physiopathology of depression. *J Psychiatry Neurosci*, 2004, **29**(3):185–93.

13. Videbech P, Ravnkilde B. Hippocampal volume and depression: a meta-analysis of MRI studies. *Am J Psychiatry*, 2004, **161**(11):1957–66.

14. Campbell S, Marriott M, Nahmias C, MacQueen GM. Lower hippocampal volume in patients suffering from depression: a meta-analysis. *Am J Psychiatry*, 2004, **161**(4):598–607.

15. Frodl T, Meisenzahl EM, Zetzsche T, Born C, Jager M, Groll C, *et al*. Larger amygdala volumes in first depressive episode as compared to recurrent major depression and healthy control subjects. *Biol Psychiatry*, 2003, **53**(4):338–44.

16. Sheline YI, Sanghavi M, Mintun MA, Gado MH. Depression duration but not age predicts hippocampal volume loss in medically healthy women with recurrent major depression. *J Neurosci*, 1999, **19**(12):5034–43.

17. Sheline YI, Gado MH, Kraemer HC. Untreated depression and hippocampal volume loss. *Am J Psychiatry*, 2003, **160**(8):1516–8.

18. Frodl T, Meisenzahl EM, Zetzsche T, Hohne T, Banac S, Schorr C, *et al*. Hippocampal and amygdala changes in patients with major depressive disorder and healthy controls during a 1-year follow-up. *J Clin Psychiatry*, 2004, **65**(4):492–9.

19. Caetano SC, Hatch JP, Brambilla P, Sassi RB, Nicoletti M, Mallinger AG, *et al*. Anatomical MRI study of hippocampus and amygdala in patients with current and remitted major depression. *Psychiatry Res*, 2004, **132**(2):141–7.

20. Vythilingam M, Vermetten E, Anderson GM, Luckenbaugh D, Anderson ER, Snow J, *et al*. Hippocampal volume, memory, and cortisol status in major depressive disorder: effects of treatment. *Biol Psychiatry*, 2004, **56**(2):101–12.

21. Dhaenen H. Imaging the serotonergic system in depression. *Eur Arch Psychiatry Clin Neurosci*, 2001, **251**(Suppl)2:II76–80.

22. Sargent PA, Kjaer KH, Bench CJ, Rabiner EA, Messa C, Meyer J, *et al*. Brain serotonin1A receptor binding measured by positron emission tomography with [11C]WAY-100635: effects of depression and antidepressant treatment. *Arch Gen Psychiatry*, 2000, **57**(2):174–80.

23. Drevets WC, Frank E, Price JC, Kupfer DJ, Greer PJ, Mathis C. Serotonin type-1A receptor imaging in depression. *Nucl Med Biol*, 2000, **27**(5):499–507.

24. Bhagwagar Z, Rabiner EA, Sargent PA, Grasby PM, Cowen PJ. Persistent reduction in brain serotonin1A receptor binding in recovered depressed men measured by positron emission tomography with [11C]WAY-100635. *Mol Psychiatry*, 2004, **9**(4):386–92.

25. Meyer JH, Wilson AA, Ginovart N, Goulding V, Hussey D, Hood K, *et al.* Occupancy of serotonin transporters by paroxetine and citalopram during treatment of depression: a [(11)C]DASB PET imaging study. *Am J Psychiatry*, 2001, **158**(11):1843–9.

26. Rosa–Neto P, Diksic M, Okazawa H, Leyton M, Ghadirian N, Mzengeza S, *et al.* Measurement of brain regional alpha-[11C]methyl-L-tryptophan trapping as a measure of serotonin synthesis in medication-free patients with major depression. *Arch Gen Psychiatry*, 2004, **61**(6):556–63.

27. Parsey RV, Oquendo MA, Zea–Ponce Y, Rodenhiser J, Kegeles LS, Pratap M, *et al.* Dopamine D(2) receptor availability and amphetamine-induced dopamine release in unipolar depression. *Biol Psychiatry*, 2001, **50**(5):313–22.

28. Kugaya A, Sanacora G, Verhoeff NP, Fujita M, Mason GF, Seneca NM, *et al.* Cerebral benzodiazepine receptors in depressed patients measured with [123I]iomazenil SPECT. *Biol Psychiatry*, 2003, **54**(8):792–9.

29. Sanacora G, Mason GF, Rothman DL, Krystal JH. Increased occipital cortex GABA concentrations in depressed patients after therapy with selective serotonin reuptake inhibitors. *Am J Psychiatry*, 2002, **159**(4):663–5.

30. Michael N, Erfurth A, Ohrmann P, Arolt V, Heindel W, Pfleiderer B. Metabolic changes within the left dorsolateral prefrontal cortex occurring with electroconvulsive therapy in patients with treatment resistant unipolar depression. *Psychol Med*, 2003, **33**(7):1277–84.

31. Vythilingam M, Charles HC, Tupler LA, Blitchington T, Kelly L, Krishnan KR. Focal and lateralized subcortical abnormalities in unipolar major depressive disorder: an automated multivoxel proton magnetic resonance spectroscopy study. *Biol Psychiatry*, 2003, **54**(7):744–50.

32. Strauss WL, Dager SR. Magnetization transfer of fluoxetine in the human brain using fluorine magnetic resonance spectroscopy. *Biol Psychiatry*, 2001, **49**(9):798–802.

33. Seminowicz DA, Mayberg HS, McIntosh AR, Goldapple K, Kennedy S, Segal Z, *et al.* Limbic-frontal circuitry in major depression: a path modeling metanalysis. *Neuroimage*, 2004, **22**(1):409–18.

34. Goldapple K, Segal Z, Garson C, Lau M, Bieling P, Kennedy S, *et al.* Modulation of cortical-limbic pathways in major depression: treatment-specific effects of cognitive behavior therapy. *Arch Gen Psychiatry*, 2004, **61**(1):34–41.

35. Mayberg HS, Liotti M, Brannan SK, McGinnis S, Mahurin RK, Jerabek PA, *et al.* Reciprocal limbic-cortical function and negative mood: converging PET findings in depression and normal sadness. *Am J Psychiatry*, 1999, **156**(5):675–82.

36. George MS, Ketter TA, Parekh PI, Horwitz B, Herscovitch P, Post RM. Brain activity during transient sadness and happiness in healthy women. *Am J Psychiatry*, 1995, **152**(3):341–51.

37. Neumeister A, Nugent AC, Waldeck T, Geraci M, Schwarz M, Bonne O, *et al.* Neural and behavioral responses to tryptophan depletion in unmedicated patients with remitted major depressive disorder and controls. *Arch Gen Psychiatry*, 2004, **61**(8):765–73.

38. Liotti M, Mayberg HS, McGinnis S, Brannan SL, Jerabek P. Unmasking disease-specific cerebral blood flow abnormalities: mood challenge in patients with remitted unipolar depression. *Am J Psychiatry*, 2002, **159**(11):1830–40.

39. van den Heuvel OA, Boellaard R, Veltman DJ, Mesina C, Lammertsma AA. Attenuation correction of PET activation studies in the presence of task-related motion. *Neuroimage*, 2003, **19**(4):1501–9.

40. Lang PJ, Greenwald MK, Bradley MM, Hamm AO. Looking at pictures: affective, facial, visceral, and behavioral reactions. *Psychophysiology*, 1993, **30**(3):261–73.

41. Ekman P, Friesen WV. Constants across cultures in the face and emotion. *J Pers Soc Psychol*, 1971, **17**(2):124–9.

42. Thomas KM, Drevets WC, Whalen PJ, Eccard CH, Dahl RE, Ryan ND, *et al*. Amygdala response to facial expressions in children and adults. *Biol Psychiatry*, 2001, **49**(4):309–16.

43. Drevets WC. Neuroimaging and neuropathological studies of depression: implications for the cognitive-emotional features of mood disorders. *Curr Opin Neurobiol*, 2001, **11**(2):240–9.

44. Sheline YI, Barch DM, Donnelly JM, Ollinger JM, Snyder AZ, Mintun MA. Increased amygdala response to masked emotional faces in depressed subjects resolves with antidepressant treatment: an fMRI study. *Biol Psychiatry*, 2001, **50**(9):651–8.

45. Fu CH, Williams SC, Cleare AJ, Brammer MJ, Walsh ND, Kim J, *et al*. Attenuation of the neural response to sad faces in major depression by antidepressant treatment: a prospective, event-related functional magnetic resonance imaging study. *Arch Gen Psychiatry*, 2004, **61**(9):877–89.

46. Davidson RJ, Irwin W, Anderle MJ, Kalin NH. The neural substrates of affective processing in depressed patients treated with venlafaxine. *Am J Psychiatry*, 2003, **160**(1):64–75.

47. Surguladze S, Brammer MJ, Keedwell P, Giampietro V, Young AW, Travis MJ, *et al*. A differential pattern of neural response toward sad versus happy facial expressions in major depressive disorder. *Biol Psychiatry*, 2005, **57**(3):201–9.

48. Kumari V, Mitterschiffthaler MT, Teasdale JD, Malhi GS, Brown RG, Giampietro V, *et al*. Neural abnormalities during cognitive generation of affect in treatment-resistant depression. *Biol Psychiatry*, 2003, **54**(8):777–91.

49. Lawrence NS, Williams AM, Surguladze S, Giampietro V, Brammer MJ, Andrew C, *et al*. Subcortical and ventral prefrontal cortical neural responses to facial expressions distinguish patients with bipolar disorder and major depression. *Biol Psychiatry*, 2004, **55**(6):578–87.

50. Dolan RJ. Emotion, cognition, and behavior. *Science*, 2002, **298**(5596):1191–4.

51. Siegle GJ, Steinhauer SR, Thase ME, Stenger VA, Carter CS. Can't shake that feeling: event-related fMRI assessment of sustained amygdala activity in response to emotional information in depressed individuals. *Biol Psychiatry*, 2002, **51**(9):693–707.

52. Elliott R, Rubinsztein JS, Sahakian BJ, Dolan RJ. The neural basis of mood-congruent processing biases in depression. *Arch Gen Psychiatry*, 2002, **59**(7):597–604.

53. Daselaar SM, Veltman DJ, Rombouts SA, Raaijmakers JG, Jonker C. Neuroanatomical correlates of episodic encoding and retrieval in young and elderly subjects. *Brain*, 2003, **126**(Pt 1):43–56.

54. Rogers MA, Kasai K, Koji M, Fukuda R, Iwanami A, Nakagome K, *et al*. Executive and prefrontal dysfunction in unipolar depression: a review of neuropsychological and imaging evidence. *Neurosci Res*, 2004, **50**(1):1–11.

55. Bechara A, Damasio AR, Damasio H, Anderson SW. Insensitivity to future consequences following damage to human prefrontal cortex. *Cognition*, 1994, **50**(1–3):7–15.

56. Austin MP, Mitchell P, Goodwin GM. Cognitive deficits in depression: possible implications for functional neuropathology. *Br J Psychiatry*, 2001, **178**:200–6.

57. Baddeley A. The fractionation of working memory. *Proc Natl Acad Sci USA*, 1996, **93**(24):13468–72.

58. Veltman DJ, Rombouts SA, Dolan RJ. Maintenance versus manipulation in verbal working memory revisited: an fMRI study. *Neuroimage*, 2003, **18**(2):247–56.

59. Shallice T. Specific impairments of planning. *Philos Trans R Soc Lond B Biol Sci*, 1982, **298**(1089):199–209.

60. Smith KA, Morris JS, Friston KJ, Cowen PJ, Dolan RJ. Brain mechanisms associated with depressive relapse and associated cognitive impairment following acute tryptophan depletion. *Br J Psychiatry*, 1999, **174**:525–9.

61. Videbech P, Ravnkilde B, Kristensen S, Egander A, Clemmensen K, Rasmussen NA, *et al*. The Danish PET/depression project: poor verbal fluency performance despite normal prefrontal activation in patients with major depression. *Psychiatry Res*, 2003, **123**(1):49–63.

62. Okada G, Okamoto Y, Morinobu S, Yamawaki S, Yokota N. Attenuated left prefrontal activation during a verbal fluency task in patients with depression. *Neuropsychobiology*, 2003, **47**(1):21–6.

63. Barch DM, Sheline YI, Csernansky JG, Snyder AZ. Working memory and prefrontal cortex dysfunction: specificity to schizophrenia compared with major depression. *Biol Psychiatry*, 2003, **53**(5):376–84.

64. Braver TS, Cohen JD, Nystrom LE, Jonides J, Smith EE, Noll DC. A parametric study of prefrontal cortex involvement in human working memory. *Neuroimage*, 1997, **5**(1):49–62.

65. Jansma JM, Ramsey NF, van der Wee NJ, Kahn RS. Working memory capacity in schizophrenia: a parametric fMRI study. *Schizophr Res*, 2004, **68**(2–3):159–71.

66. George MS, Ketter TA, Parekh PI, Rosinsky N, Ring HA, Pazzaglia PJ, *et al.* Blunted left cingulate activation in mood disorder subjects during a response interference task (the Stroop). *J Neuropsychiatry Clin Neurosci*, 1997, **9**(1):55–63.

67. Elliott R, Baker SC, Rogers RD, O'Leary DA, Paykel ES, Frith CD, *et al.* Prefrontal dysfunction in depressed patients performing a complex planning task: a study using positron emission tomography. *Psychol Med*, 1997, **27**(4):931–42.

68. Steele JD, Meyer M, Ebmeier KP. Neural predictive error signal correlates with depressive illness severity in a game paradigm. *Neuroimage*, 2004, **23**(1):269–80.

69. Pihlajamaki M, Tanila H, Hanninen T, Kononen M, Laakso M, Partanen K, *et al.* Verbal fluency activates the left medial temporal lobe: a functional magnetic resonance imaging study. *Ann Neurol*, 2000, **47**(4):470–6.

70. Airaksinen E, Larsson M, Lundberg I, Forsell Y. Cognitive functions in depressive disorders: evidence from a population-based study. *Psychol Med*, 2004, **34**(1):83–91.

71. Fossati P, Harvey PO, Le Bastard G, Ergis AM, Jouvent R, Allilaire JF. Verbal memory performance of patients with a first depressive episode and patients with unipolar and bipolar recurrent depression. *J Psychiatr Res*, 2004, **38**(2):137–44.

72. Starkman MN, Giordani B, Gebarski SS, Schteingart DE. Improvement in learning associated with increase in hippocampal formation volume. *Biol Psychiatry*, 2003, **53**(3):233–8.

73. Bremner JD, Vythilingam M, Vermetten E, Vaccarino V, Charney DS. Deficits in hippocampal and anterior cingulate functioning during verbal declarative memory encoding in midlife major depression. *Am J Psychiatry*, 2004, **161**(4):637–45.

74. Kolada JL, Bland RC, Newman SC. Obsessive-compulsive disorder. *Acta Psychiatrica Scandinavica*, 1994, **376**(Supplement):24–35.

75. Goodman WK, McDougle CJ, Price LH, Riddle MA, Pauls DL, Leckman JF. Beyond the serotonin hypothesis: a role for dopamine in some forms of obsessive-compulsive disorder? *J Clin Psychiatry*, 1990, **51**(Supplement 8):36–43.

76. McDougle CJ, Epperson CN, Pelton GH, Wasylink S, Price LH. A double-blind, placebo-controlled study of risperdone addition in serotonin reuptake inhibitor-refractory obsessive-compulsive disorder. *Arch Gen Psychiatry*, 2000, **57**:794–801.

77. American Psychiatric Association. *Diagnostic and Statistical Manual of Mental Disorders, 3rd edition.* APA, 1980.

78. McGuire PK, Bench CJ, Frith CD, Marks IM, Frackowiak RS, Dolan RJ. Functional anatomy of obsessive-compulsive phenomena. *Br J Psychiatry*, 1994, **164**(4):459–68.

79. Greenberg BD, Murphy DL, Rasmussen SA. Neuroanatomically based approaches to obsessive-compulsive disorder. Neurosurgery and transcranial magnetic stimulation. *Psychiatr Clin North Am*, 2000, **23**(3):671–86, xii.

80. Aylward EH, Harris GJ, Hoehn–Saric R, Barta PE, Machlin SR, Pearlson GD. Normal caudate nucleus in obsessive-compulsive disorder assessed by quantitative neuroimaging. *Arch Gen Psychiatry*, 1996, July, **53**(7):577–84.

81. Szeszko PR, MacMillan S, McMeniman M, Chen S, Baribault K, Lim KO, et al. Brain structural abnormalities in psycotropic drug-naive pediatric patients with obsessive-compulsive disorder. Am J Psychiatry, 2004, 161:1049–56.

82. Robinson D, Wu H, Munne RA, Ashtari M, Alvir JM, Lerner G, et al. Reduced caudate nucleus volume in obsessive-compulsive disorder. Arch Gen Psychiatry, 1995, 52(5):393–8.

83. Scarone S, Colombo C, Livian S, Abbruzzese M, Ronchi P, Locatelli M, et al. Increased right caudate nucleus size in obsessive-compulsive disorder: detection with magnetic resonance imaging. Psychiatry Research, 1992, 45(2):115–21.

84. Rosenberg DR, Keshavan MS. Toward a neurodevelopmental model of obsessive-compulsive disorder. Biol Psychiatry, 1998, 43:623–40.

85. Szeszko PR, Robinson D, Alvir JM, Bilder RM, Lencz T, Ashtari M, et al. Orbital frontal and amygdala volume reductions in obsessive-compulsive disorder. Arch Gen Psychiatry, 1999, 56(10):913–9.

86. Pujol J, Soriano–Mas C, Alonso P, Cardoner N, Menchón JM, Deus J, et al. Mapping structural brain alterations in obsessive-compulsive disorder. Arch Gen Psychiatry, 2004, 61:720–30.

87. Ashburner J, Friston KJ. Voxel-based morphometry — the methods. Neuroimage, 2000, 11:805–21.

88. Gilbert AR, Keshavan MS, Birmaher B, Nutche B, Rosenberg DR. Abnormal brain maturational trajectory in pediatric obsessive-compulsive disorder (OCD): a pilot voxel-based morphometry (VBM) study. Clinical EEG and Neuroscience, 2004, 35:223.

89. Gilbert AR, Moore GJ, Keshavan MS, Paulson LAD, Narula V, MacMaster FP, et al. Decrease in thalamic volumes of pediatric patients with obsessive-compulsive disorder who are taking paroxetine. Arch Gen Psychiatry, 2000, 57:449–56.

90. Jenike MA, Breiter HC, Baer L, Kennedy DN, Savage CR, Olivares MJ, et al. Cerebral structural abnormalities in obsessive-compulsive disorder. A quantitative morphometric magnetic resonance imaging study [see comments]. Arch Gen Psychiatry, 1996, 53(7):625–32.

91. Innis R, Baldwin R, Sybirska E, Zea Y, Laruelle M, Al–Tikriti M, et al. Single photon emission tomography imaging of monoamine reuptake sites in primate brain with [^{123}I]CIT. Eur J Pharmacology, 1991, 200:369–70.

92. Innis RB, Seibyl JP, Scanley BE, Laruelle M, Abi–Dargham A, Wallace E, et al. Single photon emission computed tomographic imaging demonstrates loss of striatal dopamine transporters in parkinson disease. Proc Natl Acad Sci, 1993, 90:11965–9.

93. Laruelle M, Baldwin RM, Malison RT, Zea–Ponce Y, Zoghbi SS, Al–Tikriti MS, et al. SPECT imaging of dopamine and serotonin transporters with [^{123}I]b-CIT: pharmacological characteristics of brain uptake in nonhuman primates. Synapse, 1993, 13:295–309.

94. Pogarell O, Hamann C, Pöpperl G, Juckel G, Choukèr M, Zaudig M, et al. Elevated brain serotonin transporter availability in patients with obsessive-compulsive disorder. Biol Psychiatry, 2003, 54:1406–13.

95. Simpson HB, Lombardo I, Slifstein M, Huang HY, Hwang DR, Abi–Dargham A, et al. Serotonin transporters in obsessive-compulsive disorder: a positron emission tomography study with [^{11}C]McN 5652. Biol Psychiatry, 2003, 54:1414–21.

96. Stengler–Wenzke K, Müller U, Angermeyer MC, Sabri O, Hesse S. Reduced serotonin transporter-availability in obsessive-compulsive disorder (OCD). European Archives of Psychiatry and Clinical Neuroscience, 2004, 254:252–5.

97. Denys D, van der Wee N, Janssen J, de Geus F, Westenberg HGM. Low level of dopaminergic D$_2$ receptor binding in obsessive-compulsive disorder. Biol Psychiatry, 2004, 55:1041–5.

98. Saxena S, Brody AL, Schwartz JM, Baxter LR. Neuroimaging and frontal-striatal circuitry in obsessive-compulsive disorder. Br J Psychiatry, 1998, 173(Suppl 35):26–37.

99. Kim CH, Koo MS, Cheon KA, Ryu YH, Lee JD, Lee HS. Dopamine transporter density of basal ganglia assessed with [^{123}] IPT SPET in obsessive-compulsive disorder. European Journal of Nuclear Medicine and Molecular Imaging, 2003, 30:1637–43.

100. Bolton J, Moore GJ, MacMillan S, Stewart CM, Rosenberg DR. Case study: caudate glutamatergic changes with paroxetine persist after medication discontinuation in pediatric OCD. *Journal of the American Academy of Child and Adolescent Psychiatry*, 2001, **40**:903–6.

101. Bartha R, Stein MB, Williamson PC, Drost DJ, Neufeld RWJ, Carr TJ, *et al.* A short ^{1}H spectroscopy and volumetric MRI study of the corpus striatum in patients with obsessive-compulsive disorder and comparison subjects. *Am J Psychiatry*, 1998, **155**:1584–1591

102. Ebert D, Speck O, König A, Berger M, Hennig J, Hohagen F. ^{1}H-magnetic resonance spectroscopy in obsessive-compulsive disorder: evidence for neuronal loss in the cingulate gyrus and the right striatum. *Psychiatry Research: Neuroimaging*, 1997, **74**:173–6.

103. Ohara K, Isoda H, Suzuki Y, Takehara Y, Ochiai M, Takeda H, *et al.* Proton magnetic resonance spectroscopy of lenticular nuclei in obsessive-compulsive disorder. *Psychiatry Research: Neuroimaging*, 1999, **92**:83–91.

104. Rosenberg DR, Amponsah A, Sullivan A, MacMillan S, Moore GJ. Increased medial thalamic choline in pediatric obsessive-compulsive disorder as detected by quantitative in vivo spectroscopic imaging. *Journal of Child Neurology*, 2001, **16**:636–41.

105. Rosenberg DR, MacMaster FP, Keshavan MS, Fitzgerald KD, Stewart CM, Moore GJ. Decrease in caudate glutamatergic concentrations in pediatric obsessive-compulsive disorder patients taking paroxetine. *Journal of the American Academy of Child and Adolescent Psychiatry*, 2000, **39**:1096–103.

106. Russell A, Cortese B, Lorch E, Ivey J, Banerjee SP, Moore GJ, *et al.* Localized functional neurochemical marker abnormalities in dorsolateral prefrontal cortex in pediatric obsessive-compulsive disorder. *Journal of Child and Adolescent Psychopharmacology*, 2003, **13**(Suppl 1):S31–S38.

107. Fitzgerald KD, Moore GJ, Paulson LA, Stewart CM, Rosenberg DR. Proton spectroscopy imaging of the thalamus in treatment-naive pediatric obsessive-compulsive disorder. *Biol Psychiatry*, 2000, **47**:174–182.

108. Carlsson ML. On the role of prefrontal cortex glutamate for the antithetical phenomenology of obsessive-compulsive disorder and attention deficit hyperactivity disorder. *Progress in Neuro-Psychophamacology and Biological Psychiatry*, 2001, **25**:5–26.

109. Shimazaki T, Iijima M, Chaki S. Anxiolytic-like activity of MGS0039, a potent group II metabotropic glutamate receptor antagonist, in a marble-burying behavior test. *European Journal of Pharmacology*, 2004, **501**:121–5.

110. Arnold PD, Rosenberg DR, Mundo E, Tharmalingam S, Kennedy JL, Richter MA. Association of a glutamate (NMDA) subunit receptor gene (GRIN2B) with obsessive-compulsive disorder: a preliminary study. *Psychopharmacology*, 2004, **174**:530–8.

111. Benazon NR, Moore GJ, Rosenberg DR. Neurochemical analyses in pediatric obsessive-compulsive disorder in patients treated with cognitive-behavioral therapy. *Journal of the American Academy of Child and Adolescent Psychiatry*, 2003, **42**:1279–85.

112. Rosenberg DR, Mirza Y, Russell A, Tang J, Smith JM, Banerjee SP, *et al.* Reduced anterior cingulate glutamatergic concentrations in childhood OCD and major depression versus healthy controls. *Journal of the American Academy of Child and Adolescent Psychiatry*, 2004, **43**:1146–53.

113. Baxter LR, Jr., Schwartz JM, Mazziotta JC, Phelps ME, Pahl JJ, Guze BH, *et al.* Cerebral glucose metabolic rates in nondepressed patients with obsessive-compulsive disorder. *Am J Psychiatry*, 1988, **145**(12):1560–3.

114. Rubin RT, Villanueva–Meyer J, Ananth J, Trajmar PG, Mena I. Regional xenon 133 cerebral blood flow and cerebral technetium 99m HMPAO uptake in unmedicated patients with obsessive-compulsive disorder and matched normal control subjects. Determination by high-resolution single-photon emission computed tomography [see comments]. *Arch Gen Psychiatry*, 1992, **49**(9):695–702.

115. Alptekin K, Degirmenci B, Kivircik B, Durak H, Yemez B, Derebek E, *et al.* Tc-99m HMPAO brain perfusion SPECT in drug-free obsessive-compulsive patients without depression. *Psychiatry Research: Neuroimaging*, 2001, **107**:51–6.

116. Baxter LR, Jr., Phelps ME, Mazziotta JC, Guze BH, Schwartz JM, Selin CE. Local cerebral glucose metabolic rates in obsessive-compulsive disorder. A comparison with rates in unipolar depression and in normal controls. *Arch Gen Psychiatry*, 1987, **44**(3):211–8.

117. Swedo SE, Schapiro MB, Grady CL, Cheslow DL, Leonard HL, Kumar A, *et al.* Cerebral glucose metabolism in childhood-onset obsessive-compulsive disorder. *Arch Gen Psychiatry*, 1989, **46**:518–23.

118. Kwon JS, Kim JJ, Lee DW, Lee JS, Lee DS, Kim MS, *et al.* Neural correlates of clinical symptoms and cognitive dysfunctions in obsessive-compulsive disorder. *Psychiatry Research: Neuroimaging*, 2003, **122**:37–47.

119. Lacerda ALT, Dalgalarrondo P, Caetano D, Camargo EE, Etchebehere ECSC, Soares JC. Elevated thalamic and prefrontal regional cerebral blood flow in obsessive-compulsive disorder: a SPECT study. *Psychiatry Research: Neuroimaging*, 2003, **123**:125–34.

120. Machlin SR, Harris GJ, Pearlson GD, Hoehn–Saric R, Jeffery P, Camargo EE. Elevated medial-frontal cerebral blood flow in obsessive-compulsive patients: a SPECT study. *Am J Psychiatry*, 1991, **148**(9):1240–2.

121. Perani D, Colombo C, Bressi S, Bonfanti A, Grassi F, Scarone S, *et al.* [^{18}F]FDG PET study in obsessive-compulsive disorder: a clinical/metabolic correlation study after treatment. *Br J Psychiatry*, 1995, **166**:244–50.

122. Saxena S, Brody AL, Ho ML, Alborzian S, Ho MK, Maidment KM, *et al.* Cerebral metabolism in major depression and obsessive-compulsive disorder occurring separately and concurrently. *Biol Psychiatry*, 2001, **50**:159–170.

123. Saxena S, Brody AL, Maidment KM, Smith E, Zohrabi N, Katz E, *et al.* Cerebral glucose metalbolism in obsessive-compulsive hoarding. *Am J Psychiatry*, 2004, **161**:1038–48.

124. Nakatani E, Nakgawa A, Ohara Y, Goto S, Uozumi N, Iwakiri M, *et al.* Effects of behavioral therapy on regional cerebral blood flow in obsessive-compulsive disorder. *Psychiatry Research: Neuroimaging*, 2003, **124**:113–20.

125. Busatto GF, Zamignani DR, Buchpiquel CA, Garrido GEJ, Glabus MF, Rocha ET, *et al.* A voxel-based investigation of regional cerebral blood flow abnormalities in obsessive-compulsive disorder using single photon emission computed tomography (SPECT). *Psychiatry Research: Neuroimaging*, 2000, **99**:15–27.

126. Baxter LR, Jr., Schwartz JM, Bergman KS, Szuba MP, Guze BH, Mazziotta JC, *et al.* Caudate glucose metabolic rate changes with both drug and behavior therapy for obsessive-compulsive disorder. *Arch Gen Psychiatry*, 1992, **49**(9):681–9.

127. Schwartz JM, Stoessel PW, Baxter LR, Jr., Martin KM, Phelps ME. Systematic changes in cerebral glucose metabolic rate after successful behavior modification treatment of obsessive-compulsive disorder. *Arch Gen Psychiatry*, 1996, **53**:109–13.

128. Rubin RT, Ananth J, Villanueva–Meyer J, Trajmar PG, Mena I. Regional ^{133}Xenon cerebral blood flow and cerebral ^{99m}Tc-HMPAO uptake in patients with obsessive-compulsive disorder before and during treatment. *Biol Psychiatry*, 1995, **38**:429–37.

129. Lucey JV, Costa DC, Blanes T, Busatto G, Pilowsky LS, Takei N, *et al.* Regional cerebral blood flow in obsessive-compulsive disordered patients at rest: differential correlates with obsessive-compulsive and anxious-avoidant dimensions. *British Journal of Psychiatry*, 1995, **167**:629–34.

130. Edmonstone Y, Austin MP, Prentice N, Dougall N, Freeman CPL, Ebmeier KP, *et al.* Uptake of ^{99m}Tc-exametazime shown by single photon emission computered tomography in obsessive-compulsive disorder compared with major depression and normal controls. *Acta Psychiatrica Scandinavica*, 1994, **90**:298–303.

131. Lucey JV, Costa DC, Adshead G, Deahl M, Busatto G, Gacinovic S, *et al.* Brain blood flow in anxiety disorders: OCD, panic disorder with agoraphobia, and post-traumatic stress disorder on 99m TcHMPAO single photon emission tomography (SPET). *British Journal of Psychiatry*, 1997, **171**:346–50.

132. Martinot JL, Allilaire JF, Mazoyer BM, Hantouche E, Huret JD, Legaut–Demare F, *et al.* Obsessive-compulsive disorder: a clinical, neuropsychological and positron emission tomography study. *Acta Psychiatr Scand*, 1990, **82**(3):233–42.

133. Saxena S, Brody AL, Ho ML, Alborzian S, Maidment KM, Zohrabi N, *et al.* Differential cerebral metabolic changes with paroxetine treatment of obsessive-compulsive disorder versus major depression. *Arch Gen Psychiatry*, 2002, **59**:250–61.

134. Mataix–Cols D, Cullen S, Lange K, Zelaya F, Andrew C, Amaro E, *et al.* Neural correlates of anxiety associated with obsessive-compulsive symptom dimensions in normal volunteers. *Biol Psychiatry*, 2003, **53**:482–93.

135. Benkelfat C, Nordahl TE, Semple WE, King AC, Murphy DL, Cohen RM. Local cerebral glucose metabolic rates in obsessive-compulsive disorder. Patients treated with clomipramine. *Arch Gen Psychiatry*, 1990, **47**(9):840–8.

136. Swedo SE, Pietrini P, Leonard HL, Schapiro MB, Rettew DC, Goldberger EL, *et al.* Cerebral glucose metabolism in childhood-onset obsessive-compulsive disorder. Revisualization during pharmacotherapy. *Arch Gen Psychiatry*, 1992, **49**(9):690–4.

137. Saxena S, Brody AL, Maidment KM, Dunkin JJ, Colgan M, Alborzian S, *et al.* Localized orbitofrontal and subcortical metabolic changes and predictors of response to paroxetine treatment in obsessive-compulsive disorder. *Neuropsychopharmacology*, 1999, **21**:683–93.

138. Hoehn–Saric R, Pearlson GD, Harris GJ, Machlin SR, Camargo EE. Effects of fluoxetine on regional cerebral blood flow in obsessive-compulsive patients. *Am J Psychiatry*, 1991, **148**:1243–5.

139. Hoehn–Saric R, Schlaepfer TE, Greenberg BD, McLeod DR, Pearlson GD, Wong SH. Cerebral blood flow in obsessive-compulsive patients with major depression: effect of treatment with sertraline or desipramine on treatment responders and non-responders. *Psychiatry Research: Neuroimaging*, 2001, **108**:89–100.

140. Kang DH, Kwon JS, Kim JJ, Youn T, Park HJ, Kim MS, *et al.* Brain glucose metabolic changes associated with neuropsychological improvements after 4 months of treatment in patients with obsessive-compulsive disorder. *Acta Psychiatrica Scandinavica*, 2003, **107**:291–7.

141. Brody AL, Saxena S, Schwartz JM, Stoessel PW, Maidment KM, Phelps ME, *et al.* FDG-PET predictors of response to behavioral therapy and pharmacotherapy in obsessive compulsive disorder. *Psychiatry Research: Neuroimaging*, 1998; **84**:1–6.

142. Whiteside SP, Port JD, Abramowitz JS. A meta-analysis of functional neuroimaging in obsessive-compulsive disorder. *Psychiatry Res*, 2004, **132**(1):69–79.

143. Phillips ML, Marks IM, Senior C, Lythgoe D, O'Dwyer AM, Meehan O, *et al.* A differential neural response in obsessive-compulsive disorder patients with washing compared with checking symptoms to disgust. *Psychological Medicine*, 2000, **30**:1037–50.

144. Rauch SL, Jenike MA, Alpert NM, Baer L, Breiter HC, Savage CR, *et al.* Regional cerebral blood flow measured during symptom provocation in obsessive-compulsive disorder using oxygen 15-labeled carbon dioxide and positron emission tomography [see comments]. *Arch Gen Psychiatry*, 1994, **51**(1):62–70.

145. Rauch SL, Shin LM, Dougherthy DD, Alpert NM, Fischman AJ, Jenike MA. Predictors of fluvoxamine response in contamination-related obsessive compulsive disorder: a PET symptom provocation study. *Neuropsychopharmacology*, 2002, **27**:782–91.

146. Breiter HC, Rauch SL, Kwong KK, Baker JR, Weisskoff RM, Kennedy DN, *et al.* Functional magnetic resonance imaging of symptom provocation in obsessive-compulsive disorder. *Arch Gen Psychiatry*, 1996, **53**(7):595–606.

147. Adler CM, McDonough–Ryan P, Sax KW, Holland SK, Arndt S, Strakowski SM. fMRI of neuronal activation with symptom provocation in unmedicated patients with obsessive-compulsive disorder. *Journal of Psychiatric Research*, 2000, **34**:317–24.

148. Shapira NA, Liu Y, He AG, Bradley MM, Lessig MC, James GA, *et al*. Brain activation by disgust-inducing pictures in obsessive-compulsive disorder. *Biol Psychiatry*, 2003, **54**:751–6.

149. Mataix–Cols D, Wooderson S, Lawrence N, Brammer MJ, Speckens A, Phillips ML. Distinct neural correlates of washing, checking, and hoarding symptom dimensions in obsessive-compulsive disorder. *Arch Gen Psychiatry*, 2004, **61**:564–76.

150. Chen XL, Xie JX, Han HB, Cui YH, Zhang BQ. MR perfusion-weighted imaging and quantitative analysis of cerebral hemodynamics with symptom provocation in unmedicated patients with obsessive-compulsive disorder. *Neuroscience Letters*, 2004, **370**:206–11.

151. van den Heuvel OA, Veltman DJ, Groenewegen HJ, Dolan RJ, Cath DC, Boellaard R, *et al*. Amygdala activity in obsessive-compulsive disorder with contamination fear: a study with oxygen-15 water positron emission tomography. *Psychiatry Res*, 2004, **132**(3):225–37.

152. Simpson HB, Tenke CE, Towey JB, Liebowitz MR, Bruder GE. Symptom provocation alters behavioral ratings and brain electrical activity in obsessive-compulsive disorder: a preliminary study. *Psychiatry Research*, 2000, **95**:149–55.

153. Cottraux J, Gerard D, Cinotti L, Froment JC, Deiber MP, Le Bars D, *et al*. A controlled positron emission tomography study of obsessive and neutral auditory stimulation in obsessive-compulsive disorder with checking rituals. *Psychiatry Res*, 1996, **60**(2–3):101–12.

154. Amaral DG, Behiea H, Kelly JL. Topographic organization of projections from the amygdala to the visual cortex in the macaque monkey. *Neuroscience*, 2003, **118**:1099–120.

155. Morris JS, Frith CD, Perrett DI, Rowland D, Young AW, Calder AJ, *et al*. A differential neural response in the human amygdala to fearful and happy facial expressions. *Nature*, 1996, **383**:812–5.

156. Morris JS, Friston KJ, Buchel C, Frith CD, Young AW, Calder AJ, *et al*. A Neuromodulatory role for the human amygdala in processing emotional facial expressions. *Brain*, 1998, **121**:47–57.

157. Phillips ML, Young AW, Senior C, Brammer MJ, Andrew C, Calder AJ, *et al*. A specific neural substrate for perceiving facial expressions of disgust. *Nature*, 1997, **389**:495–8.

158. Phillips ML, Medford N, Young AW, Williams L, Williams SCR, Bullmore ET, *et al*. Time courses of left and right amygdalar responses to fearful facial expressions. *Human Brain Mapping*, 2001, **12**:193–202.

159. Wright CI, Fischer H, Whalen PJ, McInerney SC, Shin LM, Rauch SL. Differential prefrontal cortex and amygdala habituation to repeatedly presented emotional stimuli. *Neuroreport*, 2001, **12**:379–83.

160. Ledoux J. *The emotional brain, the mysterious underpinnings of emotional life, 1st edition.* New York: Touchstone, 1996.

161. Leckman JF, Grice DE, Boardman J, Zhang H, Vitale A, Bondi C, *et al*. Symptoms of obsessive-compulsive disorder. *Am J Psychiatry*, 1997, **154**:911–17.

162. Hendler T, Goshen E, Zwas ST, Sasson Y, Gal G, Zohar J. Brain reactivity to specific symptom provocation indicates prospective therapeutic outcome in OCD. *Psychiatry Research: Neuroimaging*, 2003, **124**:87–103.

163. Purcell R, Maruff P, Kyrios M, Pantelis C. Cognitive deficits in obsessive-compulsive disorder on tests of frontal- striatal function. *Biol Psychiatry*, 1998, **43**(5):348–57.

164. Greisberg S, McKay D. Neuropsychology of obsessive-compulsive disorder: a review and treatment implications. *Clinical Psychology Review*, 2003, **23**:95–117.

165. Rauch SL, Savage CR, Alpert NM, Dougherty D, Kendrick A, Curran T, *et al*. Probing striatal function in obsessive-compulsive disorder: a PET study of implicit sequence learning. *J Neuropsychiatry Clin Neurosci*, 1997, **9**(4):568–73.

166. Rauch SL, Whalen PJ, Shin LM, Coffey BJ, Savage CR, McInerney SC, *et al.* Probing striato-thalamic function in obsessive-compulsive disorder and Tourette syndrome using neuroimaging methods. *Advances in Neurology*, 2001, **85**:207–24.

167. Deckersbach T, Savage CR, Curran T, Bohne A, Wilhelm S, Baer L, *et al.* A study of parallel implicit and explicit information processing in patients with obsessive-compulsive disorder. *Am J Psychiatry*, 2002, **159**:1780–2.

168. Pujol J, Torres L, Deus J, Cardoner N, Pifarré J, Capdevila A, *et al.* Functional magnetic resonance imaging study of frontal lobe activation during word generation in obsessive-compulsive disorder. *Biol Psychiatry*, 1999, **45**:891–7.

169. van den Heuvel OA, Veltman DJ, Groenewegen HJ, Cath DC, van Balkom AJ, van Hartskamp J, *et al.* Frontal-striatal dysfunction during planning in obsessive-compulsive disorder. *Arch Gen Psychiatry*, 2005, **62**(3):301–9.

170. van den Heuvel OA, Veltman DJ, Groenewegen HJ, Witter MP, Merkelbach J, Cath DC *et al.* Disorder-specific neuroanatomical correlates of attentional bias in obsessive-compulsive disorder, panic disorder and hypovhondriasis. *Arch Gen Psychiatry*, 2005, **62**(8):922–33.

171. Phillips ML, Drevets WC, Rauch SL, Lane R. Neurobiology of emotion perception. I: the neural basis of normal emotion perception. *Biol Psychiatry*, 2003, **54**:504–14.

172. Phillips ML, Drevets WC, Rauch SL, Lane R. Neurobiology of emotion perception. II: implications for major psychiatric disorders. *Biol Psychiatry*, 2003, **54**:515–28.

173. van der Wee N, Ramsey NF, Jansma JM, Denys DA, van Megen HJGM, Westenberg HMG, *et al.* Spatial working memory deficits in obsessive-compulsive disorder are associated with excessive engagement of the medial frontal cortex. *Neuroimage*, 2003, **20**:2271–80.

174. Ursu S, Stenger VA, Shear MK, Jones MR, Carter CS. Overactive action monitoring in obsessive-compulsive disorder: evidence from functional magnetic resonance imaging. *Psychological Science*, 2003, **14**:347–53.

175. Gehring WJ, Himle J, Nisenson LG. Action-monitoring dysfunction in obsessive-compulsive disorder. *Psychological Science*, 2000, **11**:1–6.

176. Harvey AG, Bryant RA, Tarrier N. Cognitive behaviour therapy for posttraumatic stress disorder. *Clin Psychol Rev*, 2003, **23**(3):501–22.

177. Bradley R, Greene J, Russ E, Dutra L, Westen D. A multidimensional meta-analysis of psychotherapy for PTSD. *Am J Psychiatry*, 2005, **162**(2):214–27.

178. Donnelly CL. Pharmacologic treatment approaches for children and adolescents with posttraumatic stress disorder. *Child Adolesc Psychiatr Clin N Am*, 2003, **12**(2):251–69.

179. Rauch SL, Shin LM, Segal E, Pitman RK, Carson MA, McMullin K, *et al.* Selectively reduced regional cortical volumes in post-traumatic stress disorder. *Neuroreport*, 2003, **14**(7):913–6.

180. Bremner JD, Randall P, Scott TM, Bronen RA, Seibyl JP, Southwick SM, *et al.* MRI-based measurement of hippocampal volume in patients with combat-related posttraumatic stress disorder. *Am J Psychiatry*, 1995, **152**(7):973–81.

181. Bremner JD, Randall P, Vermetten E, Staib L, Bronen RA, Mazure C, *et al.* Magnetic resonance imaging-based measurement of hippocampal volume in posttraumatic stress disorder related to childhood physical and sexual abuse — a preliminary report. *Biol Psychiatry*, 1997, **41**(1):23–32.

182. Gurvits TV, Shenton ME, Hokama H, Ohta H, Lasko NB, Gilbertson MW, *et al.* Magnetic resonance imaging study of hippocampal volume in chronic, combat-related posttraumatic stress disorder. *Biol Psychiatry*, 1996, **40**(11):1091–9.

183. De Bellis MD, Keshavan MS, Shifflett H, Iyengar S, Beers SR, Hall J, *et al.* Brain structures in pediatric maltreatment-related posttraumatic stress disorder: a sociodemographically matched study. *Biol Psychiatry*, 2002, **52**(11):1066–78.

184. Fennema–Notestine C, Stein MB, Kennedy CM, Archibald SL, Jernigan TL. Brain morphometry in female victims of intimate partner violence with and without posttraumatic stress disorder. *Biol Psychiatry*, 2002, **52**(11):1089–101.

185. Bonne O, Brandes D, Gilboa A, Gomori JM, Shenton ME, Pitman RK, *et al*. Longitudinal MRI study of hippocampal volume in trauma survivors with PTSD. *Am J Psychiatry*, 2001, **158**(8):1248–51.

186. Wignall EL, Dickson JM, Vaughan P, Farrow TF, Wilkinson ID, Hunter MD, *et al*. Smaller hippocampal volume in patients with recent-onset posttraumatic stress disorder. *Biol Psychiatry*, 2004, **56**(11):832–6.

187. Lindauer RJ, Booij J, Habraken JB, Uylings HB, Olff M, Carlier IV, *et al*. Cerebral blood flow changes during script-driven imagery in police officers with posttraumatic stress disorder. *Biol Psychiatry*, 2004, **56**(11):853–61.

188. Bremner JD, Vythilingam M, Vermetten E, Southwick SM, McGlashan T, Nazeer A, *et al*. MRI and PET study of deficits in hippocampal structure and function in women with childhood sexual abuse and posttraumatic stress disorder. *Am J Psychiatry*, 2003, **160**(5):924–32.

189. Winter H, Irle E. Hippocampal volume in adult burn patients with and without posttraumatic stress disorder. *Am J Psychiatry*, 2004, **161**(12):2194–200.

190. Gilbertson MW, Shenton ME, Ciszewski A, Kasai K, Lasko NB, Orr SP, *et al*. Smaller hippocampal volume predicts pathologic vulnerability to psychological trauma. *Nat Neurosci*, 2002, **5**(11):1242–7.

191. Vermetten E, Vythilingam M, Southwick SM, Charney DS, Bremner JD. Long-term treatment with paroxetine increases verbal declarative memory and hippocampal volume in posttraumatic stress disorder. *Biol Psychiatry*, 2003, **54**(7):693–702.

192. Villarreal G, Petropoulos H, Hamilton DA, Rowland LM, Horan WP, Griego JA, et al. Proton magnetic resonance spectroscopy of the hippocampus and occipital white matter in PTSD: preliminary results. *Can J Psychiatry*, 2002, **47**(7):666–70.

193. Mohanakrishnan Menon P, Nasrallah HA, Lyons JA, Scott MF, Liberto V. Single-voxel proton MR spectroscopy of right versus left hippocampi in PTSD. *Psychiatry Res*, 2003, 123(2):101–8. [Erratum in: *Psychiatry Res*, 2004, **130**(3):313.]

194. Bremner JD, Innis RB, Southwick SM, Staib L, Zoghbi S, Charney DS. Decreased benzodiazepine receptor binding in prefrontal cortex in combat-related posttraumatic stress disorder. *Am J Psychiatry*, 2000, **157**(7):1120–6.

195. Fujita M, Southwick SM, Denucci CC, Zoghbi SS, Dillon MS, Baldwin RM, *et al*. Central type benzodiazepine receptors in Gulf War veterans with posttraumatic stress disorder. *Biol Psychiatry*, 2004, **56**(2):95–100.

196. Bonne O, Bain E, Neumeister A, Nugent AC, Vythilingam M, Carson RE, *et al*. No change in serotonin type 1A receptor binding in patients with posttraumatic stress disorder. *Am J Psychiatry*, 2005, **162**(2):383–5.

197. Sachinvala N, Kling A, Suffin S, Lake R, Cohen M. Increased regional cerebral perfusion by 99mTc hexamethyl propylene amine oxime single photon emission computed tomography in post-traumatic stress disorder. *Mil Med*, 2000, **165**(6):473–9.

198. Bonne O, Gilboa A, Louzoun Y, Brandes D, Yona I, Lester H, *et al*. Resting regional cerebral perfusion in recent posttraumatic stress disorder. *Biol Psychiatry*, 2003, **54**(10):1077–86.

199. Seedat S, Warwick J, van Heerden B, Hugo C, Zungu–Dirwayi N, Van Kradenburg J, *et al*. Single photon emission computed tomography in posttraumatic stress disorder before and after treatment with a selective serotonin reuptake inhibitor. *J Affect Disord*, 2004, **80**(1):45–53.

200. Liberzon I, Taylor SF, Amdur R, Jung TD, Chamberlain KR, Minoshima S, *et al*. Brain activation in PTSD in response to trauma-related stimuli. *Biol Psychiatry*, 1999, **45**(7):817–26.

201. Pissiota A, Frans O, Fernandez M, von Knorring L, Fischer H, Fredrikson M. Neurofunctional correlates of posttraumatic stress disorder: a PET symptom provocation study. *Eur Arch Psychiatry Clin Neurosci*, 2002, **252**(2):68–75.

202. Bremner JD, Narayan M, Staib LH, Southwick SM, McGlashan T, Charney DS. Neural correlates of memories of childhood sexual abuse in women with and without posttraumatic stress disorder. *Am J Psychiatry*, 1999, **156**(11):1787–95.

203. Shin LM, McNally RJ, Kosslyn SM, Thompson WL, Rauch SL, Alpert NM, *et al*. Regional cerebral blood flow during script-driven imagery in childhood sexual abuse-related PTSD: A PET investigation. *Am J Psychiatry*, 1999, **156**(4):575–84.

204. Lanius RA, Williamson PC, Densmore M, Boksman K, Gupta MA, Neufeld RW, *et al*. Neural correlates of traumatic memories in posttraumatic stress disorder: a functional MRI investigation. *Am J Psychiatry*, 2001, **158**(11):1920–2.

205. Lanius RA, Williamson PC, Boksman K, Densmore M, Gupta M, Neufeld RW, *et al*. Brain activation during script-driven imagery induced dissociative responses in PTSD: a functional magnetic resonance imaging investigation. *Biol Psychiatry*, 2002, **52**(4):305–11.

206. Shin LM, Whalen PJ, Pitman RK, Bush G, Macklin ML, Lasko NB, *et al*. An fMRI study of anterior cingulate function in posttraumatic stress disorder. *Biol Psychiatry*, 2001, **50**(12):932–42.

207. Shin LM, Kosslyn SM, McNally RJ, Alpert NM, Thompson WL, Rauch SL, *et al*. Visual imagery and perception in posttraumatic stress disorder. A positron emission tomographic investigation. *Arch Gen Psychiatry*, 1997, **54**(3):233–41.

208. Rauch SL, Whalen PJ, Shin LM, McInerney SC, Macklin ML, Lasko NB, *et al*. Exaggerated amygdala response to masked facial stimuli in posttraumatic stress disorder: a functional MRI study. *Biol Psychiatry*, 2000, **47**(9):769–76.

209. Klein DF. False suffocation alarms, spontaneous panics, and related conditions: an integrative hypothesis. *Arch Gen Psychiatry*, 1993, **50**:306–17.

210. Veltman DJ, van Zijderveld GA, van Dyck R, Bakker A. Predictability, controllability, and fear of symptoms of anxiety in epinephrine-induced panic. *Biol Psychiatry*, 1998, **44**(10):1017–26.

211. Gorman JM, Liebowitz MR, Fyer AJ, Stein J. A neuroanatomical hypothesis for panic disorder. *Am J Psychiatry*, 1989, 146(2):148–61. [Comment in: *Am J Psychiatry*, 1990, **147**(1):126–7.]

212. Fontaine R, Breton G, Déry R, Fontaine S, Elic R. Temporal lobe abnormalities in panic disorder: an MRI study. *Biol Psychiatry*, 1990, **27**:304–10.

213. Vythilingam M, Anderson ER, Goddard A, Woods SW, Staib LH, Charney DS, *et al*. Temporal lobe volume in panic disorder — a quantitative magnetic resonance imaging study. *Psychiatry Research: Neuroimaging*, 2000, **99**:75–82.

214. Uchida RR, Del–Ben CM, Santos AC, Araújo D, Crippa JA, Guimaraes FS, *et al*. Decreased left temporal lobe volume of panic patients measured by magnetic resnance imaging. *Brazilian Journal of Medical and Biological Research*, 2003, **36**:925–9.

215. Massana G, Serra–Grabulosa JM, Salgado–Pineda P, Gastó C, Junqué C, Massana J, *et al*. Amygdalar atrophy in panic disorder patients detected by volumetric magnetic resonance imaging. *NeuroImage*, 2003, **19**:80–90.

216. Massana G, Serra–Grabulosa JM, Salgado–Pineda P, Gastó C, Junqué C, Massana J, *et al*. Parahippocampal gray matter density in panic disorder: a voxel-based morphometric study. *Am J Psychiatry*, 2003, **160**:566–8.

217. Dorow R, Horowski R, Paschelke G, Amin M, Braestrup C. Severe anxiety induced by FG7142, a b-carboline ligand for benzodiazepine receptors. *Lancet*, 1983, 2:98–99.

218. Nutt DJ, Cowen PJ, Little HJ. Unusual interactions of benzodiazepine receptor antagonists. *Nature*, 1982, **295**:436–8.

219. Roy–Byrne PP, Cowley DS, Greenblatt DJ, Shader RI, Hommer D. Reduced benzodiazepine sensitivity in panic disorder. *Arch Gen Psychiatry*, 1990, **47**:534–8.

220. Nutt DJ, Glue P, Lawson C, Wilson S. Flumazenil provocation of panic attacks. *Arch Gen Psychiatry*, 1990, **47**:917–25.

221. Woods SW, Charney DS, Silver JM, Krystal JH, Heninger GR. Behavioral, biochemical, and cardiovascular responses to the benzodiazepine receptor antagonist flumazenil in panic disorder. *Psychiatry Research*, 1991, **36**:115–27.

222. Kaschka W, Feistel H, Ebert D. Reduced benzodiazepine receptor binding in panic disorders measured by Iomazenil SPECT. *J Psychiatric Res*, 1995, **29**:427–34.

223. Bremner JD, Innis RB, White T, Fujita M, Silbersweig D, Goddard AW, et al. SPECT [I-123]Iomazenil measurement of the benzodiazepine receptor in panic disorder. *Biol Psychiatry*, 2000, **47**:96–106.

224. Malizia AL, Cunningham VJ, Bell CJ, Liddle PF, Jones T, Nutt DJ. Decreased brain GABAa-benzodiazepine receptor binding in panic disorder. *Arch Gen Psychiatry*, 1998, **55**:715–20.

225. Abadie P, Boulenger JP, Benali K, Barré L, Zarifian E, Baron JC. Relationships between trait and state anxiety and the central benzodiazepine receptor: a PET study. *European Journal of Neuroscience*, 1999, **11**:1470–8.

226. Maloteaux JM, Octave JN, Gossuin A, Laterre C, Trouet A. GABA induces down regulation of the ebnzodiazepine GABA receptor complex in the rat cultured neurons. *European Journal of Pharmacology*, 1987, **144**:173–83.

227. Goddard AW, Mason GF, Almai A, Rothman DL, Behar KL, Petroff OAC, et al. Reductions in occipital cortex GABA levels in panic disorder detected with ^{1}H-Magnetic Resonance Spectroscopy. *Arch Gen Psychiatry*, 2001, **58**:556–561.

228. Neumeister A, Bain E, Nugent AC, Carson RE, Bonne O, Luckenbaugh DA, et al. Reduced serotonin type 1_A receptor binding in panic disorder. *Journal of Neuroscience*, 2004, **24**:589–591.

229. Reiman EM, Raichle ME, Butler FK, Herscovitch P, Robins E. A focal brain abnormality in panic disorder, a severe form of anxiety. *Nature*, 1984, **310**:683–5.

230. Reiman EM, Raichle ME, Robins E, Butler FK, Herscovitch P, Fox PT, et al. The application of positron emission tomography to the study of panic disorder. *Am J Psychiatry*, 1986, **143**:469–77.

231. Drevets WC, Videen TO, MacLeod AK, Haller JW, Raichle ME. PET images of blood flow changes during anxiety: correction. *Science*, 1992, **256**:1696.

232. Nordahl TE, Semple WE, Gross M, Mellman TA, Stein MB, Goyer P, et al. Cerebral glucose metabolic differences in patients with panic disorder. *Neuropsychopharmacology*, 1990, **3**:261–72.

233. Nordahl TE, Stein MB, Benkelfat C, Semple WE, Andreason P, Zametkin A, et al. Regional cerebral metabolic asymmetries replicated in an independent group of patients with panic disorder. *Biol Psychiatry*, 1998, **44**:998–1006.

234. Bisaga A, Katz JL, Antonini A, Wright CE, Margouleff C, Gorman JM, et al. Cerebral glucose metabolism in women with panic disorder. *Am J Psychiatry*, 1998, **155**:1178–83.

235. De Cristofaro MTR, Sessarego A, Pupi A, Biondi F, Faravelli C. Brain perfusion abnormalities in drug-naive, lactate-sensitive panic patients: a SPECT study. *Biological Psychiatry*, 1993, **33**:505–512.

236. Eren I, Tûkel R, Polat A, Karaman R, Ünal S. Evaluation of regional cerebral blood flow changes in panic disorder with Tc99m-HMPAO SPECT. *Psychiatry Research: Neuroimaging*, 2003, **123**:135–143.

237. Lucey JV, Costa DC, Busatto G, Pilowsky LS, Marks IM, Ell PJ, et al. Caudate regional cerebral blood flow in obsessive-compulsive disorder, panic disorder and healthy controls on single photon emission computerised tomography. *Psychiatry Research: Neuroimaging*, 1997, **74**:25–33.

238. Stewart RS, Devous MD, Rush AJ, Lane L, Bonte FJ. Cerebral blood flow changes during sodium-lactate-induced panic attacks. *Am J Psychiatry*, 1988, **145**:442–9.

239. Reiman EM, Raichle ME, Robins E, Mintum MA, Fusselman MJ, Fox PT, et al. Neuroanatomical correlates of a lactate-induced anxiety attack. *Arch Gen Psychiatry*, 1989, **46**:493–500.

240. Reiman EM, Fusselman MJ, Fox PT, Raichle ME. Neuroanatomical correlates of anticipatory anxiety. *Science*, 1989, **243**:1071–4.

241. Dahl D. Systemically administered cholecystokinin affects an evoked potential in the hippocampal dentate gyrus. *Neuropeptides*, 1987, **10**:165–73.

242. Hökfelt T, Cortés R, Schalling M, Ceccatelli S, Pelto–Huikko M, Persson H, *et al.* Distribution patterns of CCK and CCK mRNA in some neuronal and non-neuronal tissues. *Neuropeptides*, 1991, **19**:31–43.

243. Lindefors N, Lindén A, Brené S, Sedvall G, Persson H. CCK peptides and mRNA in the human brain. *Progress in Neurobiology*, 1993, **40**:671–90.

244. Bradwejn J, de Montigny C. Benzodiazepines antagonize cholecystokinin-induced activation of rat hippocampal neurons. *Nature*, 1984, **312**:363–4.

245. de la Mora MP, Hernandez–Gómez AM, Méndez–Franco J, Fuxe K. Cholescystokinin-8 increases K$^+$-evoked [^{3}H] g-aminobutyric acid release in slices from rat brain areas. *European Journal of Pharmacology*, 1993, **250**:423–30.

246. de Montigny C. Cholecystokinin tetrapeptide induces panic-like attacks in healthy volunteers. Preliminary findings. *Arch Gen Psychiatry*, 1989, **46**:511–17.

247. Bradwejn J, Koszycki D, Shriqui C. Enhanced sensitivity to cholecystokinin tetrapeptide in panic disorder. Clinical and behavioral findings. *Arch Gen Psychiatry*, 1991, **48**: 603–10.

248. Bradwejn,J., Koszycki,D., Couetoux du Tertre,A., van Megen,H., den Boer,J., Westenberg,H., Annable,L., The panicogenic effects of cholecystokinin-tetrapeptide are antagonized by L-365,260, a central cholecystokinin receptor antagonist, in patients with panic disorder. *Arch Gen Psychiatry*, 1994, **51**:486–93.

249. Bradwejn J, Koszycki D. Imipramine antagonism of the panicogenic effects of cholecystokinin tetrapeptide in panic disorder patients. *Am J Psychiatry*, 1994, **151**:261–3.

250. van Megen HJGM, Westenberg HGM, den Boer JA, Slaap B, Scheepmakers A. Effect of the selective serotonin reuptake inhibitor fluvoxamine on CCK-4 induced panic attacks. *Psychopharmacology*, 1997, **129**:357–64.

251. Benkelfat C, Bradwejn J, Meyer E, Ellenbogen M, Milot S, Gjedde A, *et al.* Functional neuroanatomy of CCK$_4$-induced anxiety in normal healthy volunteers. *Am J Psychiatry*, 1995, **152**:1180–4.

252. Javanmard M, Shlik J, Kennedy SH, Vaccarino FJ, Houle S, Bradwejn J. Neuroanatomic correlates of CCK-4-induced panic attacks in healthy humans: a comparison of two time points. *Biol Psychiatry*, 1999, **45**:872–82.

253. Boshuisen ML, Ter Horst GJ, Paans AMJ, Reinders AATS, den Boer JA. rCBF differences between panic disorder patients and control subjects during anticipatory anxiety and rest. *Biol Psychiatry*, 2002, **52**:126–35.

254. Boshuisen ML. *The anxious brain: neuroimaging in panic and anxiety* (thesis/dissertation). 2003.

255. Southwick SM, Krystal JH, Morgan CA, Johnson D, Nagy LM, Nicolaou A, *et al.* Abnormal noradrenergic function in post-traumatic stress disorder. *Arch Gen Psychiatry*, 1993, **50**:266–274.

256. Charney DS, Heninger GR, Breier A. Noradrenergic function in panic disorder. *Arch Gen Psychiatry*, 1984, **41**:751–63.

257. Charney DS, Woods SW, Goodman WK, Heninger GR. Neurobiological mechanisms of panic anxiety: biochemical and behavioral correlates of yohimbine-induced panic attacks. *Am J Psychiatry*, 1987, **144**:1030–6.

258. Hoehn–Saric R, Merchant AF, Keyser ML, Smith VK. Effect of clonidine on anxiety disorders., *Arch Gen Psychiatry*, 1981, **38**:1278–82.

259. Charney DS, Heninger GR. Abnormal regulation of noradrenergic function in panic disorders. Effects of clonidine in healthy subjects and patients with agoraphobia and panic disorder. *Arch Gen Psychiatry*, 1986, **43**:1042–54.

260. Nutt DJ. Altered central alpha2-adrenoreceptor sensitivity in panic disorder. *Arch Gen Psychiatry*, 1989, **46**:165–9.

261. Goddard AW, Woods SW, Sholomskas DE, Goodman WK, Charney DS, Heninger GR. Effects of the serotonin reuptake inhibitor fluoxamine on yohimbine-induced anxiety in panic disorder. *Psychiatry Research*, 1993, **48**:119–133.

262. Cameron OG, Zubieta JK, Grunhaus L, Minoshima S. Effects of yohimbine on cerebral blood flow, symptoms, and physiological functions in humans. Psychosomatic Medicine, 2000, **62**:549–59.

263. Woods SW, Koster K, Krystal JK, Smith EO, Zubal IG, Hoffer PB, *et al*. Yohimbine alters regional cerebral blood flow in panic disorder. *The Lancet*, 1988, **2**:678.

264. Meyer JH, Swinson R, Kennedy SH, Houle S, Brown GM. Increased left posterior parietal-temporal cortex activation after D-fenfluramine in women with panic disorder. *Psychiatry Research: Neuroimaging*, 2000, **98**:133–43.

265. Bystritsky A, Pontillo D, Powers M, Sabb FW, Craske MG, Bookheimer SY. Functional MRI changes during panic anticipation and imagery exposure. *NeuroReport*, 2001, **12**:3953–7.

266. Maddock RJ, Buonocore MH, Kile SJ, Garrett AS. Brain regions showing increased activation by threat-related words in panic disorder. *NeuroReport*, 2003, **14**:325–8.

267. Potts NL, Davidson JR, Krishnan KR, Doraiswamy PM. Magnetic resonance imaging in social phobia. *Psychiatry Res*, 1994, **52**(1):35–42.

268. Rauch SL, Wright CI, Martis B, Busa E, McMullin KG, Shin LM, *et al*. A magnetic resonance imaging study of cortical thickness in animal phobia. *Biol Psychiatry*, 2004, **55**(9):946–52.

269. Tiihonen J, Kuikka J, Bergstrom K, Lepola U, Koponen H, Leinonen E. Dopamine reuptake site densities in patients with social phobia. *Am J Psychiatry*, 1997, **154**(2):239–42. [Comment in: *Am J Psychiatry*, 2001, **158**(2):327–8.]

270. Schneier FR, Liebowitz MR, Abi–Dargham A, Zea–Ponce Y, Lin SH, Laruelle M. Low dopamine D(2) receptor binding potential in social phobia. *Am J Psychiatry*, 2000, **157**(3):457–9.

271. Phan KL, Fitzgerald DA, Cortese BM, Seraji–Bozorgzad N, Tancer ME, Moore GJ. Anterior cingulate neurochemistry in social anxiety disorder: 1H-MRS at 4 Tesla. *Neuroreport*, 2005, **16**(2):183–6.

272. Stein MB, Leslie WD. A brain single photon-emission computed tomography (SPECT) study of generalized social phobia. *Biol Psychiatry*, 1996, **39**(9):825–8.

273. Van der Linden G, van Heerden B, Warwick J, Wessels C, van Kradenburg J, Zungu–Dirwayi N, *et al*. Functional brain imaging and pharmacotherapy in social phobia: single photon emission computed tomography before and after treatment with the selective serotonin reuptake inhibitor citalopram. *Prog Neuropsychopharmacol Biol Psychiatry*, 2000, **24**(3):419–38.

274. Carey PD, Warwick J, Niehaus DJ, van der Linden G, van Heerden BB, Harvey BH, *et al*. Single photon emission computed tomography (SPECT) of anxiety disorders before and after treatment with citalopram. *BMC Psychiatry*, 2004, **4**(1):30.

275. Tillfors M, Furmark T, Marteinsdottir I, Fischer H, Pissiota A, Langstrom B, *et al*. Cerebral blood flow in subjects with social phobia during stressful speaking tasks: a PET study. *Am J Psychiatry*, 2001, **158**(8):1220–6.

276. Tillfors M, Furmark T, Marteinsdottir I, Fredrikson M. Cerebral blood flow during anticipation of public speaking in social phobia: a PET study. *Biol Psychiatry*, 2002, **52**(11):1113–9.

277. Van Ameringen M, Mancini C, Szechtman H, Nahmias C, Oakman JM, Hall GB, *et al*. A PET provocation study of generalized social phobia. *Psychiatry Res*, 2004, **132**(1):13–8.

278. Birbaumer N, Grodd W, Diedrich O, Klose U, Erb M, Lotze M, *et al*. fMRI reveals amygdala activation to human faces in social phobics. *Neuroreport*, 1998, **9**(6):1223–6.

279. Schneider F, Weiss U, Kessler C, Muller–Gartner HW, Posse S, Salloum JB, *et al*. Subcortical correlates of differential classical conditioning of aversive emotional reactions in social phobia. *Biol Psychiatry*, 1999, **45**(7):863–71.

280. Stein MB, Goldin PR, Sareen J, Zorrilla LT, Brown GG. Increased amygdala activation to angry and contemptuous faces in generalized social phobia. *Arch Gen Psychiatry*, 2002, **59**(11):1027–34.

281. Fischer H, Furmark T, Wik G, Fredrikson M. Brain representation of habituation to repeated complex visual stimulation studied with PET. *Neuroreport*, 2000, **11**(1):123–6.

282. Paquette V, Levesque J, Mensour B, Leroux JM, Beaudoin G, Bourgouin P, *et al.* 'Change the mind and you change the brain': effects of cognitive-behavioral therapy on the neural correlates of spider phobia. *Neuroimage*, 2003, **18**(2):401–9.

283. Dilger S, Straube T, Mentzel HJ, Fitzek C, Reichenbach JR, Hecht H, *et al.* Brain activation to phobia-related pictures in spider phobic humans: an event-related functional magnetic resonance imaging study. *Neurosci Lett*, 2003, **348**(1):29–32.

284. Veltman DJ, Tuinebreijer WE, Winkelman D, Lammertsma AA, Witter MP, Dolan RJ, *et al.* Neurophysiological correlates of habituation during exposure in spider phobia. *Psychiatry Res*, 2004, **132**(2):149–58.

285. Wright CI, Martis B, McMullin K, Shin LM, Rauch SL. Amygdala and insular responses to emotionally valenced human faces in small animal specific phobia. *Biol Psychiatry*, 2003, **54**(10):1067–76.

286. Straube T, Mentzel HJ, Glauer M, Miltner WH. Brain activation to phobia-related words in phobic subjects. *Neurosci Lett*, 2004, **372**(3):204–8.

287. Martis B, Wright CI, McMullin KG, Shin LM, Rauch SL. Functional magnetic resonance imaging evidence for a lack of striatal dysfunction during implicit sequence learning in individuals with animal phobia. *Am J Psychiatry*, 2004, **161**(1):67–71.

288. Remijnse PL, van den Heuvel OA, Veltman DJ. Neuroimaging in obsessive-compulsive disorder. *Current Medical Imaging Reviews*, 2005, **1**(3):331–51.

289. Gorman JM, Kent JM, Sullivan GM, Coplan JD. Neuroanatomical hypothesis of panic disorder, revised. *Am J Psychiatry*, 2000, **157**:493–505.

290. Rauch SL, Wright CI. Neuroimaging studies of amygdala function in anxiety disorders. *Annals of the New York Academy of Sciences*, 2003, **985**:389–410.

291. Mataix–Cols D, Rauch SL, Baer L, Eisen JL, Shera DM, Goodman WK *et al.* Symptom stability in adult obsessive-compulsive disorder: data from a naturalistic two-year follow-up study. *Am J Psychiatry*, 2002, **159**:263–8.

9

Stroke

Steven C. Cramer

1. Stroke and stroke recovery

Stroke remains a major source of morbidity and mortality. Approximately 1 in 15 deaths in the US is attributable to stroke, making this the third leading cause of death after heart disease and cancer. However, approximately 85% of patients survive the stroke, living an average of seven years thereafter. Most are left with significant disability[1,2].

Stroke can affect any aspect of brain function. The nature of post-stroke deficits can vary widely, as can severity. In the weeks and months following a stroke, most patients show spontaneous improvement in behaviours affected by stroke[3–5]. However, this recovery is highly variable and generally incomplete. As a result, stroke is the leading cause of adult disability in the US and many other countries.

A number of investigations have examined the brain events that underlie spontaneous recovery of function after stroke. The majority has focussed on motor or language recovery. A number of brain mapping techniques has been used to investigate recovery, each with its relative strengths. FMRI has been the tool for many of these, given its good temporal and excellent spatial resolution.

This chapter concentrates on recovery of motor function, one of the major sources of impairment in stroke patients. However, findings in motor recovery overlap substantially with investigations of recovery in other brain systems such as language[6].

2. The biology of stroke recovery

A number of changes arise in the brain over the weeks following a stroke. These have been described at multiple levels. Cellular and molecular studies in animals undergoing an experimental unilateral infarct have characterized neurogenesis, angiogenesis, inflammation, excitability, and cellular growth, many of which evolve bilaterally during the days to weeks that follow a unilateral insult. A body of evidence suggests that many of these events contribute to spontaneous recovery of function after a stroke[7]. In animal studies, exogenous interventions have been found that amplify these molecular events and simultaneously improve behavioural outcome. Examples include amphetamine[8], growth factors[9,10], cellular therapies[11,12], brain stimulation[13–15], increased environmental complexity[16,17], and physical activity leve1[18].

Thus, there are discrete molecular brain events that arise days to weeks after an infarct. These brain events likely underlie spontaneous recovery and can be therapeutically augmented in association with improved behavioural outcome in animals. Stroke deficits remain the most common cause of disability in adults living in the US and many other countries.

There is a great need to translate results of animal studies into improved therapeutics for human patients with stroke. To do so requires an understanding of the biology of recovery in humans. The cellular-molecular measurements obtained in animal studies are not easily duplicated in human patients, where brain tissue is uncommonly available for examination. However, human brain mapping with techniques such as FMRI are providing insights important to this goal. Human studies are also of value because of the limitations of animal models in this context[19]. For example, rodent studies are of limited value because most of these creatures are quadrupeds with vastly different brain organization from humans, such as relative size of basal ganglia and white matter. Primate studies have been instructive, however size and pathogenesis of brain injury has limited overlap with spontaneous human cerebrovascular disease. Animal models often lack the heterogeneity of injury found in the human condition; animals generally have a more uniform pre-infarct behavioural status; animals are generally at a much younger point in the life span; most, if not all, human stroke risk factors are absent in animal models; cognitive/affective features important to all aspects of recovery usually have limited correspondence with the human condition; and medical complications that affect a majority of human stroke patients are generally absent in animal studies. There is no human like humans to understand humans.

Functional imaging in human subjects may be of value in the area of stroke recovery because these data provide biological insights that are sometimes not otherwise available. Molecular events are generally difficult to obtain in humans. Behavioural changes are easier to measure but do not consistently correspond tightly with the molecular/physiological events that comprise therapeutic targets. For example, a wide range of brain events and behavioural strategies can produce the same behavioural phenotype. Also, behavioural assessments generally often do not provide mechanistic insights or distinguish patient subgroups with biologically distinct therapeutic targets. Functional imaging, which exists between the molecular and behavioural levels, provides insights into brain changes at the systems level.

For example, functional imaging can provide improved insight into anatomical measures. Human[20,21] and experimental animal[22,23] studies of brain infarction have consistently found that behavioural deficits correlate significantly with acute or with chronic measurement of infarct volume. However, these correlations are sometimes limited, especially chronically, as this approach to understanding brain injury assumes an equivalency of cortical function akin to theories of cerebral mass action[24]. Introduction of FMRI measures into analysis of injury can improve the correlation between injury and behavioural effects[25], and thus this approach may have improved value for predicting stroke outcome as opposed to using anatomical scans to measure total stroke volume (Fig. 9.1). Use of a method such as structural or perfusion imaging characterizes injury but provides limited insight as to how this injury will influence final behavioral deficits from injury.

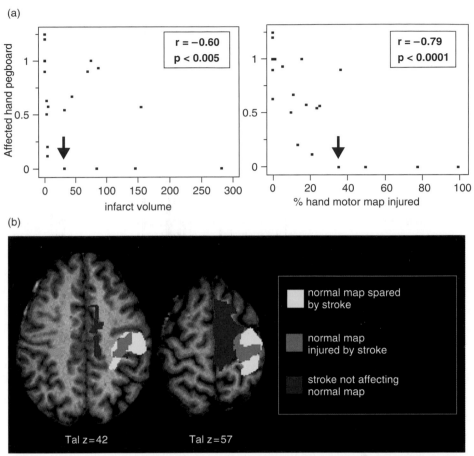

Fig. 9.1 (**a**) Infarct volume (top left) and fraction of hand motor map injured by stroke (top right); each show a significant inverse relationship with pegboard performance by the affected hand . (normalized to pegboard results for the unaffected hand). However, correlation is stronger and more significant in the latter case. Note that injury to >37% of the hand motor map was associated with total loss of hand motor function. The arrow indicates the patient whose images are displayed below. (**b**) Images from a patient whose stroke was mild to moderate in size (33 cm^3) but injured 35% of the hand motor area and was associated with total loss of hand motor function. (Reproduced with permission from Oxford University Press[25])

There are a broad range of neurological settings in which functional imaging has been found useful when behavioural exam or anatomical brain imaging provide limited insight. For example, when neurological exam is normal, expression of genetic risk for Alzheimer's disease[26] can nevertheless be measured when a memory task is performed during FMRI. When neuropsychological testing is normal, FMRI of frontal lobe activation during a memory task performance describes effects of HIV status on the brain[27]. Decreases in cortical metabolism by positron emission tomography (PET) scanning are linked with cognitive deficits in patients with traumatic brain injury even when anatomical MRI is unrevealing[28].

When stroke renders a patient hemiplegic, and exam is thus silent, functional MRI permits measurement of activity across brain motor networks[29]. Even in patients without a neurological diagnosis, functional brain imaging studies suggest that the same behavioural phenotype can arise from varying patterns of brain activity; for example, some elderly patients might activate a greater fraction of their cognitive reserve to maintain normal function[30].

Human brain mapping with FMRI and other techniques therefore hold great potential for implementation of therapeutics that target stroke recovery. Potential roles for functional imaging might include gaining insights into the nature of the biological targets for an individual patient with stroke, triaging patients according to features of brain function, and providing a surrogate marker of treatment effects. The goal is to use brain mapping to extract key neurophysiological data for improved clinical decision making. This goal has precedence in medical practice. For example, when a patient presents with a ventricular tachyarrhythmia or a refractory epileptic disorder, current practice often incorporates electrophysiological data to guide specific decisions in treatment[31,32]. With further study, brain mapping techniques such as FMRI might provide information useful for decision making in treatment of stroke recovery for the individual patient. Examples of using brain mapping for improved decision making are emerging. For example, in one study[33], FMRI was used to localize the stroke hemisphere's hand motor area in patients with chronic stroke. This information was then used to guide targeted subthreshold cortical stimulation.

When considering clinical measures for the study of stroke recovery, it is important to remember that restorative neurotherapeutics emphasizes specific brain systems. This is true at the behavioural level, where reinforcing specific behaviours is critical to successful therapeutic effect on outcome[34]. This is also true for functional imaging, where a specific behaviour is used to activate the brain. Thus, the global clinical measures used in acute stroke trials are, in themselves, insufficient to capture system-directed therapies or to interpret many studies of functional activation after stroke.

3. Methodological considerations and sources of bias

Many patterns of altered brain function have been described during the study of patients with stroke. These have been exhaustively compiled elsewhere[6,35–38].

Initial functional imaging studies were cross-sectional and observational in nature. Subsequent studies have examined stroke patient subpopulations, increased sample size, correlated features of brain activation with clinical measures, and performed serial studies during the period of behavioural gains post-stroke. However, the overall understanding of changes in brain function after stroke, and the relationship between these changes and clinical measures, remains limited. This is, in part, because of the relative dearth of such investigations.

However, at least three groups of issues limit the current understanding of brain events underlying spontaneous return of function following a stroke. The first is the heterogeneity of stroke, its causes, injury patterns, effects, and therapies. There are a great number of variables that likely modify brain function after stroke (see Table 9.1).

Table 9.1 Clinical variables that potentially influence stroke recovery and its measurement by functional imaging

Stroke topography	Medical co-morbidities
Time post-stroke	Pre-stroke disability
Age	Pre-stroke experience and education
Hemispheric dominance	Type of post-stroke therapy
Side of brain affected	Amount post-stroke therapy
Depression	Acute stroke interventions
Injury to other brain network nodes	Medications during stroke recovery period
Infarct volume	Medications at time of brain mapping
Initial stroke deficits	Final clinical status
Arterial patency	Stroke mechanism

(Reproduced with permission from Lippincott, Williams and Wilkins[143])

Some of these are also important to the study of brain function in health, such as age, hemispheric dominance, and medical comorbidity. Others are also important to the study of brain function in the setting of acute stroke, such as infarct volume, concomitant depression, and pre-stroke disability. Each is a source of variance that can reduce power in functional imaging studies of stroke recovery.

A second group of issues pertains to the divergence of investigative approaches — small differences in the lack of standardized methods for studying and reporting brain function across studies. For example, squeezing vs. finger tapping activates different motor circuits[39,40]. Differences in force[41–43], frequency[44–47], amplitude[48], or complexity[49–51] of finger movements can substantially impact activation in multiple brain sensorimotor areas. A similar degree of variability exists in clinical assessments used to measure stroke recovery[52,53]. This situation in stroke recovery contrasts with that found in multiple sclerosis, where the Multiple Sclerosis Functional Composite[54] is routinely included; and in spinal cord injury, where the American Spinal Injury Association (ASIA) motor score, ASIA pinprick sensory score, ASIA light touch sensory score, and ASIA Impairment Scale[55] are routinely reported. Adoption of a standardized approach to be included in studies of stroke recovery might reduce the impact of this latter issue.

A third group of issues pertains to brain and vascular changes common in patients with stroke. Vascular disease can modify neuronal-vascular coupling. Available data suggest this is most important with highly advanced stenosis or occlusion of the cerebral arteries[56–61]. Moreover, advanced large cerebral artery narrowing itself can be associated with reorganization of brain function[62]. Further studies are needed in this area. Also, brain injury such as stroke can affect the intrinsic T2* property of brain tissue — the underlying measurement in BOLD FMRI. Recent data from our lab (below) suggest that this might be important. Multimodal assessment of brain function may be useful in addressing these concerns in contexts where they are most significant. Methods such as electroencephalography and magnetoencephalography have reduced spatial resolution in comparison to FMRI; however, temporal resolution is improved. These vascular issues might not have the same impact upon findings with these methods.

4. Changes in brain function described after stroke

Despite these factors, a number of findings emerge from overview of functional imaging studies after stroke. Reorganization of brain motor function after stroke has been framed in the context of sensorimotor integration[63,64], attention[65–68], learning[69–71], and complexity[16,72].

4.1 Changes in networks

The earliest finding was a change in multiple nodes within relevant distributed networks[73]. This has been replicated repeatedly. Clearly, altered function within one area changes function within interconnected areas within a distributed brain network after stroke, similar to multifocal, distant changes in brain function reported after a focal brain perturbation in the motor system of healthy subjects[74–76]. A number of animal studies have been concordant with results in humans (see for example[77–84]). Figure 9.2 presents a model that compiles these findings.

4.2 Changes in laterality

One finding that might be of particular importance to understanding stroke recovery in humans is a reduction in the laterality of brain activity[85–89]. This issue has also received considerable attention in the study of normal ageing[90] and has also been discussed in a number of other contexts including epilepsy[91], traumatic brain injury[92], and multiple sclerosis[93]. Early reports emphasized a less lateralized pattern of activation after stroke than normal (i.e. the effect of stroke is to increase the extent to which both hemispheres are recruited rather than just the contralateral hemisphere). For example, a language task or a right-hand motor task that activates the left hemisphere in healthy controls will activate relevant regions within both the right and the left hemispheres in patients with a left hemisphere stroke.

A number of factors have been found to modify the extent to which stroke is associated with reduced laterality. Examples include time after stroke (laterality often increases towards normal as patients recover[94–99]), hemispheric dominance (motor-task performance with the non-dominant hand is less lateralized than with the dominant hand in both health and after stroke[89,100,101]), and topography of injury (reduced laterality may be more common with a cortical, rather than subcortical, infarct[96,102]). Other factors relevant to laterality in normal subjects are also likely to be important after stroke, such as task complexity (more complex tasks are a less lateralized brain event[103–105]), subject age (reduced laterality with increased age[90]), task familiarity (repeating the same behaviour can reduce laterality[106]), proximal vs. distal (more proximal motor tasks show reduced laterality compared to distal tasks[39,107,108]), and perhaps gender[109]. The motor cortex site of activation during movement of the ipsilateral hand is different from that activated during

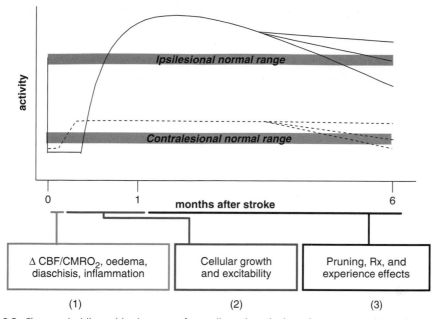

Fig. 9.2 Changes in bilateral brain areas after unilateral stroke have been grouped into three time periods. (**1**) In the initial hours–days after a stroke, brain function and behaviour can be globally deranged[144], and few restorative structural changes have started. (**2**) A period of growth then begins lasting several weeks. Structural and functional changes in the contralesional hemisphere precede those of the ipsilesional hemisphere, and, at such times, activity in relevant contralesional areas can even exceed activity in the lesion hemisphere. This growth-related period may be a key target for certain restorative therapies. (**3**) Subsequently, there is pruning, reduction in functional overactivations, and establishment of a static pattern of brain activity and behaviour. The final pattern may nevertheless remain accessible to plasticity-inducing, clinically meaningful, interventions[145–147]. An excess of growth followed by pruning has precedence in human neurobiology, being a recapitulation of normal developmental events[148]. Supra- and subnormal activity levels in the ipsilesional and contralesional hemispheres correlate with features of behavioural outcome in specific patient populations, as described above. (Reproduced with permission from Lippincott, Williams and Wilkins[143])

movement of the contralateral hand (Fig. 9.3), the latter possibly representing premotor cortex activity, often on the anterior precentral gyrus[110].

Several studies suggest that increased activity in the non-stroke hemisphere after stroke (i.e. reduced laterality) reflects greater injury and/or deficits. This is particularly emphasized in the serial FMRI study by Fujii *et al*.[97] and by TMS studies[111,112]. TMS studies have further suggested possible mechanisms for this finding. In the primary motor cortex, stroke hemisphere inhibition upon the non-stroke hemisphere is reduced[113], and non-stroke hemisphere inhibition upon the stroke hemisphere is increased[114].

Reduced laterality might not merely reflect more severe stroke or passive changes in inhibition, however. Some studies suggest that changes in laterality of brain function

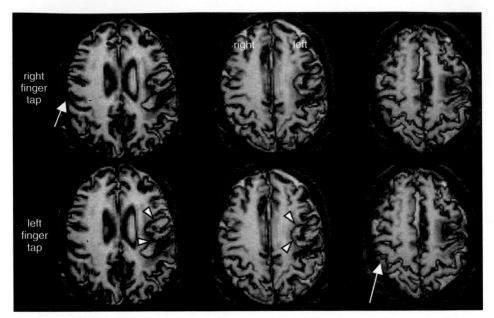

Fig. 9.3 Images are presented from a stroke patient with excellent recovery 14 months after a left fronto-parieto-temporal cortical embolus. White arrows indicate right hemisphere sensorimotor cortex activation; the long arrow is contralateral to finger movement and the short arrow is ipsilateral. Activation significant at p < 0.001 is presented on contiguous axial slices, arranged with images at left ventral to those at right. The arrowheads indicate the infarct location. In the unaffected right hemisphere, the activation site seen during right (recovered) finger tapping is lateral, anterior, and ventral to the activation site seen during left finger tapping. Note the absence of activation in stroke hemisphere primary sensorimotor cortex during tapping by either hand. Note too that the site of right hemisphere activation during right finger movement (top row, activation is ipsilateral to movement) is different from the site activated during left finger movement (bottom row, activation is contralateral to movement). (Reproduced with permission from the American Physiological Society[110])

might nonetheless be important to whatever behavioural recovery is achieved after stroke[98,115–118], even if the final behaviour is less than normal. A number of cases have been published where brain activation is mostly or completely restricted to the non-stroke hemisphere, contralateral to results in controls[89,110,119,120] (Fig. 9.3).

4.3 Changes in activation site

Shifts in the site of activation have also been reported after stroke, in all manner of direction, by FMRI, PET, and TMS. The most common changes described have been a ventral or a posterior shift in the contralateral (stroke hemisphere) activation site during unilateral motor task performance by the stroke-affected hand. Weiller *et al.* described a ventral shift in the centre of activation during motor-task performance in recovered patients whose stroke affected the posterior aspect of the internal capsule, suggesting that topographic shifts in cortical activation site might reflect survival of selected corticospinal tract fibres[86].

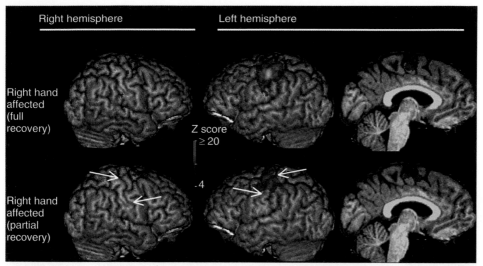

Fig. 9.4 Group maps from patients with stroke affecting the right arm (left brain) show a difference in activation site and size varying with level of recovery. The Talairach coordinates for centre of activation for the activation cluster in the left primary sensorimotor cortex in those with complete recovery were 31, -21, 50; this was ventral compared to those with partial recovery among whom the centre of activation was located at 30, -19, 54. In addition, patients with full recovery, as opposed to those with partial recovery, showed 2.7-fold larger contralateral sensorimotor activation, with negligible differences in the supplementary motor area, despite no differences in finger-tapping force or in surface EMG recordings. White arrows indicate the central sulcus. (Reproduced with permission from Lippincott, Williams and Wilkins[101])

An FMRI study also reported the same finding among patients with complete motor recovery, as compared to patients with partial recovery[101] (Fig. 9.4). This suggests that, at least for hand motor recovery, a ventral shift might be associated with better recovery of function. A posterior shift in activation site has been described in motor studies of stroke recovery across multiple imaging modalities[121–124], and has also been described in the motor system of patients with multiple sclerosis[93] or spinal cord injury[125,126]. In most studies of stroke patients, a posterior shift did not correlate with clinical status; however, a recent study suggests that the degree of posterior shift is linearly related to the degree of recovery, at least for proximal movements[108].

4.4 Changes in activation size

Studies have described changes in activation size in many brain areas in the setting of stroke recovery. Several studies have emphasized increased activation over time within several areas within the stroke-affected hemisphere, accompanied by decreased activation over time in several areas particularly within the non-stroke hemisphere[94,98,99,127,128], consistent with TMS studies[129,130]. TMS studies converge on the conclusion that progressive expansion in the area of the excitable primary motor cortex within the stroke hemisphere during the period of stroke recovery is a feature of patients with superior motor

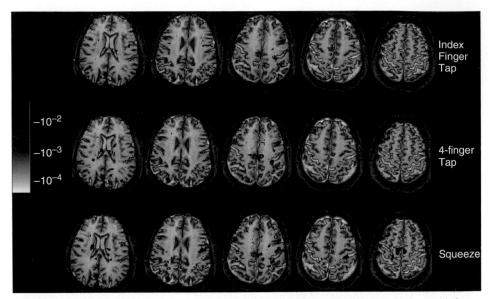

Fig. 9.5 Activation is shown in selected axial brain slices during each right-hand motor task from a 69-year-old healthy control. Images are in radiological orientation, with the left hemisphere on the right side. The activation volume in the left primary sensorimotor cortex is largest for squeezing as compared to 4-finger tapping which, in turn, was larger than index-finger tapping. Across all control subjects, contralateral sensorimotor cortex activation volume was significantly larger during squeezing vs. index-finger tapping. Note too that right sensorimotor cortex activation was only seen during squeezing. (Reproduced with permission from Sage Publications Inc.[39])

outcomes[129,131]. Importantly, while clinical status reaches a plateau in three months or less for many functions such as motor status[3,132], brain reorganization might continue to evolve for months beyond this[128,130]. The task used to probe activation can significantly influence the volume of activation. For example, contralateral activation volume during right hand squeezing is significantly larger than the volume during right index finger tapping (Fig. 9.5)[39].

4.5 Correlations between behaviour and changes in brain activation

In some serial functional imaging studies, the correlate of better clinical outcome has been increased activation in key stroke hemisphere areas[94,97–99,101], but in other studies, the correlate has been reduction in such activation[95,133]. These differences across FMRI studies might arise from several sources. Several methodological issues might contribute, such as divergence in time after stroke at which investigations are performed, in the task used to activate the brain, in the patient populations enrolled, or in other variables. Indeed, when our lab applied the same FMRI probe, tapping affected the index finger at 2 Hz (driven by auditory metronome) across a 25 degree range of motion with eyes closed, shoulder adducted, and elbow extended, at 1.5 Tesla field strength, we found that activation volume *decreased* with stroke[101] and *increased* with spinal cord injury[134] as compared to age-matched controls. Together, these observations suggest that a particular brain mapping method will have the best clinical validity when applied to a specific patient population.

Also, for behaviours arising from a lateralized, *primary* cortex-driven brain area, increased activation in the primary cortex correlates with *better* outcome[101,129] (Fig. 9.4), indicating preservation of key substrate with optimal connections for supporting the behaviour of interest. However, in other brain areas such as *secondary* motor areas, greater activation correlates with *poorer* outcome as, in this case, greater activation represents a compensatory event that is generally not able to support full return of behaviour due to the nature of anatomical connections in these areas (Fig. 9.6)[135]. One unifying conclusion across these studies is that the best outcomes are associated with the greatest return to the normal state of brain function[135].

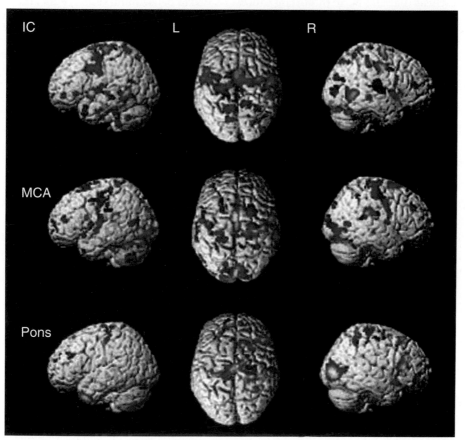

Fig. 9.6 These images display brain voxels in which there was a negative (linear) correlation between recovery from stroke and task-related BOLD signal within different stroke subtypes. Results are surface-rendered onto a canonical brain. The brain is shown (from left to right) from the left side, from above (left hemisphere on the left), and from the right. All voxels are significant at P < 0.05, corrected for multiple comparisons across the whole brain. (Reproduced with permission from Oxford University Press.[135])

4.6 Changes along the infarct rim

Increased activity along the rim of a cortical infarct has been described in FMRI and PET studies[89,102,136]. Butz *et al*.[137] found peri-infarct low-frequency activity in the majority of patients with cortical stroke, the functional significance of which was unclear. These observations might correspond to the increased levels of growth-related proteins found along the rim of experimental infarcts introduced into animals[8,138]. However, the intrinsic T2* property of brain tissue, changes in which underlie activation in BOLD FMRI, can change with stroke. Recent data from our lab suggest that the area surrounding an infarct might have increased T2* signal compared to normal brain tissue, the impact of which upon BOLD FMRI could be important.

4.7 Diaschisis

Diaschisis may also be an important process related to behavioural recovery after stroke. Brain areas connected to, but spatially distant from, the region of infarction show numerous changes post-stroke[99,139–141]. For example, we found several patients with a behavioural deficit early after stroke associated with failure to activate the brain area underlying that behaviour despite normal resting cerebral blood flow in the area and lack of injury to the area; behavioural recovery was associated with restitution of brain activity[99]. While numerous methods have been used to describe diaschisis, this process may be directly measured using FDG-PET[118,142].

5. Summary

Functional imaging of stroke recovery is a unique source of information that might be useful in the development of restorative treatments. A number of features of brain function change after stroke. Current studies have defined many of the most common events. Key challenges for the future are to develop standardized approaches to help address certain questions, determine the psychometric qualities of these measures, and define the clinical utility of these methods.

References

1. Gresham G, Duncan P, Stason W, Adams H, Adelman A, Alexander D, *et al. Post-stroke rehabilitation*. Rockville, MD: US Department of Health and Human Services. Public Health Service, Agency for Health Care Policy and Research. 1995.
2. Rathore S, Hinn A, Cooper L, Tyroler H, Rosamond W. Characterization of incident stroke signs and symptoms: Findings from the atherosclerosis risk in communities study. *Stroke*. 2002;**33**:2718–21.
3. Duncan P, Goldstein L, Matchar D, Divine G, Feussner J. Measurement of motor recovery after stroke. *Stroke*. 1992;**23**:1084–9.
4. Hier D, Mondlock J, Caplan L. Recovery of behavioral abnormalities after right hemisphere stroke. *Neurology*. 1983;**33**:345–50.
5. Kertesz A, McCabe P. Recovery patterns and prognosis in aphasia. *Brain*. 1977;**100** Pt 1:1–18.
6. Baron J, Cohen L, Cramer S, Dobkin B, Johansen–Berg H, Loubinoux I, *et al*. Neuroimaging in stroke recovery: a position paper from the first international workshop on neuroimaging and stroke recovery. *Cerebrovasc Dis*. 2004;**18**:260–7.

7. Cramer S, Chopp M. Recovery recapitulates ontogeny. *Trends Neurosci.* 2000;**23**:265–71.

8. Stroemer R, Kent T, Hulsebosch C. Enhanced neocortical neural sprouting, synaptogenesis, and behavioral recovery with d-amphetamine therapy after neocortical infarction in rats. *Stroke.* 1998;**29**:2381–95.

9. Kawamata T, Dietrich W, Schallert T, Gotts J, Cocke R, Benowitz L, *et al.* Intracisternal basic fibroblast growth factor (bfgf) enhances functional recovery and upregulates the expression of a molecular marker of neuronal sprouting following focal cerebral infarction. *Proc Natl Acad Sci.* 1997;**94**:8179–84.

10. Ren J, Kaplan P, Charette M, Speller H, Finklestein S. Time window of intracisternal osteogenic protein-1 in enhancing functional recovery after stroke. *Neuropharmacology.* 2000;**39**:860–5.

11. Chen J, Li Y, Katakowski M, Chen X, Wang L, Lu D, *et al.* Intravenous bone marrow stromal cell therapy reduces apoptosis and promotes endogenous cell proliferation after stroke in female rat. *J Neurosci Res.* 2003;**73**:778–86.

12. Mahmood A, Lu D, Chopp M. Intravenous administration of marrow stromal cells (mscs) increases the expression of growth factors in rat brain after traumatic brain injury. *J Neurotrauma.* 2004;**21**:33–9.

13. Kleim J, Bruneau R, VandenBerg P, MacDonald E, Mulrooney R, Pocock D. Motor cortex stimulation enhances motor recovery and reduces peri-infarct dysfunction following ischemic insult. *Neurol Res.* 2003;**25**:789–93.

14. Adkins–Muir D, Jones T. Cortical electrical stimulation combined with rehabilitative training: Enhanced functional recovery and dendritic plasticity following focal cortical ischemia in rats. *Neurol Res.* 2003;**25**:780–8.

15. Plautz E, Barbay S, Frost S, Friel K, Dancause N, Zoubina E, *et al.* Post-infarct cortical plasticity and behavioral recovery using concurrent cortical stimulation and rehabilitative training: A feasibility study in primates. *Neurol Res.* 2003;**25**:801–10.

16. Johansson B, Belichenko P. Neuronal plasticity and dendritic spines: effect of environmental enrichment on intact and postischemic rat brain. *J Cereb Blood Flow Metab.* 2002;**22**:89–96.

17. Johansson B, Ohlsson A. Environment, social interaction, and physical activity as determinants of functional outcome after cerebral infarction in the rat. *Exp Neurol.* 1996;**139**:322–7.

18. Jones T, Chu C, Grande L, Gregory A. Motor skills training enhances lesion-induced structural plasticity in the motor cortex of adult rats. *J Neurosci.* 1999;**19**:10153–63.

19. Cramer S. Clinical issues in animal models of stroke and rehabilitation. *Ilar J.* 2003;**44**:83–84

20. Saver J, Johnston K, Homer D, Wityk R, Koroshetz W, Truskowski L, Haley E. Infarct volume as a surrogate or auxiliary outcome measure in ischemic stroke clinical trials. The ranttas investigators. *Stroke.* 1999;**30**:293–8.

21. Brott T, Marler J, Olinger C, Adams H, Tomsick T, Barsan W, *et al.* Measurements of acute cerebral infarction: lesion size by computed tomography. *Stroke.* 1989;**20**:871–5.

22. Lyden P, Lonzo L, Nunez S, Dockstader T, Mathieu–Costello O, Zivin J. Effect of ischemic cerebral volume changes on behavior. *Behav Brain Res.* 1997;**87**:59–67.

23. Rogers D, Campbell C, Stretton J, Mackay K. Correlation between motor impairment and infarct volume after permanent and transient middle cerebral artery occlusion in the rat. *Stroke.* 1997;**28**:2060–5; discussion 2066.

24. Lashley K. In search of the engram. *Society of Experimental Biology.* 1950;Symposium **4**:454–82.

25. Crafton K, Mark A, Cramer S. Improved understanding of cortical injury by incorporating measures of functional anatomy. *Brain.* 2003;**126**:1650–9.

26. Bookheimer S, Strojwas M, Cohen M, Saunders A, Pericak–Vance M, Mazziotta J, *et al.* Patterns of brain activation in people at risk for alzheimer's disease. *N Engl J Med.* 2000;**343**:450–6.

27. Ernst T, Chang L, Jovicich J, Ames N, Arnold S. Abnormal brain activation on functional mri in cognitively asymptomatic hiv patients. *Neurology*. 2002;**59**:1343–9.

28. Fontaine A, Azouvi P, Remy P, Bussel B, Samson Y. Functional anatomy of neuropsychological deficits after severe traumatic brain injury. *Neurology*. 1999;**53**:1963–8.

29. Cramer S, Mark A, Barquist K, Nhan H, Stegbauer K, Price R, et al. Motor cortex activation is preserved in patients with chronic hemiplegic stroke. *Ann Neurol*. 2002;**52**:607–16.

30. Scarmeas N, Zarahn E, Anderson K, Hilton J, Flynn J, Van Heertum R, et al. Cognitive reserve modulates functional brain responses during memory tasks: a pet study in healthy young and elderly subjects. *Neuroimage*. 2003;**19**:1215–27.

31. Wetzel U, Hindricks G, Dorszewski A, Schirdewahn P, Gerds–Li J, Piorkowski C, et al. Electroanatomic mapping of the endocardium. Implication for catheter ablation of ventricular tachycardia. *Herz*. 2003;**28**:583–90.

32. Sheth R. Epilepsy surgery. Presurgical evaluation. *Neurol Clin*. 2002;**20**:1195–215.

33. Cramer S, Benson R, Himes D, Burra V, Janowsky J, Weinand M, et al. Use of functional mri to guide therapy in a clinical stroke trial. *Stroke*. 2005;(in press).

34. Feeney D, Gonzalez A, Law W. Amphetamine, halperidol, and experience interact to affect the rate of recovery after motor cortex injury. *Science*. 1982;**217**:855–7.

35. Calautti C, Baron J. Functional neuroimaging studies of motor recovery after stroke in adults: A review. *Stroke*. 2003;**34**:1553–66.

36. Chen R, Cohen L, Hallett M. Nervous system reorganization following injury. *Neuroscience*. 2002;**111**:761–73.

37. Rijntjes M, Weiller C. Recovery of motor and language abilities after stroke: the contribution of functional imaging. *Prog Neurobiol*. 2002;**66**:109–22.

38. Cramer S, Bastings E. Mapping clinically relevant plasticity after stroke. *Neuropharmacology*. 2000;**39**:842–51.

39. Cramer S, Nelles G, Schaechter J, Kaplan J, Finklestein S, Rosen B. A functional mri study of three motor tasks in the evaluation of stroke recovery. *Neurorehabil Neural Repair*. 2001;**15**:1–8.

40. Ehrsson H, Fagergren A, Jonsson T, Westling G, Johansson R, Forssberg H. Cortical activity in precision- versus power-grip tasks: an FMRI study. *J Neurophysiol*. 2000;**83**:528–36.

41. Dettmers C, Fink G, Lemon R, Stephan K, Passingham R, Silbersweig D, et al. Relation between cerebral activity and force in the motor areas of the human brain. *J Neurophys*. 1995;**74**:802–15.

42. Cramer S, Weisskoff R, Schaechter J, Nelles G, Foley M, Finklestein S, et al. Motor cortex activation is related to force of squeezing. *Hum Brain Mapp*. 2002;**16**:197–205.

43. Ward N, Frackowiak R. Age-related changes in the neural correlates of motor performance. *Brain*. 2003;**126**:873–88.

44. Blinkenberg M, Bonde C, Holm S, Svarer C, Andersen J, Paulson O, et al. Rate dependence of regional cerebral activation during performance of a repetitive motor task: a pet study. *J Cereb Blood Flow Metab*. 1996;**16**:794–803.

45. VanMeter J, Maisog J, Zeffiro T, Hallett M, Herscovitch P, Rapoport S. Parametric analysis of functional neuroimages: Application to a variable-rate motor task. *Neuroimage*. 1995;**2**:273–83.

46. Schlaug G, Sanes J, Thangaraj V, Darby D, Jancke L, Edelman R, et al. Cerebral activation covaries with movement rate. *Neuroreport*. 1996;**7**:879–83.

47. Rao S, Bandettini P, Binder J, Bobholz J, Hammeke T, Stein E, et al. Relationship between finger movement rate and functional magnetic resonance signal change in human primary motor cortex. *J Cereb Blood Flow Metab*. 1996;**16**:1250–4.

48. Waldvogel D, van Gelderen P, Ishii K, Hallett M. The effect of movement amplitude on activation in functional magnetic resonance imaging studies. *J Cereb Blood Flow Metab*. 1999;**19**:1209–12.

49. Sadato N, Campbell G, Ibanez V, Deiber M, Hallett M. Complexity affects regional cerebral blood flow change during sequential finger movements. *J Neurosci*. 1996;**16**:2691–700.

50. Gerloff C, Corwell B, Chen R, Hallett M, Cohen L. The role of the human motor cortex in the control of complex and simple finger movement sequences. *Brain*. 1998;**121**(Pt 9):1695–709.

51. Rao S, Binder J, Bandettini P, Hammeke T, Yetkin F, Jesmanowicz A, *et al.* Functional magnetic resonance imaging of complex human movements. *Neurology*. 1993;**43**:2311–18

52. Uchino K, Billheimer D, Cramer S. Entry criteria and baseline characteristics predict outcome in acute stroke trials. *Stroke*. 2001;**32**:909–16.

53. Duncan P, Jorgensen H, Wade D. Outcome measures in acute stroke trials: a systematic review and some recommendations to improve practice. *Stroke*. 2000;**31**:1429–38.

54. Cutter G, Baier M, Rudick R, Cookfair D, Fischer J, Petkau J, *et al.* Development of a multiple sclerosis functional composite as a clinical trial outcome measure. *Brain*. 1999;**122**:871–82.

55. Ditunno J, Young W, Donovan W. The international standards booklet for neurological and functional classification of spinal cord injury. American Spinal Injury Association. *Paraplegia*. 1994;**32**:70–80.

56. Hamzei F, Knab R, Weiller C, Rother J. The influence of extra- and intracranial artery disease on the bold signal in FMRI. *Neuroimage*. 2003;**20**:1393–1399

57. Rossini P, Altamura C, Ferretti A, Vernieri F, Zappasodi F, Caulo M, *et al.* Does cerebrovascular disease affect the coupling between neuronal activity and local haemodynamics? *Brain*. 2004;**127**:99–110.

58. Bilecen D, Radu E, Schulte A, Hennig J, Scheffler K, Seifritz E. FMRI of the auditory cortex in patients with unilateral carotid artery steno-occlusive disease. *J Magn Reson Imaging*. 2002;**15**:621–7.

59. Hund–Georgiadis M, Mildner T, Georgiadis D, Weih K, von Cramon D. Impaired hemodynamics and neural activation? A FMRI study of major cerebral artery stenosis. *Neurology*. 2003;**61**:1276–9.

60. Carusone L, Srinivasan J, Gitelman D, Mesulam M, Parrish T. Hemodynamic response changes in cerebrovascular disease: Implications for functional mr imaging. *AJNR Am J Neuroradiol*. 2002;**23**:1222–8.

61. Cramer S, Mark A, Maravilla K. Preserved cortical function with reduced cerebral blood flow after stroke. *Stroke*. 2002;**33**:418.

62. Krakauer JW, Radoeva PD, Zarahn E, Wydra J, Lazar RM, Hirsch J, *et al.* Hypoperfusion without stroke alters motor activation in the opposite hemisphere. *Ann Neurol*. 2004;**56**:796–802.

63. Pavlides C, Miyashita E, Asanuma H. Projection from the sensory to the motor cortex is important in learning motor skills in the monkey. *J Neurophysiol*. 1993;**70**:733–41.

64. Bornschlegl M, Asanuma H. Importance of the projection from the sensory to the motor cortex for recovery of motor function following partial thalamic lesion in the monkey. *Brain Res*. 1987;**437**:121–30.

65. Baker J, Donoghue J, Sanes J. Gaze direction modulates finger movement activation patterns in human cerebral cortex. *J Neurosci*. 1999;**19**:10044–52.

66. Stefan K, Wycislo M, Classen J. Modulation of associative human motor cortical plasticity by attention. *J Neurophysiol*. 2004;**92**:66–72.

67. Immink MA, Wright DL. Motor programming during practice conditions high and low in contextual interference. *J Exp Psychol Hum Percept Perform*. 2001;**27**:423–37.

68. Li Y, Wright DL. An assessment of the attention demands during random- and blocked-practice schedules. *Q J Exp Psychol A*. 2000;**53**:591–606.

69. Karni A, Meyer G, Jezzard P, Adams M, Turner R, Ungerleider L. Functional mri evidence for adult motor cortex plasticity during motor skill learning. *Nature*. 1996;**377**:155–8.

70. Kleim J, Barbay S, Cooper N, Hogg T, Reidel C, Remple M, *et al.* Motor learning-dependent synaptogenesis is localized to functionally reorganized motor cortex. *Neurobiol Learn Mem*. 2002;**77**:63–77.

71. Nudo R, Plautz E, Frost S. Role of adaptive plasticity in recovery of function after damage to motor cortex. *Muscle Nerve*. 2001;**24**:1000–19.

72. Chen R, Gerloff C, Hallett M, Cohen L. Involvement of the ipsilateral motor cortex in finger movements of different complexities. *Ann Neurol.* 1997;**41**:247–54.

73. Brion J–P, Demeurisse G, Capon A. Evidence of cortical reorganization in hemiparetic patients. *Stroke.* 1989;**20**:1079–84.

74. Siebner H, Peller M, Willoch F, Minoshima S, Boecker H, Auer C, *et al.* Lasting cortical activation after repetitive tms of the motor cortex: a glucose metabolic study. *Neurology.* 2000;**54**:956–63.

75. Lee L, Siebner H, Rowe J, Rizzo V, Rothwell J, Frackowiak R, *et al.* Acute remapping within the motor system induced by low-frequency repetitive transcranial magnetic stimulation. *J Neurosci.* 2003;**23**:5308–18.

76. Ilmoniemi R, Virtanen J, Ruohonen J, Karhu J, Aronen H, Naatanen R, *et al.* Neuronal responses to magnetic stimulation reveal cortical reactivity and connectivity. *Neuroreport.* 1997;**8**:3537–40.

77. Jones T, Schallert T. Overgrowth and pruning of dendrites in adult rats recovering from neocortical damage. *Brain Res.* 1992;**581**:156–60.

78. Jones T, Kleim J, Greenough W. Synaptogenesis and dendritic growth in the cortex opposite unilateral sensorimotor cortex damage in adult rats: a quantitative electron microscopic examination. *Brain Res.* 1996;**733**:142–8.

79. Dijkhuizen R, Singhal A, Mandeville J, Wu O, Halpern E, Finklestein S, *et al.* Correlation between brain reorganization, ischemic damage, and neurologic status after transient focal cerebral ischemia in rats: a functional magnetic resonance imaging study. *J Neurosci.* 2003;**23**:510–17.

80. Biernaskie J, Corbett D. Enriched rehabilitative training promotes improved forelimb motor function and enhanced dendritic growth after focal ischemic injury. *J Neurosci.* 2001;**21**:5272–80.

81. Kolb B. *Plasticity and recovery in adulthood. Brain plasticity and behavior.* Mahwah, NJ: Lawrence Erlbaum and Associates; 1995:95–112.

82. Nudo R, Wise B, SiFuentes F, Milliken G. Neural substrates for the effects of rehabilitative training on motor recovery after ischemic infarct. *Science.* 1996;**272**:1791–4.

83. Xerri C, Merzenich M, Peterson B, Jenkins W. Plasticity of primary somatosensory cortex paralleling sensorimotor skill recovery from stroke in adult monkeys. *J Neurophysiol.* 1998;**79**:2119–48.

84. Liu Y, Rouiller E. Mechanisms of recovery of dexterity following unilateral lesion of the sensorimotor cortex in adult monkeys. *Exp Brain Res.* 1999;**128**:149–59.

85. Chollet F, DiPiero V, Wise R, Brooks D, Dolan R, Frackowiak R. The functional anatomy of motor recovery after stroke in humans: A study with positron emission tomography. *Ann Neurol.* 1991;**29**:63–71.

86. Weiller C, Ramsay S, Wise R, Friston K, Frackowiak R. Individual patterns of functional reorganization in the human cerebral cortex after capsular infarction. *Ann Neurol.* 1993;**33**:181–9.

87. Cao Y, D'Olhaberriague L, Vikingstad E, Levine S, Welch K. Pilot study of functional mri to assess cerebral activation of motor function after poststroke hemiparesis. *Stroke.* 1998;**29**:112–22.

88. Seitz R, Hoflich P, Binkofski F, Tellmann L, Herzog H, Freund H–J. Role of the premotor cortex in recovery from middle cerebral artery infarction. *Arch Neurol.* 1998;**55**:1081–8.

89. Cramer S, Nelles G, Benson R, Kaplan J, Parker R, Kwong K, *et al.* A functional mri study of subjects recovered from hemiparetic stroke. *Stroke.* 1997;**28**:2518–27.

90. Cabeza R. Hemispheric asymmetry reduction in older adults: the Harold model. *Psychol Aging.* 2002;**17**:85–100.

91. Detre J. FMRI: applications in epilepsy. *Epilepsia.* 2004;**45**(Suppl 4):26–31.

92. Christodoulou C, DeLuca J, Ricker J, Madigan N, Bly B, Lange G, *et al.* Functional magnetic resonance imaging of working memory impairment after traumatic brain injury. *J Neurol Neurosurg Psychiatry.* 2001;**71**:161–8.

93. Lee M, Reddy H, Johansen–Berg H, Pendlebury S, Jenkinson M, Smith S, *et al.* The motor cortex shows adaptive functional changes to brain injury from multiple sclerosis. *Ann Neurol.* 2000;**47**:606–13.

94. Marshall R, Perera G, Lazar R, Krakauer J, Constantine R, DeLaPaz R. Evolution of cortical activation during recovery from corticospinal tract infarction. *Stroke.* 2000;**31**:656–61.

95. Calautti C, Leroy F, Guincestre J, Baron J. Dynamics of motor network overactivation after striatocapsular stroke: a longitudinal PET study using a fixed-performance paradigm. *Stroke.* 2001;**32**:2534–42.

96. Feydy A, Carlier R, Roby–Brami A, Bussel B, Cazalis F, Pierot L, *et al.* Longitudinal study of motor recovery after stroke: recruitment and focusing of brain activation. *Stroke.* 2002;**33**:1610–17.

97. Fujii Y, Nakada T. Cortical reorganization in patients with subcortical hemiparesis: neural mechanisms of functional recovery and prognostic implication. *J Neurosurg.* 2003;**98**:64–73.

98. Heiss W, Kessler J, Thiel A, Ghaemi M, Karbe H. Differential capacity of left and right hemispheric areas for compensation of poststroke aphasia. *Ann Neurol.* 1999;**45**:430–8.

99. Nhan H, Barquist K, Bell K, Esselman P, Odderson I, Cramer S. Brain function early after stroke in relation to subsequent recovery. *J Cereb Blood Flow Metab.* 2004;**24**:756–63.

100. Kim S–G, Ashe J, Hendrich K, Ellermann J, Merkle H, Ugurbil K, *et al.* Functional magnetic resonance imaging of motor cortex: hemispheric asymmetry and handedness. *Science.* 1993;**261**:615–17.

101. Zemke A, Heagerty P, Lee C, Cramer S. Motor cortex organization after stroke is related to side of stroke and level of recovery. *Stroke.* 2003;**34**:E23–28.

102. Luft A, Waller S, Forrester L, Smith G, Whitall J, Macko R, *et al.* Lesion location alters brain activation in chronically impaired stroke survivors. *Neuroimage.* 2004;**21**:924–35.

103. Wexler B, Fulbright R, Lacadie C, Skudlarski P, Kelz M, Constable R, *et al.* An FMRI study of the human cortical motor system response to increasing functional demands. *Magn Reson Imaging.* 1997;**15**:385–96.

104. Just M, Carpenter P, Keller T, Eddy W, Thulborn K. Brain activation modulated by sentence comprehension. *Science.* 1996;**274**:114–16.

105. Shibasaki H, Sadato N, Lyshkow H, Yonekura Y, Honda M, Nagamine T, *et al.* Both primary motor cortex and supplementary motor area play an important role in complex finger movement. *Brain.* 1993:1387–98.

106. Lohmann H, Deppe M, Jansen A, Schwindt W, Knecht S. Task repetition can affect functional magnetic resonance imaging-based measures of language lateralization and lead to pseudoincreases in bilaterality. *J Cereb Blood Flow Metab.* 2004;**24**:179–87.

107. Colebatch J, Deiber M–P, Passingham R, Friston K, Frackowiak R. Regional cerebral blood flow during voluntary arm and hand movements in human subjects. *J Neurophys.* 1991;**65**:1392–401.

108. Cramer S, Crafton K. Changes in lateralization and somatotopic organization after cortical stroke. *Stroke.* 2004;**35**:240.

109. Vikingstad EM, George KP, Johnson AF, Cao Y. Cortical language lateralization in right handed normal subjects using functional magnetic resonance imaging. *J Neurol Sci.* 2000;**175**:17–27.

110. Cramer S, Finklestein S, Schaechter J, Bush G, Rosen B. Distinct regions of motor cortex control ipsilateral and contralateral finger movements. *J Neurophysiology.* 1999;**81**:383–7.

111. Turton A, Wroe S, Trepte N, Fraser C, Lemon R. Contralateral and ipsilateral emg responses to transcranial magnetic stimulation during recovery of arm and hand function after stroke. *Electroenceph Clin Neurophys.* 1996;**101**:316–28.

112. Netz J, Lammers T, Homberg V. Reorganization of motor output in the non-affected hemisphere after stroke. *Brain.* 1997;**120**:1579–86.

113. Shimizu T, Hosaki A, Hino T, Sato M, Komori T, Hirai S, *et al.* Motor cortical disinhibition in the unaffected hemisphere after unilateral cortical stroke. *Brain.* 2002;**125**:1896–907.

114. Murase N, Duque J, Mazzocchio R, Cohen L. Influence of interhemispheric interactions on motor function in chronic stroke. *Ann Neurol.* 2004;**55**:400–9.

115. Johansen–Berg H, Rushworth M, Bogdanovic M, Kischka U, Wimalaratna S, Matthews P. The role of ipsilateral premotor cortex in hand movement after stroke. *Proc Natl Acad Sci USA*. 2002;**99**:14518–23.

116. Cardebat D, Demonet J, De Boissezon X, Marie N, Marie R, Lambert J, *et al.* Behavioral and neurofunctional changes over time in healthy and aphasic subjects: a PET language activation study. *Stroke*. 2003;**34**:2900–6.

117. Thulborn K, Carpenter P, Just M. Plasticity of language-related brain function during recovery from stroke. *Stroke*. 1999;**30**:749–754

118. Cappa S, Perani D, Grassi F, Bressi S, Alberoni M, Franceschi M, *et al.* A PET follow-up study of recovery after stroke in acute aphasics. *Brain Lang*. 1997;**56**:55–67.

119. Gold B, Kertesz A. Right hemisphere semantic processing of visual words in an aphasic patient: an FMRI study. *Brain Lang*. 2000;**73**:456–65.

120. Buckner R, Corbetta M, Schatz J, Raichle M, Petersen S. Preserved speech abilities and compensation following prefrontal damage. *Proc Natl Acad Sci USA*. 1996;**93**:1249–53.

121. Rossini PM, Caltagirone C, Castriota–Scanderbeg A, Cicinelli P, Del Gratta C, Demartin M, *et al.* Hand motor cortical area reorganization in stroke: a study with FMRI, MEG and TCS maps. *Neuroreport*. 1998;**9**:2141–6.

122. Cramer S, Moore C, Finklestein S, Rosen B. A pilot study of somatotopic mapping after cortical infarct. *Stroke*. 2000;**31**:668–71.

123. Pineiro R, Pendlebury S, Johansen–Berg H, Matthews P. Functional mri detects posterior shifts in primary sensorimotor cortex activation after stroke: evidence of local adaptive reorganization? *Stroke*. 2001;**32**:1134–9.

124. Calautti C, Leroy F, Guincestre J, Baron J. Displacement of primary sensorimotor cortex activation after subcortical stroke: a longitudinal PET study with clinical correlation. *Neuroimage*. 2003;**19**:1650–4.

125. Turner J, Lee J, Schandler S, Cohen M. An FMRI investigation of hand representation in paraplegic humans. *Neurorehabil Neural Repair*. 2003;**17**:37–47.

126. Green J, Sora E, Bialy Y, Ricamato A, Thatcher R. Cortical sensorimotor reorganization after spinal cord injury: An electroencephalographic study. *Neurology*. 1998;**50**:1115–21.

127. Nelles G, Spiekermann G, Jueptner M, Leonhardt G, Muller S, Gerhard H, *et al.* Evolution of functional reorganization in hemiplegic stroke: a serial positron emission tomographic activation study. *Ann Neurol*. 1999;**46**:901–9.

128. Tombari D, Loubinoux I, Pariente J, Gerdelat A, Albucher J, Tardy J, *et al.* A longitudinal FMRI study: in recovering and then in clinically stable sub-cortical stroke patients. *Neuroimage*. 2004;**23**:827–39.

129. Traversa R, Cicinelli P, Bassi A, Rossini P, Bernardi G. Mapping of motor cortical reorganization after stroke. A brain stimulation study with focal magnetic pulses. *Stroke*. 1997;**28**:110–17.

130. Traversa R, Cicinelli P, Oliveri M, Giuseppina Palmieri M, Filippi M, Pasqualetti P, *et al.* Neurophysiological follow-up of motor cortical output in stroke patients. *Clin Neurophysiol*. 2000;**111**:1695–703.

131. Cicinelli P, Traversa R, Rossini P. Post-stroke reorganization of brain motor output to the hand: a 2–4 month follow-up with focal magnetic transcranial stimulation. *Electroencephalogr Clin Neurophysiol*. 1997;**105**:438–50.

132. Nakayama H, Jorgensen H, Raaschou H, Olsen T. Recovery of upper extremity function in stroke patients: the Copenhagen stroke study. *Arch Phys Med Rehabil*. 1994;**75**:394–8.

133. Ward N, Brown M, Thompson A, Frackowiak R. Neural correlates of motor recovery after stroke: a longitudinal FMRI study. *Brain*. 2003;**126**:2476–96.

134. Cramer S, Fray E, Tievsky A, Parker R, Riskind P, Stein M, *et al.* Changes in motor cortex activation after recovery from spinal cord inflammation. *Mult Scler*. 2001;**7**:364–70.

135. Ward N, Brown M, Thompson A, Frackowiak R. Neural correlates of outcome after stroke: A cross-sectional FMRI study. *Brain*. 2003;**126**:1430–48.

136. Rosen H, Petersen S, Linenweber M, Snyder A, White D, Chapman L, *et al*. Neural correlates of recovery from aphasia after damage to left inferior frontal cortex. *Neurology*. 2000;**55**:1883–94.

137. Butz M, Gross J, Timmermann L, Moll M, Freund H, Witte O, *et al*. Perilesional pathological oscillatory activity in the magnetoencephalogram of patients with cortical brain lesions. *Neurosci Lett*. 2004;**355**:93–6.

138. Li Y, Jiang N, Powers C, Chopp M. Neuronal damage and plasticity identified by map-2, gap-43 and cyclin d1 immunoreactivity after focal cerebral ischemia in rat. *Stroke*. 1998;**29**:1972–81.

139. Baron J, D'Antona R, Pantano P, Serdaru M, Samson Y, Bousser M. Effects of thalamic stroke on energy metabolism of the cerebral cortex. A positron tomography study in man. *Brain*. 1986;**109**:1243–59.

140. Seitz R, Azari N, Knorr U, Binkofski F, Herzog H, Freund H. The role of diaschisis in stroke recovery. *Stroke*. 1999;**30**:1844–50.

141. Witte O, Stoll G. Delayed and remote effects of focal cortical infarctions: secondary damage and reactive plasticity. *Adv Neurol*. 1997;**73**:207–27.

142. Heiss W, Emunds H, Herholz K. Cerebral glucose metabolism as a predictor of rehabilitation after ischemic stroke. *Stroke*. 1993;**24**:1784–8.

143. Cramer S. Functional imaging in stroke recovery. *Stroke*. 2004;**35**:2695–8.

144. Grotta J, Bratina P. Subjective experiences of 24 patients dramatically recovering from stroke. *Stroke*. 1995;**26**:1285–8.

145. Pariente J, Loubinoux I, Carel C, Albucher J, Leger A, Manelfe C, *et al*. Fluoxetine modulates motor performance and cerebral activation of patients recovering from stroke. *Ann Neurol*. 2001;**50**:718–29.

146. Carey J, Kimberley T, Lewis S, Auerbach E, Dorsey L, Rundquist P, *et al*. Analysis of FMRI and finger tracking training in subjects with chronic stroke. *Brain*. 2002;**125**:773–88.

147. Liepert J, Bauder H, Wolfgang H, Miltner W, Taub E, Weiller C. Treatment-induced cortical reorganization after stroke in humans. *Stroke*. 2000;**31**:1210–16.

148. Chugani H, Phelps M, Mazziotta J. Positron emission tomography study of human brain functional development. *Ann Neurol*. 1987;**22**:487–97.

10

Parkinson's disease

Thomas Eckert, Dennis Zgaljardic, and
David Eidelberg

1. Overview and treatment issues

Idiopathic Parkinson's disease (PD) is a relatively common neurological disorder with
a prevalence rate of 1–3% in people over the age of 65 years[1]. Given the increasing age of our
population, it is expected that the prevalence of PD in the general population will rise
steadily over time. The clinical syndrome of parkinsonism is characterized by the existence
of at least two of the following symptoms: bradykinesia, rigidity, or tremor. Although clinical
signs of parkinsonism can be observed in conditions such as multiple system atrophy
(MSA), progressive supranuclear palsy (PSP), and Alzheimer's disease (AD), as well as
medication-induced syndromes, it is most commonly observed in patients with classical PD.

1.1 Pathology

Neuropathologically, PD is characterized by neurodegeneration of dopamine-containing
neurons in the substantia nigra pars compacta (SNc). However, the onset of parkinsonian
symptoms manifests only after histopathologically advanced stages have been reached.
In addition to SNc neurodegeneration, another hallmark of postmortem diagnosis in
presymptomatic and symptomatic stages of PD is the development of specific
eosinophilic inclusion bodies (i.e. Lewy bodies). Lewy bodies contain an aggregated form
of the normal presynaptic protein, a-synuclein. The occurrence of Lewy bodies in post-
mortem investigation is not solely confined to PD, as they are present in other syndromes
such as MSA and Hallervorden–Spatz disease. However, the pattern and distribution of
Lewy bodies in such syndromes differ from PD.

Due to the progressive nature of the disease, the pathology of PD involves degeneration
of multiple neuronal systems that are dependent on the stage of the disease. Braak and
colleagues (2003) described six pathological stages of disease progression in PD[2]. These
pathological stages are defined by their varying degree of cortical involvement in addition
to the above-mentioned pathologies. Stage 1 is characterized by the existence of inclusion
bodies and neuronal damage confined to the dorsal IX/X motor nucleus and/or intermediate
reticular zone. Stage 2 features damage in caudal raphe nuclei, gigantocellular nucleus,
and coeruleus-subcoeruleus complex. Stage 3 involves further progression with degeneration of midbrain structures. In Stage 4, the first cortical areas presenting with a-synuclein-
containing lesions are evident within the temporal mesocortex and the allocortex.

This is followed by Stage 5, which includes pathology within higher-order sensory association areas of the neocortex and prefrontal areas. Finally, Stage 6 of PD involves first-order sensory association areas of the neocortex and premotor areas. Occasionally at this stage, there is also involvement of primary sensory and motor areas. It has been reported that neuronal damage can also be observed in peripheral neuronal systems such as the preganglionic peripheral sympathetic innervation of the heart.

1.2 Clinical disease progression

Hoehn and Yahr (1967) evaluated 856 patients with parkinsonism[3], providing the only available data regarding the course of the disease in untreated patients. Based on their findings, these authors described five clinical stages of disease progression. Stage I is characterized by unilateral symptoms. Although quite common in early PD, tremor is present in only 60% of PD patients; 40% present with bradykinesia and rigidity as the primary findings. Stage II is defined by bilateral symptomatology, although most patients will show unilateral dominant symptoms throughout the course of the disease. Poewe and Wenning (1998)[4] described the latencies of the spread of symptoms between body parts. In patients presenting with unilateral symptoms to the upper extremities, the spread of symptoms to the ipsilateral lower extremity occurred after 0.8–1.4 years; the onset of bilateral involvement occurred between 2.1 and 3.4 years. Stage III is defined by the development of postural instability. Patients in Stages IV and V are considered to be in the advanced stages of PD. Patients in Stage IV experience severe disability but maintain the ability to stand and ambulate unassisted. In Stage V, patients are typically confined to a bed or need a wheelchair to ambulate.

In an attempt to identify clinical features that predict differences in disease progression, tremor-dominant PD has been described as a positive predictor of slower disease progression compared to the akinetic rigid subtype. Preserved cognition and young onset are also associated with a better prognosis. On average, patients with PD reach Stage IV after 9.0 ± 7.2 years. Although 34% of PD patients with a disease duration of 10 years and longer were still classified as Stage I or II, 37% reached Stage III, IV, or even V within the first five years of diagnosis.

Hoehn and Yahr also evaluated the extent of motor disability and incidence of death in a longitudinal study with a group of 271 patients. They discovered that 28% of these patients became either severely disabled or had died within five years of disease onset, rising up to 61% at 10 years and 90% at 15 years. Of note, one must acknowledge that the patients studied originally by Hoehn and Yahr were not diagnosed using validated clinical diagnostic criteria. Therefore, it is likely that these studies included a significant number of patients with atypical parkinsonian syndromes.

Hoehn and Yahr (1969)[90] also performed the first study assessing the progression of motor symptoms in PD patients following dopamine treatment. In comparison to the untreated patients with PD in the original cohort, the treated group lasted approximately 3–5 years longer in each disease stage. Levodopa treatment was also associated with specific side-effects, such as motor fluctuations, dyskinesias, wearing off, dystonia, visual hallucinations, and psychotic symptoms. These treatment complications were present, generally, in later stages of the disease. Following the introduction of dopaminergic treatment, patients can experience a period of positive benefit and symptom relief. This period, also known as the 'drug honeymoon', can last for approximately two years. Over time, patients can develop the medication side-effects mentioned above. In general, 50% of patients develop motor fluctuations approximately five years following initial treatment. In recent years, there has been a shift towards the development of new therapies to ameliorate disease progression[5, 6].

1.3 Disturbances of the motor system

The extrapyramidal system consists of the basal ganglia and its input and output circuitry (i.e. basal ganglia-thalamocortical circuits)[7]. In addition to this motor circuit, there is an oculomotor, prefrontal, and limbic circuit all working in parallel. The basal ganglia consist of the putamen, the internal and external segments of the globus pallidus (GPe and GPi, respectively), the caudate nucleus, the subthalamic nucleus (STN), and the substantia nigra pars compacta and reticulata (SNc and SNr, respectively). Functionally, the basal ganglia consist of input and output structures. The striatum, consisting of the caudate nucleus and the putamen, represents the main input structure of the basal ganglia. It receives information from the entire cerebral cortex. The GPi and SNr are the major output structures of the basal ganglia. Their inhibitory neurons project to specific nuclei of the thalamus, which in turn project with excitatory neurons to prefrontal cortical areas. A complex processing system links the input and output structures of the basal ganglia. The motor circuit is believed to consist of a direct and indirect pathway (see Fig. 10.1). The direct pathway maintains a monosynaptic inhibitory connection between the putamen and the output nuclei of the basal ganglia (GPi and SNr). The indirect pathway projects inhibitory signals from the putamen to the external segment of the globus pallidus (GPe). This pathway continues to the subthalamic nucleus (STN), which projects excitatory signals to the output nuclei, GPi, and SNr. Hypokinetic disorders, such as PD, are thought to result in an increase of the indirect pathway. The dopaminergic deficit in PD leads to an over-inhibition of the GPe, which in turn disinhibits the STN. Consequently, this increases the excitatory output of the STN, which over-stimulates the GPi and the SNr. As a result of this over-stimulation, the inhibitory signals over-inhibit the thalamus, which subsequently reduces its excitatory output to cortical structures.

This model, which was initially derived from animal studies, represents the basis of our understanding of how stereotaxic interventions in GPi STN can improve the hypokinetic symptoms of PD[8]. External inhibition of the STN through electrical stimulation decreases the over-stimulation of the basal ganglia output structures and, therefore, normalizes the overactive indirect pathway. The development of neural pathway mapping using functional imaging techniques such as positron emission tomography (PET) and FMRI has facilitated the testing of hypotheses concerning the pathophysiology of PD and its response to treatment. These *in vivo* approaches have been especially valuable in the study of cognitive function in PD and related disorders.

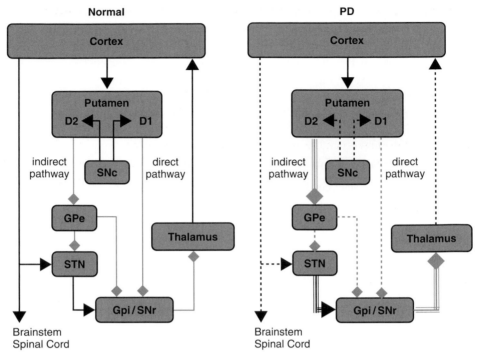

Fig. 10.1 Basal ganglia motor loop model (see text). D2 = dopamine D2-receptor mediated; D1 = dopamine D1-receptor mediated; SNc = substantia nigra pars compacta; SNr = substantia nigra pars reticularis; GPi = internal segment of the globus pallidus; GPe = external segment of the globus pallidus; STN = subthalamic nucleus. Arrow indicates excitatory and rectangle inhibitory output; single line indicates steady state; dotted line, decreased output; and triple line, increased output.

1.4 Disturbances of cognitive function

Dementia is defined as an impairment of multiple cognitive domains (including memory) that are related to a specific medical condition such as PD. The dementia typically associated with PD is of a subcortical type and occurs in approximately one-third of patients with the disease, although prevalence rates can vary, ranging from 4–93%[9]. The presence of cortical deficits in demented PD patients, such as impaired learning, aphasia, and/or apraxia may result from additional pathology indicative of Alzheimer's disease, dementia with Lewy bodies, or both[10]. Demented patients with PD primarily exhibit impairments in declarative memory (with relatively intact recognition), executive and visuospatial functions, speech and language, as well as mood[11].

Non-demented patients with PD may exhibit a similar, though milder, neuropsychological profile. The cognitive impairments exhibited by non-demented patients typically resemble a dysexecutive syndrome with secondary memory and visuospatial processing difficulties[12,13]. However, select deficits have been documented in most cognitive domains[14]. PD patients who later develop dementia are typically older at disease onset

(>60 years), experience depressive symptomatology, and have a tendency to demonstrate substandard performance on neuropsychological tests of visuospatial skills, cognitive flexibility, and word-list generation[11].

1.4.1 Memory

Memory deficits exhibited by patients with PD are characterized by impairments of delayed recall (due to poor retrieval), temporal ordering, and conditional associative learning[9]. PD patients tend to maintain normal rates of memory decay, demonstrate preserved encoding of information and recognition, and benefit from external cueing. This profile contrasts with that of patients with AD, who exhibit increased forgetting (due to impaired encoding), poor recognition, and an inability to benefit from external cueing.

1.4.2 Visuospatial skills

Visuospatial deficits are frequently reported in PD. Non-demented patients with PD may not essentially exhibit a pure visuospatial deficit (e.g. orientation and distance, judgement of direction, visual analysis and synthesis). Nonetheless, neuropsychological task performance can be compromised if tests are timed or incorporate either a motor or a frontal/executive element[14]. In contrast, demented PD patients tend to exhibit impaired visuospatial performance in comparison to non-demented patients and age-matched healthy control subjects on tasks that do not incorporate a timed motor and/or frontal/executive component.

1.4.3 Speech and language

Deficits in the motor aspects of speech are common in patients with PD. Deficits in speech output have been attributed to vocal-motor deficits (dysarthria) involving a reduction of speech volume and pitch. Demented patients are usually more likely to exhibit impairments of speech intonation, length of utterance, and spontaneity[15]. Confrontation naming performance is reduced in demented patients with PD, albeit significantly better than performances of other demented patient groups. Further, verbal fluency, especially with phonemic cueing, is impaired in PD patients and has typically been attributed to executive dysfunction (e.g. set-shifting or strategy initiation), rather than to a breakdown of lexical stores, as reported in patients with AD.

1.4.4 Executive dysfunction

Executive dysfunction is regarded as the primary cognitive sequela of PD. PD patients, with or without dementia, are known to exhibit impairments in working memory, planning, response-monitoring, set-shifting, and attentional control. These impairments can be described in terms of the difficulties PD patients may experience in developing their own plan of action or initiating goal-directed behaviour, as well as maintaining adequate levels of processing resources necessary for concept formation and self-monitoring behaviour. In theory, a mechanism or central processor within the prefrontal cortex distributes mental resources according to processing demands so as to govern non-routine behaviours[16]. This process is believed to influence inhibitory resources, allowing for the suppression of routine behaviours in favour of more goal-appropriate ones.

For instance, patients with frontal dysfunction, as in PD[17], may exhibit normal behaviour in familiar settings, but may find it difficult to adapt when confronted with a novel environment or stimulus. Furthermore, poor performance on standardized neuropsychological tests may stem from imposing greater resource demands such as relying heavily on internally generated information and exceeding available resources, thereby preventing efficient strategy formation in these patients[18]. As a result, patients may find it difficult to inhibit irrelevant resources while performing a task, which may lead to excessive cognitive load. This, in turn, reduces cognitive processing speed and results, potentially, in an inability to select and execute mental strategies efficiently.

1.4.5 Mood disturbances in PD

Among the psychiatric sequelae associated with PD, depression and apathy are most common. Prevalence rates of depression are approximately 40%. Depression in PD does not appear to be associated with a reaction to the disease. Typically, PD patients have been shown to have greater prevalence of depression compared to demographically-matched normal control subjects with corresponding levels of physical disability and/or motor limitations. In some cases, the mood disturbance has preceded motor symptomatology. Diagnosis of depression in patients with PD can be difficult because PD symptomatology tends to resemble depressive symptomatology (e.g. motor retardation, insomnia, a lack of energy, early morning awakenings, fatigue, and weight loss) or are masked by deficits in emotional processing[14]. Apathy is characterized as indifference to environmental, emotional, and/or physical states. Reported prevalence estimates of apathy in PD currently range from 16.5–42% and are typically lower than rates for depression. The aetiology of apathy in PD has yet to be systematically assessed, although studies have shown that individuals with PD do exhibit greater levels of apathy in comparison to age-matched physically disabled patients. In addition, comparisons of subjective and/or clinical ratings show that PD patients with high levels of apathy have a greater incidence of cognitive deficits, especially for executive functions.

1.5 Genetics

PD is generally considered to be a sporadic disease. The growing area of genetics in PD has been reviewed recently[19]. A familial association in some cases was noted as early as 1890. In the current day, approximately 15% of PD patients have an affected relative. Inherited forms of PD generally have an earlier disease onset. Several genetic mutations have been identified in association with PD. It has been proposed that altered gene products can result in impaired protein degradation, and that the accumulation of inappropriately folded proteins leads to the characteristic dopaminergic degeneration found in PD. In accordance with this notion, the a-synuclein (PARK1) and DJ-1 (PARK7) mutations have been shown to cause abnormal protein conformations and overwhelm the main cellular protein degradation system. By contrast, the parkin (PARK2) and UCH-L1 (PARK5) mutations appear to undermine the cell's ability to detect and degrade the inappropriately folded proteins[19]. Although a number of genes associated with PD have already been identified, it is very likely that more will emerge as new familial clusters are identified.

The discovery of new PD-associated genes may rely on the use of functional brain imaging to detect a preclinical/subclinical endophenotype in clinically unaffected family members[20].

1.6 Differential diagnosis

The clinical syndrome of parkinsonism is a feature of a number of different diseases. It occurs as a side-effect to various neuroleptic medications, as well as in a number of neurodegenerative diseases. The most common alternative diagnoses for patients with parkinsonism include multiple system atrophy (MSA), progressive supranuclear palsy (PSP), and corticobasal degeneration (CBGD). An autopsy study revealed that only about 75% of patients with parkinsonism prove to have PD at neuropathological examination[21]. The accurate ability to diagnose patients with parkinsonism is of importance because prognosis and treatment options vary between PD patients and those with atypical parkinsonism. The life expectancy of PD patients approximates their unaffected contemporaries. However, the life expectancy of patients with atypical parkinsonian syndromes is comparatively low, resembling that of PD patients of the pre-levodopa era. Similarly, PD patients respond well to dopaminergic medication and benefit from neurosurgical approaches such as deep brain stimulation (DBS). By contrast, patients with atypical parkinsonian syndromes may present with an initial positive response to dopaminergic treatment that diminishes with disease progression. Likewise, their response to stereotaxic surgery is often disappointing[22].

Because a definitive diagnosis of PD is difficult to achieve clinically in the early stages of the disease, it is likely that randomized trials of neuroprotective agents routinely include patients with atypical parkinsonian disorders. In addition, surgical therapies for PD are increasingly being considered at earlier disease stages. Thus, correct early diagnosis of PD will become increasingly relevant to the study of new therapies.

The growing awareness of occurrence of these different parkinsonian syndromes in the last 20 years has led to the development of clinical classification criteria for the various disorders. Clinically, early stage idiopathic PD is characterized by an unilateral presentation with ongoing responsiveness to dopaminergic medication. The occurrence of the characteristic resting tremor is about 60% in PD, with motor fluctuations and dystonic posturing occurring in later stages[23].

To improve clinical diagnosis in patients with parkinsonism, criteria have been developed for PD[23], MSA[24], and PSP[25]. Nevertheless when based solely upon clinical criteria, the diagnosis of these parkinsonian syndromes is inaccurate, even at early disease stages. Although diagnostic accuracy increases with disease duration, definite diagnosis for parkinsonian syndromes can only be achieved following neuropathological examination. Nonetheless, several techniques have been employed to increase diagnostic accuracy *in vivo*. Electrophysiological investigations such as sphincter electromyography, autonomic function tests, and clonidine-growth hormone test have revealed controversial results in various studies. By contrast, the application of imaging methods for this purpose has proved promising[26]. These imaging methods and their application in the differential diagnosis of parkinsonian disorders are discussed below.

1.7 **Therapeutics in Parkinson's disease**

An important feature of PD compared to other disorders with parkinsonism is its consistent responsiveness to pharmacological treatment with dopaminergic medication. The discovery of the dopamine deficiency in PD[27] was followed by groundbreaking studies reporting clinical improvement in PD patients following the oral application of levodopa[28,29]. Dopamine does not cross the blood-brain barrier. However, levodopa, a dopamine precursor, can be made available to dopamine-depleted brain structures and improve PD signs and symptoms. In the early days of dopaminergic treatment, very high doses of levodopa had to be administered effectively to reduce rigidity and bradykinesia. However, because of the peripheral conversion of levodopa to dopamine, side-effects were common. As a means to remedy the peripheral conversion of levodopa to dopamine, oral levodopa is now combined with dopa-decarboxylase (DDC)-inhibitors such as carbidopa or benserazid, as well as catechol-O-methyltransferase (COMT) inhibitors, such as entacapone and tolcapone. A number of combination fast-, normal-, or controlled-release medications combining levodopa and a DDC-inhibitor, as well as COMT inhibitors, represent the basis of pharmacological treatment in PD.

Another approach to restore the dopaminergic deficit in PD relies upon dopamine agonist therapy. There are two main groups of dopamine agonists: ergot derivates (e.g. bromocriptine, cabergoline, a-dihydroergocriptine, pergolide, lisuride) and non-ergot derivates (e.g. pramipexole, ropinerole). Dopamine agonists are generally considered to be somewhat less effective than levodopa in the reduction of akinesia and rigidity. However, these agents have the advantage of having a long half-life with the benefit of reducing motor fluctuations. On the other hand, dopamine agonists may have significant short-term side-effects such as nausea, daytime sleepiness, and visual hallucinations.

The development of agents targeting disease progression has become the current focus of pharmacological research. To investigate the neuroprotective effects of selegiline and tocopherol, a multicentre, large, double-blind study (DATATOP) was performed[30]. The findings suggested that while there was no observable neuroprotective effect for tocopherol, the initiation of levodopa treatment could be delayed by selegiline. However, this potential neuroprotective effect was not sustained after two years of treatment. The neuroprotective effects of various dopamine agonists have also been investigated[5,31]. A major issue in neuroprotective trials for PD surrounds the objective assessment of disease progression. The clinical evaluation of parkinsonism can be influenced by symptomatic treatment effects. Therefore, a need exists to develop surrogate imaging markers for the assessment of changes in disease severity over time[32]. Ideally, these methods should be independent of symptomatic treatment effects and should be appropriate for repeated measures in individual subjects.

Deep brain stimulation (DBS) and stereotactic ablation of basal ganglia are alternatives to pharmacological therapy for the treatment of PD[33]. The implantation of deep brain electrodes allows for non-permanent interference in basal ganglia function. Stimulator adjustments can be made 'on-line' in order to optimize motor performance and minimize side-effects. Stereotactic ablation of various basal ganglia structures including the internal globus pallidus (GPi), the ventral intermediate nucleus of the thalamus (Vim), and the subthalamic nucleus (STN) have been investigated for their effect on motor symptoms in PD. While the Vim appears to be the superior target for intractable tremor in PD and essential tremor, the STN has proven to be the target of choice for the combined treatment of bradykinesia, rigidity, and tremor as well as for the long-term complications of dyskinisia and dystonia[34]. Additional neurosurgical approaches have attempted to target the dopaminergic deficit within the basal ganglia directly by implanting embryonic tissue into the putamen. Recent double-blinded clinical trials using foetal dopaminergic cells failed to disclose statistically significant clinical benefit despite consistent increases in PET signal[35,36] (see below).

2. Parkinson's disease: imaging approaches for diagnosis and therapy

2.1 Routine structural imaging

Routine structural imaging with computerized tomography (CT) and magnetic resonance imaging (MRI) does not reveal consistent pathological changes in patients with idiopathic PD. However, these techniques can be used to exclude certain atypical causes of parkinsonism, such as normal pressure hydrocephalus, lower body parkinsonism due to arteriovascular disease, or hemiparkinsonism/hemiatrophy syndrome. Routine MRI has also been used in the diagnosis of atypical parkinsonian syndromes. For instance, the constellation of putaminal atrophy, a hyperintense putamenal rim in T2 sequences, and infratentorial signal changes is consistent with the diagnosis of MSA. MR imaging of PSP patients has revealed atrophy of the globus pallidus, as well as focal atrophy in frontal and temporal regions. Nevertheless, even though these changes were demonstrated to have high specificity, they have been reported to occur in only 50% of patients[37].

A number of researchers have employed inversion recovery sequences or modified T2-sequences to visualize changes in the substantia nigra in PD patients. These methods may discriminate PD patients from healthy control subjects. However, these techniques are less promising for the differential diagnosis of parkinsonian syndromes. A rather novel approach in structural brain imaging has been the recent application of ultrasound to the midbrain of PD patients (Berg *et al.* 2001[91]). Visualization of the substantia nigra using ultrasound has revealed an increased echogenicity in early-stage PD patients compared to healthy controls.

2.2 Functional imaging in Parkinson's disease

2.2.1 Imaging of the presynaptic dopaminergic system with PET and SPECT

Radiotracer imaging (RTI) of the dopaminergic system, with positron emission tomography (PET) and single photon emission computerized tomography (SPECT) are conceptually quite similar. PET has better spatial resolution than SPECT, although it is generally less available for routine clinical use. However, PET has recently become more widespread, less reliant upon on-site radiotracer production, and is less costly.

Nonetheless, PET is widely used for research purposes, and its clinical applicability is growing, especially in North America.

PET and SPECT methods can be divided into the quantification of presynaptic and postsynaptic dopaminergic function. Presynaptic dopaminergic imaging techniques assess either: (1) the uptake and conversion from fluorodopa to fluorodopamine by the aromatic acid decarboxylase (AADC) [using [18F]fluorodopa PET (FDOPA)]; (2) the density of monoamine containing synaptic vesicles [using [11C]dihydrotetrabenazine PET (DTBZ)]; or (3) the expression of the dopamine transporter (DAT) on the cell surface facilitating the release and reabsorption of dopamine in the nigrostriatal intersynaptic cleft using [123I]-2b-carbomethyl-3b-(4-iodophenyl) tropane (β-CIT) and related radiola- belled cocaine derivates for PET or SPECT imaging[38]. Each of these RTI methods reflects different aspects of monoaminergic nerve terminal function.

Radiotracer imaging of the presynaptic nigrostriatal dopaminergic system has been used extensively to assess disease severity and progression in PD. FDOPA PET and β-CIT SPECT have revealed a 4–13% annual reduction in baseline putamenal uptake compared with 0–2.5% in healthy controls[39,40]. This technique has also been used to estimate the duration of the preclinical period in PD[41]. Striatal FDOPA measurements have been correlated with dopamine cell counts measured in postmortem specimens[42]. The rate of striatal DAT binding decline in PD may be associated with age of onset[1,38,43].

A specific concern is the measurement of neuroprotective effects of potential drugs to retard disease progression in PD[32]. The role of RTI in this way is to enhance the statistical power of randomized, blinded studies. This will potentially reduce the number of subjects needed while providing an objective outcome measure of the neuroprotective response.

There have been two large studies that investigated disease progression in patients receiving levodopa versus those receiving dopamine agonists[5,31]. Both studies demonstrated better clinical performance in the levodopa group. However, the rate of disease progression assessed by RTI was reduced only with dopamine agonists. A similar discordance occurred in the subsequent ELLDOPA trial[6]. Subjects treated with high-dose levodopa had the best clinical outcome even after up to four weeks of medication washout, despite more rapidly progressing PD as assessed by β-CIT SPECT.

These results raise questions regarding the use of RTI as a surrogate marker for neuro- protection trials in PD[32]. The nigrostriatal system is influenced by a number of other neuronal systems and neurotransmitters, and is far more complex than might be sug- gested from RTI studies targeting individual enzymes/receptor systems. All of these imaging techniques require simplified assumptions for acquisition and analysis of data and can be affected by factors other than the primary biological process under study. Thus, the correspondence between tracer uptake and tissue biology is insufficient for the application of RTI as a surrogate marker in neurodegenerative trials.

A critical issue in this regard is the possible occurrence of temporal up- and downregu- lation of neuropeptides and receptors, which might influence imaging results. A PET study comparing FDOPA, DTBZ, and a DAT ligand in the same group of PD patients, revealed a relative upregulation of DDC and downregulation of DAT[44]. This suggests that surviv- ing neurons synthesize more dopamine and also take up less from the synaptic cleft.

External dopaminergic treatment may change the proportion of available dopamine at the synaptic level, which is likely to influence the regulation of these enzymes.

At the time of writing, the effect of medication on RTI assessments of presynaptic dopaminergic functioning has not been investigated thoroughly. Guttman and colleagues (2001) reported significantly decreased binding of [11C] RTI-32 after treatment with levodopa and decreased, though not significantly, DAT binding following treatment with pramipexole[45]. Similar changes may have contributed to the group differences observed in the CALM PD study. However, further investigations with greater sample sizes need to be performed before firm conclusions can be drawn. Functional changes of up- or down-regulation of neuropeptides or receptors are likely to be time-regulated. Therefore, the duration of medication washout can be critical to the results of an imaging study of this type. Another problem in evaluating PD disease progression with RTI is the simplifying assumption that the loss of nigrostriatal neurons is the single pathological process at play. Nigral cell loss might be the main pathology in PD, but it appears to be only one of several pathways leading to clinical symptoms and disability in PD, especially at advanced stages of disease.

FDOPA PET has also been used as an imaging marker in foetal tissue transplantation trials. In these trials, FDOPA has been applied to provide additional information about graft survival and function. Early reports from small groups of patients receiving foetal tissue implantation described significant increases of FDOPA uptake in the putamen indicating survival of transplanted neurons. Subsequently, 39 patients with advanced PD underwent FDOPA imaging at baseline and at 12 months in the first double-blind, placebo-controlled surgical trial of human embryonic dopaminergic tissue transplantation. The primary clinical outcome of this study (i.e. the change of patient-rated global clinical impression at 12 months) was not significantly different between the transplantation and the sham surgery group[35]. However, in contrast to that, FDOPA PET revealed an increase of 40% in putamenal FDOPA uptake[43]. A second double-blind, placebo-controlled foetal transplantation trial showed similar results, which revealed a trend toward improvement in the Unified Parkinsons' Disease Rating Scale (UPDRS) motor score and a significant increase in putamenal FDOPA uptake[36].

FDOPA imaging demonstrates that foetal tissue transplantation leads to an increase in dopaminergic function in the striatum. However, this approach does not provide information about the integration of grafted neurons into the host. Indeed, abnormal connectivity of engrafted cells might lead to the development of 'runaway' dyskinesias in certain transplant recipients[46].

2.2.2 Imaging of the postsynaptic dopamine receptor with PET and SPECT

Imaging of the postsynaptic dopaminergic system in parkinsonian syndromes has been performed with radiotracer binding to the dopamine D2-receptor. These studies have been conducted mainly with [11C]-raclopride (RAC) for PET imaging and [123I]-(S)-2-hydroxy-3-iodo-6-methoxy-[(1-ethyl-2-pyrrolidinyl)methyl] benzamide (IBZM) for SPECT. Postsynaptic dopaminergic imaging in parkinsonian disorders is of particular interest for differential diagnosis of PD and atypical parkinsonian disorders.

Although the presynaptic nigrostriatal dopaminergic system is affected in most parkinsonian syndromes, the postsynaptic system is mainly impacted in MSA, PSP, and CBGD patients, even at early disease stages. Thus, this technique is applicable to differentiate patients with classical PD from those with atypical parkinsonian syndromes. However, it does not allow for the discrimination of PD patients from healthy controls, and between the various atypical parkinsonian disorders.

2.2.3 Glucose metabolism

Imaging of brain glucose metabolism using [18F]-fluorodeoxyglucose (FDG) and PET has revealed characteristic metabolic changes in patients with PD[47–49]. Network analysis of resting FDG PET has revealed specific disease-related spatial covariance patterns associated with PD and other movement disorders. The Parkinson's disease-related pattern (PDRP) is characterized by metabolic increases in the putamen/GP, ventral thalamus, and brainstem covarying with decreases in premotor cortex and parietal association regions (see Fig. 10.2)[50]. This metabolic topography has been validated in multiple independent populations of

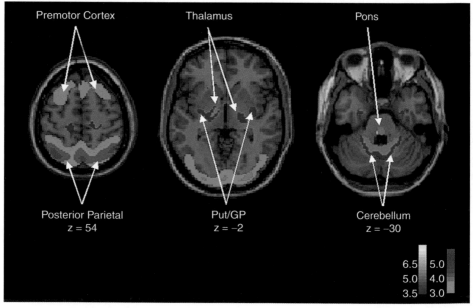

Fig. 10.2 This Parkinson's disease-related metabolic covariance pattern (PDRP) was identified by network analysis of [18F]-fluorodeoxyglucose (FDG) PET scans from 20 PD patients and 20 age-matched normal volunteer subjects[50]. The PDRP is characterized by pallidal, thalamic, pontine, and cerebellar hypermetabolism associated with metabolic decrements in the lateral premotor and posterior parietal areas. The display represents voxels that contribute significantly to the network at p = 0.001 and are shown to be reliable by bootstrap estimation (p < 0.0001). (Voxels with positive region weights (metabolic increases) are colour coded from red to yellow; those with negative region weights (metabolic decreases) are colour coded from blue to purple. The numbers under each slice are in millimetres, relative to the anterior-posterior commissure line.)

unmedicated PD patients[51–53]. The PDRP is detectable early in the disease course, increases with disease progression, and correlates consistently with advancing motor disability[54]. PDRP activity correlates with nigrostriatal dopamine deficiency as determined by FDOPA PET and with internal pallidal (GPi) single-unit activity recorded during surgery[55].

PDRP expression can be quantified on a single-case basis[56,57]. The activity of the PDRP and other disease-related networks can be assessed by this method before and during the application of different therapeutic methods as a means of monitoring treatment effects. This approach has been applied to compare metabolic responses to PD treatment under a variety of conditions such as levodopa infusion and stereotaxic lesioning and stimulation of GPi and STN (see Fig. 10.3 and reviews[50,54]).

Although these interventions suppressed PDRP activity, there were differences in the magnitude of PDRP reduction depending on the anatomical target (GPi or STN) or mode of treatment (ablation or DBS) (see Fig. 10.3). The STN appears to be the superior target to the GPi[34]. In most instances, the degree of network suppression correlated with UPDRS measures of treatment response (e.g. [58,59]).

Neuroimaging-based assessment of treatment effects through the quantification of network changes might also be applicable to other movement disorders. Reproducible

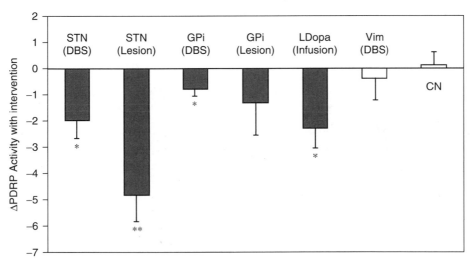

Fig. 10.3 Relative changes of PDRP network modulation during anti-parkinsonian therapy with levodopa infusion and unilateral ventral pallidotomy, pallidal and STN DBS, and subthalamotomy (*filled bars*). For the surgical interventions, Δ PDRP reflects changes in network activity in the operated hemispheres. With levodopa infusion, the PDRP changes were averaged across hemispheres. The control data (*open bars*) represent: (1) Δ PDRP values in the *unoperated* contralateral hemispheres (CN) of the surgical patients scanned in the unmedicated state; and (2) PDRP changes with unilateral Vim thalamic stimulation for tremor-predominant PD. (Asterisks represent p values with respect to the untreated condition (paired Student's *t* test): * = $p < 0.01$; ** = $p < 0.005$.)

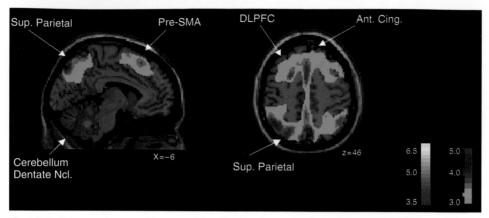

Fig. 10.4 This covariance pattern was identified in the network analysis of FDG PET scans from 15 non-demented PD patients with mild–moderate motor symptoms (H&Y Stage 3.3). This metabolic network (identified using the same PCA methodology as the PDRP) was characterized by relative hypometabolism of prefrontal, preSMA, and superior parietal regions, associated with cerebellar metabolic increases. (The display represents voxels that contribute significantly to the network at p = 0.001. Voxels with positive region weights (metabolic increases) are colour coded from red to yellow; those with negative region weights (metabolic decreases) are colour coded from blue to purple. The numbers under each slice are in millimetres, relative to the anterior-posterior commissure line.)

metabolic patterns have also been identified in Huntington's disease[60] and in torsion dystonia[61,62].

The relationship between brain metabolism and neuropsychological performance has recently been investigated (see[17] for review). Mentis *et al.* (2002) used multivariate analysis in resting FDG PET data to identify spatial covariance patterns associated with the cognitive and psychiatric manifestations of PD[63]. The cognitive pattern (see Fig. 10.4) was associated with verbal learning and visuospatial ability. It was characterized by hypermetabolism in the medial and anterior temporal lobe, and with relative hypometabolism in the lateral parieto-occipito-temporal and medial parietal regions. A second pattern was associated with mood disturbance. It was characterized by hypermetabolism in the cerebellum and medial occipital lobe, and with hypometabolism in the dorsolateral prefrontal, orbitofrontal, and anterior cingulate regions. Similarly, Lozza *et al.* (2004) identified a cognitive pattern in patients with PD using FDG PET that was related to working memory and planning/organization abilities[53]. The time course of expression of these patterns during disease progression and their modulation by therapy is a topic of ongoing research.

Apart from its ability to monitor treatment effects and disease progression, disease-related changes of glucose metabolism appear to be a useful diagnostic tool in the differential diagnosis of parkinsonian syndromes. Using Statistical Parametric Mapping (SPM), it was possible to predict the probable clinical diagnosis over two years in about 90% of the patients[64]. The study included a high number of early disease stage patients with ambiguous diagnosis at the time of imaging. Thus, this method has the potential to differentiate patients with different parkinsonian disorders at early clinical stages. This single-case approach is likely to be applicable to other imaging modalities including perfusion-based MRI and SPECT (e.g.[52]).

2.2.4 Perfusion SPECT

SPECT imaging of cerebral perfusion has been used to evaluate functional changes in patients with parkinsonian syndromes scanned at rest. For instance, computed scores for the PDRP identified previously using PET in 22 MSA patients scanned with Tc99m ECD accurately discriminated these subjects from PD patients of similar age and severity[52]. Van Laere et al. (2004) also evaluated patients with PD and MSA using this SPECT method[65]. However, data analysis revealed hypoperfusion of the basal ganglia in both MSA and PD. It is not clear whether these findings relate to technical differences between the SPECT populations or to demographic effects. Given that PDRP expression can separate PD and MSA in both SPECT groups (Eckert et al. (2007)[88], it is likely that the disease-related topography is fundamentally similar when assessed by either PET or SPECT. Uncoupling of cerebral blood flow and metabolism at the level of the basal ganglia is also possible. Such an effect may have a bearing on network computations in perfusion MRI data.

2.2.4 Perfusion PET

It is not fully known how these resting-state changes in PD relate to alterations in brain function during motor performance. PET studies utilizing ^{15}O-labelled water ($H_2^{15}O$) to measure brain activation responses, or FMRI to assess changes in blood oxygen level dependent (BOLD) signal have investigated disease-related activation differences. PET and FMRI have been employed for a number of different motor and cognitive tasks performed in the untreated state and following therapy. Because PET imaging has been in use longer than FMRI, the majority of activation studies in PD employed this approach.

Motor activation Comparison of motor activation responses in PD patients to that of healthy controls has typically revealed relative declines in the supplementary motor area (SMA) and dorsolateral prefrontal cortex (DLPFC), with increases in lateral premotor, parietal, and cerebellar regions (see[66] for review). It should also be noted that most of the activation studies have applied paradigms that incorporate timing cues. Thus, the temporal initiation of movements is a particular problem in PD patients. While healthy individuals perform temporally self-initiated movements faster than movements with timing cues, it is the opposite in PD patients. This also confirms the clinical observation that PD patients improve movement if they employ external visual or auditory cueing.

An early study in the field of treatment-related changes in motor activation responses investigated the effect of apomorphine infusion on externally paced joystick movements. Metabolic increases were found in the SMA following apomorphine infusion[67]. Applying a similar paradigm, Limousin and colleagues (1997) described increases of brain perfusion in the SMA of PD patients during STN DBS[68]. An investigation of the effect of GPi stimulation on cerebral blood flow during motor performance revealed a significant enhancement of motor activation responses in SMA and anterior cingulate cortex[69]. The increase of these changes correlated with on-line measures of task performance. While performing the same motor task during levodopa infusion, PD patients demonstrated activation increases in the posterior putamen, ventral thalamus, and pons contralateral to the dominant right hand[70]. Thus, GPi DBS and levodopa infusion resulted in comparable clinical improvement during task performance; the changes in activation with therapy varied on a regional level. This demonstrates the potential use of functional imaging to identify the neural basis by which different therapeutic methods mediate their clinical effect. Overall, these studies reveal a relative normalization of cerebral blood flow characteristic to motor performance during treatment. However, the investigation of pathological activation changes during treatment is not trivial, as performance characteristics need to be carefully monitored. If performance parameters such as power, frequency, and speed are not controlled across patients and in between scans, potentially erroneous group differences are likely to result. Thus, the investigation of activation changes in PD patients during treatment may provide valuable knowledge concerning the underlying pathology of the disease. However, the application of this approach as a component of pharmacological treatment trials appears to be less rewarding.

Cognition Network analysis has also been applied to brain activation studies[18,71,72]. While performing a motor sequence learning task, target acquisition is normally mediated by an activation pattern characterized by increases in the left dorsolateral prefrontal cortex, rostral supplementary motor area/anterior cingulate cortex, and left striatum during the acquisition phase of sequence learning[71,73]. The retrieval phase of sequence learning is characterized by a different activation pattern involving the right dorsolateral prefrontal cortex and posterior parietal association areas. The network pattern associated with target retrieval in control subjects accurately predicts learning in unmedicated PD patients[73]. Interestingly, therapy with pallidal deep brain stimulation produces an increase in the expression of the retrieval network activity (and improved learning), while levodopa infusion produces a decline in the expression of this network (and impaired learning). A significant correlation was noted between the change in network activity and the treatment responses[71], suggesting the use of this pattern as a marker for the effects of therapy on non-motor features of PD[50].

2.2.2 Magnetic resonance tomography

Diffusion-weighted imaging Diffusion-weighted imaging (DWI) sequences represent a relatively new imaging technique that is available on most standard MRI scanners. DWI determines the random movements of water molecules that are aligned with fibre tracts in the central nervous system. The application of different field gradients with various degrees of diffusion sensitization allows for the quantification of diffusion by the calculation of the apparent diffusion coefficient (ADC) in the brain tissue. Within the central nervous system, the movement of water molecules occurs mainly along the fibre tracts. While diffusion vertical to these fibre tracts is limited in healthy tissue, pathological processes such as neuronal loss and gliosis increase the mobility of water molecules by destruction of these fibre tracts. As a result, the ADC measured by DWI increases in such pathological structures. This method has been applied for the differential diagnosis of patients with classical PD, MSA, and PSP[74]. These investigators found ADC increases in the globus pallidus, putamen, and caudate nucleus in MSA and PSP patients compared to classical PD. This finding suggests that ADC can differentiate patients with PD from those with atypical parkinsonian syndromes. However, this method was unable to differentiate patients with PSP from those with MSA.

MR spectroscopy Proton magnetic resonance spectroscopy (MRS) represents one of the first functional MRI applications. Measuring the content of certain chemical metabolites of the brain within a certain voxel, this method provides insight into metabolic changes using MRI. The four main metabolites measured by MRS are N-acetylaspartate (NAA) as the major contributor, followed by compounds containing choline (Cho), creatine-phosphocreatine (Cre), and lactate (Lac). NAA is thought to be a neuron-specific molecule because of its absence in mature glial cell cultures and tumours of glial cell origin. On the other hand, Cho and Cre are thought to be contained in all tissues. Most studies compare ratios of NAA to Cho, and NAA to Cre to evaluate NAA decreases as a marker for neuronal loss. Studies have reported decreases of NAA in the lentiform nucleus in patients with atypical parkinsonian syndromes compared to those with PD[75]. Nonetheless, while MRS revealed group differences in the lentiform nucleus, findings were not applicable for differential diagnosis of single patients. This may partially be explained by methodological considerations. To acquire sufficient spectra with a good signal-to-noise ratio, large regions or long scanning times become necessary. As patients cannot tolerate long periods of time in the scanner, the chosen regions of interest (ROIs) are quite large (approximately 20x20x20 mm). Such ROIs often contain surrounding tissue that limits the relevant signal acquired.

Magnetization transfer imaging Magnetization transfer imaging (MTI) is a functional imaging technique that relies on the transfer of energy between highly-bound protons within structures such as myelin and the very mobile protons of free water. Conventional MRI sequences instead visualize mobile water protons only. This difference enables MTI to gain further information regarding the lipid layers of neurons, which is not revealed by other MR sequences. The amount of magnetization transfer can be quantified as the magnetization transfer ratio. This ratio has shown to correlate with the degree of myelinization and axonal density. MTI has mainly been used for evaluation of pathological lesions in multiple sclerosis. Assessment of magnetization transfer ratio in patients with PD, MSA, PSP, and healthy control subjects using a ROI-based approach revealed decreases matching the pathological changes of the underlying diseases[76]. When compared to normal control subjects, magnetization transfer ratios were significantly decreased in the substantia nigra of patients with PD, MSA, and PSP. Moreover, significant decreases were found in the putamen of MSA patients when compared to PD and normal controls, and in the globus pallidus of PSP patients compared to PD, MSA, and normal controls. A comparison of imaging diagnosis to probable clinical diagnosis on an individual basis showed an overall correct classification of 75%. Compared to MRS, MTI has an advantage in that ROIs can be manually adjusted so that minimal surrounding tissue will be included in the analysis. Quantitative MTI methods might be valuable in assessing disease progression in PD.

Perfusion MRI Perfusion MRI is another method used to evaluate regional brain function *in vivo*. Cerebral blood flow is closely correlated with energy metabolism (e.g. glucose metabolism) arising from presynaptic activity and the maintenance of membrane potentials. Perfusion-weighted MR obtained by arterial spin labelling (ASL)[77] has shown to be a valuable non-invasive tool for the quantitative measurement of resting cerebral blood flow (CBF). Perfusion-weighted MRI can be repeated frequently without concern for the effects of radiation or other tracer toxicity because no exogenous tracer is employed. Resting CBF measurements acquired with ASL are stable for minutes to weeks, making it a valuable technique for assessing disease progression and treatment effects. Furthermore, ASL allows for functional neuroimaging with the increased resolution of an MRI acquisition modality. Thus, CBF assessed by this means may correspond more closely to the underlying network pathology of disease. Moreover, the success of this method in Alzheimer's disease[78], as well as recent technical advances, indicates its potential for the study of network expression in large PD populations. This attribute may also enhance the utility of MR-based patterns as potential disease biomarkers. While this method has not been assessed regarding its ability to reveal metabolic changes in parkinsonian disorders, this topic is currently under investigation.

2.3 FMRI in Parkinson's disease

2.3.1 Motor activation studies

As mentioned above, the investigation of motor and cognitive disturbances are the main focus of functional imaging in PD patients. The current theory of the motor disturbances in PD is based on the basal ganglia loop model (see Fig. 10.1). While most motor activation studies in PD have been conducted with PET, several recent studies have utilized MRI to quantify BOLD signal changes during task performance.

The first FMRI study investigating motor activation in PD patients was performed by Sabatini and colleagues (2000)[79]. Employing a motor block paradigm with complex sequential finger movements in moderately affected PD patients, the authors confirmed previously described changes with increased activation in premotor and parietal areas, and with decreases in the SMA and DLPFC (Fig. 10.5a). In addition to these changes, they also noted increased activation in the sensorimotor cortex and the caudal SMA (Fig. 10.5b). The authors attributed these new findings, at least in part, to the very complex motor design.

The finding of increased activation in the sensorimotor cortex was confirmed by Haslinger and colleagues (2001)[80]. The authors employed a modification of the earlier PET paradigm using an event-related design in which patient and control subjects executed joystick movements in freely chosen directions after auditory timing cues. The authors found a similar group difference in activation responses as in the prior study, and confirmed the presence of increased activation responses in premotor, parietal, and sensorimotor areas. They also demonstrated relative normalization of these changes after levodopa treatment.

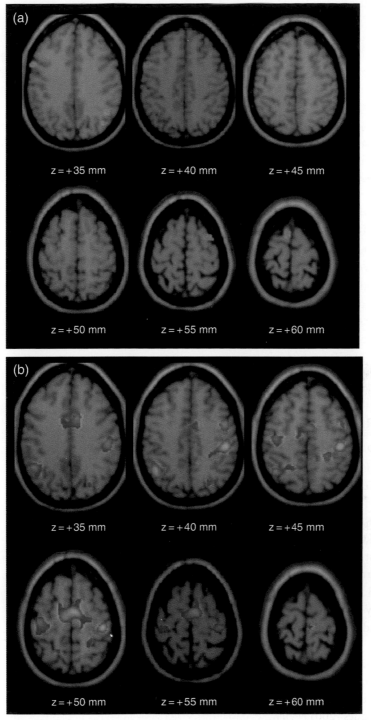

Fig. 10.5 Area of relative overactivity in (**a**) normal controls compared to PD patients and (**b**) PD patients compared to normal controls during a complex sequential hand movement, superimposed onto a stereotaxically normalized MRI brain scan. (z = location of area of activation above commissural plane; threshold = p < 0.001) (Reproduced with permission from Oxford University Press[79].)

In a subsequent PD motor FMRI study, Buhmann and colleagues (2003)[81] employed a simple finger opposition task in very early untreated PD patients. In contrast to the prior studies, these investigators noted reduced activation in the sensorimotor area of PD patients. Moreover, activation increased following the administration of levodopa. Based on these findings, the authors suggested that the previously reported increased sensorimotor activation might be an expression of long-term changes to dopaminergic treatment. Although long-term cortical reorganization changes after dopaminergic medication is a possibility, we note that about half of the patients reported by Haslinger (2001)[80] had not been on dopaminergic medication before imaging and that the rest of those patients had mild disease.

Increased BOLD response in the primary motor cortex (PMC) in PD patients compared to control subjects during motor paradigms is also supported by our own findings. We examined BOLD response changes in early untreated PD patients performing a simple self-paced motor paradigm and found increased activation of the primary sensorimotor cortex in PD patients compared to controls (Eckert *et al.* (2006)[89]. We found relative increases of BOLD response in the contralateral sensorimotor cortex and in the ipsilateral and contralateral premotor areas (see Fig. 10.6) that agree with the results

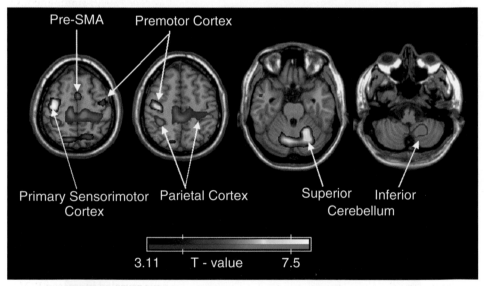

Fig. 10.6 Between-group analysis for the comparison between early PD patients (n = 9, H&Y Stages 1 and 2) who have never been on dopaminergic treatment and healthy, age-matched control subjects (n = 9) performing a simple, temporary, self-initiated activation paradigm consisting of fist opening and closing of the left hand with a frequency of 1 Hz. Analysis was performed using SPM99 (Wellcome Institute, London) using a fixed effect model. The display represents voxels that contribute significantly to the network at p < 0.05, corrected, extent threshold 30 voxels. Voxels with positive region weights (metabolic increases) are colour coded from red to yellow; those with negative region weights (metabolic decreases) are colour coded from blue to purple. Colour-coded T-values are displayed onto four axial slices of a normalized T1-weighted template image. (T. Eckert, personal communication)

published by Sabatini and colleagues (2000) and Haslinger and colleagues (2001). We also noted increased activation in the ipsilateral superior cerebellum as previously described with PET, but also relative reductions in the ipsilateral inferior cerebellum of PD patients. Moreover, we also found increased activation of pre-SMA in PD during the performance of simple, temporally self-initiated movements. This increased pre-SMA activation is likely to be an effect of our self-initiated paradigm in contrast to other paradigms employing mainly auditory paced movements. The differences in SMA activation between self-paced and cued movements underscore the importance of temporal initiation in the activation of the medial frontal cortex. Further well-controlled FMRI investigations at high field may shed light on the basis for these apparent disparities.

2.3.2 Cognitive changes in PD

Performing complex movements is a process of learning movement sequences, optimizing movement, and retrieving this information for movement performance. Using FMRI in an elderly sample of healthy normal controls, Honey *et al.* (2003) found that dopaminergic drugs modulated striatal connectivity[82]. Specifically, sulpiride, a D2 receptor antagonist, increased connectivity between the caudate and other circuit components while performing an object-location learning task. This finding appears to mimic the enhanced connectivity reported in parkinsonian patients (e.g. [83]). Mattay *et al.* (2002) simultaneously analysed dopaminergic modulation on motor and non-motor (i.e. working memory) functions (in early onset PD patients) using FMRI[84]. The cortical motor regions activated during a motor task demonstrated greater activation while patients were in the 'on' state. By contrast, the regions subserving working memory showed greater activation during the 'off' state. The latter positively correlated with an increase in task performance errors. Their findings suggest that two distinct cortical networks exist in PD that are differentially modulated by dopamine, which is associated with impaired prefrontal cortical information processing[71].

Lastly, Grossman and colleagues (2003) found that non-demented PD patients had reduced recruitment of striatal regions when asked to process sentences with high demands on working memory[85]. The authors suggest that impaired syntactic performance in PD may be attributed to cognitive resource limitations including impaired information processing speed. In order to maintain equivalent levels of sentence comprehension as controls, the PD group exhibited greater recruitment of other cortical regions to compensate for depleted working memory resources[18,72].

In summary, the above-mentioned motor FMRI studies have revealed increased BOLD response in premotor and parietal cortical areas in PD patients compared to normal controls. These findings most likely represent compensatory pathways that are engaged in promoting adequate motor performance. However, other regional activation responses in PD are not as consistent. Indeed, the finding of increased BOLD response in the primary motor cortex in all but one of the FMRI studies of PD patients[81] is not easily interpreted. This discrepancy is likely to be a result of variations in the respective paradigms and the selection of patients. Another brain region with inconsistent findings is the SMA. While BOLD response decreases are described during the performance of temporally cued movements in the SMA, the performance of temporally self-triggered movements resulted in increased local BOLD response in early PD patients. Because the cueing of movements is known to affect motor performance in PD patients, further investigations in this regard will be potentially enlightening.

Other FMRI studies in PD have examined various aspects of the cognitive pathways. These studies indicate that pathways mediating information processing can be modulated by dopaminergic treatment. More studies will be needed to explore fully the pathophysiological basis of motor and non-motor behaviour and neural responses in PD.

2.3.3 Pros and cons of FMRI

In summary, FMRI is a promising technique for the assessment of PD and related disorders. FMRI is a safe procedure that can be repeated many times in a given subject. By contrast, PET imaging requires the intravenous application of dose-limited radioactive tracers. Furthermore, FMRI enables the investigator to perform event-related designs that are more difficult to accomplish with PET. Applying event-related designs has the advantage of examining the temporal aspects of brain activation, and also the ability to avoid exhaustion effects in the analysis. This seems to be of particular importance in the assessment of PD patients, particularly in more advanced disease stages. However, unlike PET, MRI is susceptible to magnetic effects such as heating of metallic implants in DBS studies. Local heating around the electrodes might not only influence brain function but can possibly destroy brain tissue. Pilot studies using FMRI in DBS patients have been performed indicating that this approach might not be harmful, at least with externalized wires[86,87].

Acknowledgements

This work was supported by NIH RO1 NS 35069. Dr Eidelberg was supported by NIH K24 NS 02101. The authors wish to thank Ms Toni Flanagan for valuable editorial assistance.

References

1. Feigin A, Eidelberg D (2002). The natural history of Parkinson's disease. In: (Factor SA, Weiner WJ, editors) *Parkinson's Disease: Diagnosis and Clinical Management*, pp. 109–13. Demos Medical Publishing Inc., New York.

2. Braak H, Del Tredici K, Rub U, de Vos RA, Jansen Steur EN, Braak E (2003). Staging of brain pathology related to sporadic Parkinson's disease. *Neurobiol Aging* **24**, 197–211.

3. Hoehn MM, Yahr MD (1967). Parkinsonism: onset, progression and mortality. *Neurology* **17**, 427–42.

4. Poewe WH, Wenning GK (1998). The natural history of Parkinson's disease. *Ann Neurol* **44**, S1–9.

5. Whone AL, Watts RL, Stoessl AJ, Davis M, Reske S, Nahmias C, *et al.* (2003). Slower progression of Parkinson's disease with ropinirole versus levodopa: the REAL-PET study. *Ann Neurol* **54**, 93–101.

6. Fahn S, Oakes D, Shoulson I, Kieburtz K, Rudolph A, Lang A, *et al.* (2004). Levodopa and the progression of Parkinson's disease. *N Engl J Med* **351**, 2498–508.

7. DeLong MR (2000). The basal ganglia. In: (Kandel ER, Schwartz JH, Jessell TM, editors) *Principles of Neural Science*, 4th edn, pp. 853–67. McGraw–Hill, New York.

8. Lozano AM, Dostrovsky J, Chen R, Ashby P (2002). Deep brain stimulation for Parkinson's disease: disrupting the disruption. *Lancet Neurol* **1**, 225–31.

9. Lichter DG (2000). Movement disorders and frontal-subcortical circuits. In: (Lichter DJ, Cummings JL, editors) *Frontal-subcortical circuits in psychiatric and neurological disorders*, pp. 260–313. The Guildford Press, New York.

10. Tröster AI, Woods SP (2003). Neuropsychological aspects of Parkinson's disease and parkinsonian syndromes. In: (Pahwa R, Lyons KE, Koller WC, editors) *Handbook of Parkinson's disease*, pp. 127–57. Marcel Decker, New York.

11. Emre M (2003). What causes mental dysfunction in Parkinson's disease? *Mov Disord* **18** Suppl 6, S63–71.

12. Cummings JL (1993). Frontal-subcortical circuits and human behavior. *Arch Neurol* **50**, 873–80.

13. Dubois B, Pillon B (1997). Cognitive deficits in Parkinson's disease. *J Neurol* **244**, 2–8.

14. Zgaljardic DJ, Borod JC, Foldi NS, Mattis P (2003). A review of the cognitive and behavioral sequelae of Parkinson's disease: relationship to frontostriatal circuitry. *Cogn Behav Neurol* **16**, 193–210.

15. Cummings JL, Darkins A, Mendez M, Hill MA, Benson DF (1988). Alzheimer's disease and Parkinson's disease: comparison of speech and language alterations. *Neurology* **38**, 680–4.

16. Taylor AE, Saint–Cyr JA (1995). The neuropsychology of Parkinson's disease. *Brain Cogn* **28**, 281–96.

17. Carbon M, Marie RM (2003). Functional imaging of cognition in Parkinson's disease. *Curr Opin Neurol* **16**, 475–80.

18. Mentis MJ, Dhawan V, Nakamura T, Ghilardi MF, Feigin A, Edwards C, *et al.* (2003). Enhancement of brain activation during trial-and-error sequence learning in early PD. *Neurology* **60**, 612–9.

19. Vila M, Przedborski S (2004). Genetic clues to the pathogenesis of Parkinson's disease. *Nat Med* **10** Suppl, S58–62.

20. Khan NL, Valente EM, Bentivoglio AR, Wood NW, Albanese A, Brooks DJ, *et al.* (2002). Clinical and subclinical dopaminergic dysfunction in PARK6-linked parkinsonism: an 18F-dopa PET study. *Ann Neurol* **52**, 849–53.

21. Hughes AJ, Daniel SE, Kilford L, Lees AJ (1992). Accuracy of clinical diagnosis of idiopathic Parkinson's disease: a clinico-pathological study of 100 cases. *J Neurol Neurosurg Psychiatry* **55**, 181–4.

22. Tarsy D, Apetauerova D, Ryan P, Norregaard T (2003). Adverse effects of subthalamic nucleus DBS in a patient with multiple system atrophy. *Neurology* **61**, 247–9.

23. Gelb DJ, Oliver E, Gilman S (1999). Diagnostic criteria for Parkinson disease. *Arch Neurol* **56**, 33–9.

24. Gilman S, Low PA, Quinn N, Albanese A, Ben–Shlomo Y, Fowler CJ, *et al.* (1999). Consensus statement on the diagnosis of multiple system atrophy. *J Neurol Sci* **163**, 94–8.

25. Litvan I, Agid Y, Calne D, Campbell G, Dubois B, Duvoisin RC, *et al.* (1996). Clinical research criteria for the diagnosis of progressive supranuclear palsy (Steele–Richardson–Olszewski syndrome): report of the NINDS-SPSP international workshop. *Neurology* **47**, 1–9.

26. Eckert T, Eidelberg D (2004). The role of functional neuroimaging in the differential diagnosis of idiopathic Parkinson's disease and multiple system atrophy. *Clin Auton Res* **14**, 84–91.

27. Ehringer H, Hornykiewicz O (1960). Distribution of noradrenaline and dopamine (3-hydroxytyramine) in the human brain and their behavior in diseases of the extrapyramidal system. *Klin Wochenschr* **38**, 1236–9.

28. Birkmayer W, Hornykiewicz O (1961). The L-3,4-dioxyphenylalanine (DOPA)-effect in Parkinson-akinesia. *Wien Klin Wochenschr* **73**, 787–8.

29. Cotzias GC, Van Woert MH, Schiffer LM (1967). Aromatic amino acids and modification of parkinsonism. *N Engl J Med* **276**, 374–9.

30. Shoulson I (1998). DATATOP: a decade of neuroprotective inquiry. Parkinson Study Group. Deprenyl and tocopherol antioxidative therapy of Parkinsonism. *Ann Neurol* **44**, S160–6.

31. Parkinson Study Group (2002). Dopamine transporter brain imaging to assess the effects of pramipexole vs levodopa on Parkinson disease progression. *Jama* **287**, 1653–61.

32. Ravina B, Eidelberg D, Ahlskog JE, Albin RL, Brooks DJ, Carbon M, *et al.* (2005). The role of radiotracer imaging in Parkinson disease. *Neurology* **64**, 208–15.

33. Benabid AL (2003). Deep brain stimulation for Parkinson's disease. *Curr Opin Neurobiol* **13**, 696–706.

34. Hamani C, Saint–Cyr JA, Fraser J, Kaplitt M, Lozano AM (2004). The subthalamic nucleus in the context of movement disorders. *Brain* **127**, 4–20.

35. Freed CR, Greene PE, Breeze RE, Tsai WY, DuMouchel W, Kao R, *et al.* (2001). Transplantation of embryonic dopamine neurons for severe Parkinson's disease. *N Engl J Med* **344**, 710–9.

36. Olanow CW, Goetz CG, Kordower JH, Stoessl AJ, Sossi V, Brin MF, *et al.* (2003). A double-blind controlled trial of bilateral fetal nigral transplantation in Parkinson's disease. *Ann Neurol* **54**, 403–14.

37. Schrag A, Good CD, Miszkiel K, Morris HR, Mathias CJ, Lees AJ, *et al.* (2000). Differentiation of atypical parkinsonian syndromes with routine MRI. *Neurology* **54**, 697–702.

38. Dhawan V, Eidelberg D (2001). SPECT imaging in Parkinson's disease. *Adv Neurol* **86**, 205–13.

39. Brooks DJ (2003). Imaging end points for monitoring neuroprotection in Parkinson's disease. *Ann Neurol* **53**, S110–8.

40. Marek K, Jennings D, Seibyl J (2003). Dopamine agonists and Parkinson's disease progression: what can we learn from neuroimaging studies. *Ann Neurol* **53**, S160–6.

41. Morrish PK, Rakshi JS, Bailey DL, Sawle GV, Brooks DJ (1998). Measuring the rate of progression and estimating the preclinical period of Parkinson's disease with [18F]dopa PET. *J Neurol Neurosurg Psychiatry* **64**, 314–9.

42. Snow B, Tooyama I, McGeer E, Yamada T, Calne D, Takahashi H, *et al.* (1993). Human positron emission tomographic [18F]fluorodopa studies correlate with dopamine cell counts and levels. *Ann Neurol* **34**, 324–30.

43. Nakamura T, Dhawan V, Chaly T, Fukuda M, Ma Y, Breeze R, *et al.* (2001). Blinded positron emission tomography study of dopamine cell implantation for Parkinson's disease. *Ann Neurol* **50**, 181–7.

44. Lee CS, Samii A, Sossi V, Ruth TJ, Schulzer M, Holden JE, *et al.* (2000). In vivo positron emission tomographic evidence for compensatory changes in presynaptic dopaminergic nerve terminals in Parkinson's disease. *Ann Neurol* **47**, 493–503.

45. Guttman M, Stewart D, Hussey D, Wilson A, Houle S, Kish S (2001). Influence of L-dopa and pramipexole on striatal dopamine transporter in early PD. *Neurology* **56**, 1559–64.

46. Ma Y, Feigin A, Dhawan V, Fukuda M, Shi Q, Greene P, *et al.* (2002). Dyskinesia after fetal cell transplantation for parkinsonism: a PET study. *Ann Neurol* **52**, 628–34.

47. Eidelberg D, Moeller JR, Dhawan V, Spetsieris P, Takikawa S, Ishikawa T, *et al.* (1994). The metabolic topography of parkinsonism. *J Cereb Blood Flow Metab* **14**, 783–801.

48. Eidelberg D, Moeller JR, Ishikawa T, Dhawan V, Spetsieris P, Chaly T, *et al.* (1995). Early differential diagnosis of Parkinson's disease with 18F-fluorodeoxyglucose and positron emission tomography. *Neurology* **45**, 1995–2004.

49. Eidelberg D, Edwards C, Mentis M, Dhawan V, Moeller J (2000). Movement disorders: Parkinson's disease. In: (Mazziotta JC, Toga AW, Frackowiak R, editors) *Brain Mapping: The Disorders.* Academic Press, San Diego.

50. Carbon M, Eidelberg D (2002). Modulation of regional brain function by deep brain stimulation: studies with positron emission tomography. *Curr Opin Neurol* **15**, 451–5.

51. Moeller JR, Nakamura T, Mentis MJ, Dhawan V, Spetsieres P, Antonini A, *et al.* (1999). Reproducibility of regional metabolic covariance patterns: comparison of four populations. *J Nucl Med* **40**, 1264–9.

52. Feigin A, Antonini A, Fukuda M, De Notaris R, Benti R, Pezzoli G, *et al.* (2002). Tc-99m ethylene cysteinate dimer SPECT in the differential diagnosis of parkinsonism. *Mov Disord* **17**, 1265–70.

53. Lozza C, Baron JC, Eidelberg D, Mentis MJ, Carbon M, Marie RM (2004). Executive processes in Parkinson's disease: FDG-PET and network analysis. *Hum Brain Mapp* **22**, 236–45.

54. Eckert T, Eidelberg D (2005). Neuroimaging and therapeutics in movement disorders. *Neurorx* **2**, 361–71.

55. Eidelberg D, Moeller JR, Kazumata K, Antonini A, Sterio D, Dhawan V, *et al.* (1997). Metabolic correlates of pallidal neuronal activity in Parkinson's disease. *Brain* **120**, 1315–24.

56. Eidelberg D, Moeller JR, Ishikawa T, Dhawan V, Spetsieris P, Chaly T, *et al.* (1995). Assessment of disease severity in parkinsonism with fluorine-18-fluorodeoxyglucose and PET. *J Nucl Med* **36**, 378–83.

57. Asanuma K, Tang C, Ma Y, Dhawan V, Mattis P, Edwards C, Kaplitt MG, Feigin A, Eidelberg D (2006). Network modulation in the treatment of Parkinson's disease. *Brain* **129**(Pt 10), 2667–2678.

58. Fukuda M, Mentis MJ, Ma Y, Dhawan V, Antonini A, Lang AE, *et al.* (2001). Networks mediating the clinical effects of pallidal brain stimulation for Parkinson's disease: a PET study of resting-state glucose metabolism. *Brain* **124**, 1601–9.

59. Feigin A, Fukuda M, Dhawan V, Przedborski S, Jackson–Lewis V, Mentis MJ, *et al.* (2001). Metabolic correlates of levodopa response in Parkinson's disease. *Neurology* **57**, 2083–8.

60. Feigin A, Leenders KL, Moeller JR, Missimer J, Kuenig G, Spetsieris P, *et al.* (2001). Metabolic network abnormalities in early Huntington's disease: an [(18)F]FDG PET study. *J Nucl Med* **42**, 1591–5.

61. Eidelberg D, Moeller JR, Antonini A, Kazumata K, Nakamura T, Dhawan V, *et al.* (1998). Functional brain networks in DYT1 dystonia. *Ann Neurol* **44**, 303–12.

62. Carbon M, Su S, Dhawan V, Raymond D, Bressman S, Eidelberg D (2004). Regional metabolism in primary torsion dystonia: effects of penetrance and genotype. *Neurology* **62**, 1384–90.

63. Mentis MJ, McIntosh AR, Perrine K, Dhawan V, Berlin B, Feigin A, *et al.* (2002). Relationships among the metabolic patterns that correlate with mnemonic, visuospatial, and mood symptoms in Parkinson's disease. *Am J Psychiatry* **159**, 746–54.

64. Eckert T, Barnes A, Dhawan V, Frucht S, Gordon MF, Feigin A, Eidelberg D (2005). FDG PET in the differential diagnosis of parkinsonian disorders. *NeuroImage*, **26**, 912–921.

65. Van Laere K, Santens P, Bosman T, De Reuck J, Mortelmans L, Dierckx R (2004). Statistical parametric mapping of (99m)Tc-ECD SPECT in idiopathic Parkinson's disease and multiple system atrophy with predominant parkinsonian features: correlation with clinical parameters. *J Nucl Med* **45**, 933–42.

66. Thobois S, Jahanshahi M, Pinto S, Frackowiak R, Limousin-Dowsey P (2004). PET and SPECT functional imaging studies in Parkinsonian syndromes: from the lesion to its consequences. *Neuroimage* **23**, 1–16.

67. Jenkins IH, Fernandez W, Playford ED, Lees AJ, Frackowiak RS, Passingham RE, *et al.* (1992). Impaired activation of the supplementary motor area in Parkinson's disease is reversed when akinesia is treated with apomorphine. *Ann Neurol* **32**, 749–57.

68. Limousin P, Greene J, Pollak P, Rothwell J, Benabid AL, Frackowiak R (1997). Changes in cerebral activity pattern due to subthalamic nucleus or internal pallidum stimulation in Parkinson's disease. *Ann Neurol* **42**, 283–91.

69. Fukuda M, Mentis M, Ghilardi MF, Dhawan V, Antonini A, Hammerstad J, *et al.* (2001). Functional correlates of pallidal stimulation for Parkinson's disease. *Ann Neurol* **49**, 155–64.

70. Feigin A, Ghilardi MF, Fukuda M, Mentis MJ, Dhawan V, Barnes A, *et al.* (2002). Effects of levodopa infusion on motor activation responses in Parkinson's disease. *Neurology* **59**, 220–6.

71. Carbon M, Ghilardi MF, Feigin A, Fukuda M, Silvestri G, Mentis MJ, *et al.* (2003). Learning networks in health and Parkinson's disease: reproducibility and treatment effects. *Hum Brain Mapp* **19**, 197–211.

72. Mentis MJ, Dhawan V, Feigin A, Delalot D, Zgaljardic D, Edwards C, *et al.* (2003). Early stage Parkinson's disease patients and normal volunteers: comparative mechanisms of sequence learning. *Hum Brain Mapp* **20**, 246–58.

73. Nakamura T, Ghilardi MF, Mentis M, Dhawan V, Fukuda M, Hacking A, *et al.* (2001). Functional networks in motor sequence learning: abnormal topographies in Parkinson's disease. *Hum Brain Mapp* **12**, 42–60.

74. Seppi K, Schocke MF, Esterhammer R, Kremser C, Brenneis C, Mueller J, *et al.* (2003). Diffusion-weighted imaging discriminates progressive supranuclear palsy from PD, but not from the parkinson variant of multiple system atrophy. *Neurology* **60**, 922–7.

75. Davie CA, Wenning GK, Barker GJ, Tofts PS, Kendall BE, Quinn N, *et al.* (1995). Differentiation of multiple system atrophy from idiopathic Parkinson's disease using proton magnetic resonance spectroscopy. *Ann Neurol* **37**, 204–10.

76. Eckert T, Sailer M, Kaufmann J, Schrader C, Peschel T, Bodammer N, *et al.* (2004). Differentiation of idiopathic Parkinson's disease, multiple system atrophy, progressive supranuclear palsy, and healthy controls using magnetization transfer imaging. *Neuroimage* **21**, 229–35.

77. Barbier EL, Lamalle L, Decorps M (2001). Methodology of brain perfusion imaging. *J Magn Reson Imaging* **13**, 496–520.

78. Alsop DC, Detre JA, Grossman M (2000). Assessment of cerebral blood flow in Alzheimer's disease by spin-labeled magnetic resonance imaging. *Ann Neurol* **47**, 93–100.

79. Sabatini U, Boulanouar K, Fabre N, Martin F, Carel C, Colonnese C, *et al.* (2000). Cortical motor reorganization in akinetic patients with Parkinson's disease: a functional MRI study. *Brain* **123**, 394–403.

80. Haslinger B, Erhard P, Kampfe N, Boecker H, Rummeny E, Schwaiger M, *et al.* (2001). Event-related functional magnetic resonance imaging in Parkinson's disease before and after levodopa. *Brain* **124**, 558–70.

81. Buhmann C, Glauche V, Sturenburg HJ, Oechsner M, Weiller C, Buchel C (2003). Pharmacologically modulated FMRI–cortical responsiveness to levodopa in drug-naive hemiparkinsonian patients. *Brain* **126**, 451–61.

82. Honey GD, Suckling J, Zelaya F, Long C, Routledge C, Jackson S, *et al.* (2003). Dopaminergic drug effects on physiological connectivity in a human cortico-striato-thalamic system. *Brain* **126**, 1767–81.

83. Lewis SJ, Dove A, Robbins TW, Barker RA, Owen AM (2003). Cognitive impairments in early Parkinson's disease are accompanied by reductions in activity in frontostriatal neural circuitry. *J Neurosci* **23**, 6351–6.

84. Mattay VS, Tessitore A, Callicott JH, Bertolino A, Goldberg TE, Chase TN, *et al.* (2002). Dopaminergic modulation of cortical function in patients with Parkinson's disease. *Ann Neurol* **51**, 156–64.

85. Grossman M, Cooke A, DeVita C, Lee C, Alsop D, Detre J, *et al.* (2003). Grammatical and resource components of sentence processing in Parkinson's disease: an FMRI study. *Neurology* **60**, 775–81.

86. Stefurak T, Mikulis D, Mayberg H, Lang AE, Hevenor S, Pahapill P, *et al.* (2003). Deep brain stimulation for Parkinson's disease dissociates mood and motor circuits: a functional MRI case study. *Mov Disord* **18**, 1508–16.

87. Hesselmann V, Sorger B, Girnus R, Lasek K, Maarouf M, Wedekind C, *et al.* (2004). Intraoperative functional MRI as a new approach to monitor deep brain stimulation in Parkinson's disease. *Eur Radiol* **14**, 686–90.

88. Eckert T, Van Laere K, Lewis DE, Edwards C, Santens P, Eidelberg D (2007). Quantification of PD-related network expression with ECD SPECT. *European Journal of Nuclear Medicine and Molecular Imaging* **34**(4), 496–501.

89. Eckert T, Peschel T, Heinze HJ, Rotte M (2006). Increased pre-SMA activation in early PD patients during simple self-initiated hand movements. *J Neurol* **253**(2), 199–207.

90. Yahr MD, Duvoisin RC, Schear MJ, Barrett RE, Hoehn MM (1969). Treatment of parkinsonism with levodopa. *Arch Neurol* **21**(4), 343–354.

91. Berg D, Siefker C, Becker G (2001). Echogenicity of the substantia nigra in Parkinson's disease and its relation to clinical findings. *J Neurol* **248**(8), 684–689.

11

Multiple sclerosis

Massimo Filippi and Maria A. Rocca

1. Introduction

Multiple sclerosis (MS) is the most common chronic inflammatory demyelinating disease affecting the central nervous system (CNS) of young adults in the western countries, leading, in the majority of the cases, to severe and irreversible clinical disability[1,2]. Since its clinical introduction, conventional magnetic resonance imaging (cMRI — dual-echo and post-contrast T1-weighted scans) has greatly improved our ability to diagnose MS and to monitor its evolution, either natural or modified by treatment[3,4]. CMRI-derived measures have indeed shown several advantages over clinical assessment, including their more objective nature and increased sensitivity to MS-related changes[3,4]. Nevertheless, the magnitude of the relationship between cMRI measures of disease activity or burden and the clinical manifestations of the disease is weak[5,6] (Fig. 11.1). This necessarily limits the role of cMRI for the understanding of MS pathophysiology and monitoring of experimental treatment.

Several factors are likely to be responsible for this clinical/MRI discrepancy. First, dual-echo imaging lacks specificity with regard to the heterogeneous pathological substrates of individual lesions[3,5] and, as a consequence, does not allow an accurate quantification of tissue damage. Specifically, oedema, inflammation, demyelination, remyelination, gliosis, and axonal loss[7,8] all lead to a similar appearance of hyperintensity on T2-weighted images. This is a major issue now that there is compelling evidence that: (a) inflammatory demyelination is not enough to explain 'fixed' neurological deficits in MS[5,6,9]; (b) irreversible axonal damage does occur in inflamed MS lesions[7,8,10,11]; and (c) axonal damage is the main contributor to the clinical manifestations of the disease and to its clinical worsening over time[10,11]. Secondly, T2-weighted images do not delineate tissue damage occurring in the normal-appearing white matter (NAWM), which usually represents a large portion of the brain tissue from MS patients and which is known to be damaged in MS patients. Post-mortem studies have shown subtle changes in the NAWM from MS patients, which not only include diffuse astrocytic hyperplasia, patchy oedema, and perivascular cellular infiltration, but also axonal damage[12–14]. Finally, dual-echo imaging does not provide an accurate picture of gray matter (GM) damage, which several pathological studies have shown to be prominent in MS[15–17] and which is likely to be associated with some clinical manifestations of the disease, such as cognitive impairment and fatigue.

These limitations of dual-echo imaging are only partially overcome by the use of post-contrast T1-weighted scans. Gadolinium (Gd)-enhanced T1-weighted images allow to

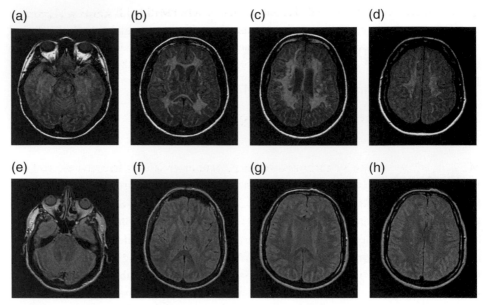

Fig. 11.1 Axial PD-weighted MR images of the brain from two patients with secondary progressive MS and severe clinical disability. In the first patient **(a)–(d)**, conventional imaging shows several hyperintense lesions suggestive of multifocal white matter pathology. The extent of these lesions and the involvement of specific brain regions might help to explain clinical disability in this patient. In the second patient **(e)–(h)**, conventional imaging shows few hyperintense lesions. The application of modern MR-based techniques, capable of measuring 'occult' CNS pathology, might help to explain clinical disability of this other patient.

distinguish active from inactive lesions, since enhancement occurs as a result of increased blood-brain barrier (BBB) permeability[5] and corresponds to areas with on-going inflammation[18]. However, the activity of the lesions, as demonstrated on post-contrast T1-weighted imaging, still does not provide information on tissue damage. Chronically hypointense areas on T1-weighted images correspond to areas where severe tissue disruption has occurred[19], and their extent is correlated with the clinical severity of the disease and its evolution over time[19,20]. Still, measuring the extent of T1-hypointense lesions may not correspond to the severity of intrinsic lesion pathology and provides no information about NAWM and GM damage.

Recently, several non-conventional MRI techniques have been developed and applied in an attempt to improve our understanding of the evolution of MS[21]. These techniques, including magnetization transfer (MT) MRI, diffusion-weighted (DW) MRI, and proton MR spectroscopy (^{1}H-MRS) may provide quantitative information about MS micro- and macroscopic lesion burdens with a higher pathological specificity to the most destructive aspects of the disease (i.e. severe demyelination and axonal loss) than cMRI. In addition, their application in longitudinal studies is progressively improving our ability to monitor reparative mechanisms, such as resolution of oedema, remyelination, reactive gliosis, and recovery from sublethal axonal injury. Finally, FMRI holds substantial promise to define the role of adaptive cortical reorganization with the potential to limit the clinical consequences of irreversible MS tissue damage. This chapter provides an update of the current 'state-of-the-art' of the application of structural, metabolic, and functional MR-based techniques to the study of MS pathophysiology.

2. Structural and metabolic imaging methods

2.1 MT MRI

MT MRI is based on the interactions between protons in a relatively free environment and those where motion is restricted. Off-resonance irradiation is applied, which saturates the magnetization of the less mobile protons, but this is transferred to the mobile protons, thus reducing the signal intensity from the observable magnetization. Thus, a low MT ratio (MTR) indicates a reduced capacity of the macromolecules in the CNS to exchange magnetization with the surrounding water molecules, reflecting damage to myelin or to the axonal membrane (Fig. 11.2). MT MRI has several advantages over cMRI in the assessment of MS. First, it provides quantitative information with a high specificity to demyelination and axonal loss — the more disabling substrates of MS pathology. Secondly, it enables us to assess the 'invisible' disease burden in the brain tissue which does not show macroscopic abnormalities on cMRI. Thirdly, with the application of MTR histogram analysis, it provides, from a single procedure, multiple parameters influenced by both the macro- and microscopic lesion burdens, which might also be used as paraclinical measures of MS evolution, either natural or modified by treatment. A post-mortem study[22] has provided the most compelling evidence that a marked reduction

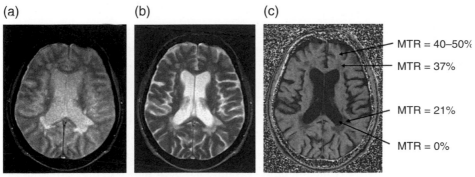

Fig. 11.2 Axial gradient echo images of the brain without (**a**) and with (**b**) a magnetization transfer (MT) pulse applied. The MT pulse saturates the magnetization of the less mobile protons, but this is transferred to the mobile protons, thus reducing the signal intensity from the observable magnetization. In (**c**), the corresponding MT ratio (MTR) map obtained from images (a) and (b) is shown. Since the degree of signal loss depends on the density of the macromolecules in a given tissue, a low MTR indicates a reduced capacity of the macromolecules in the CNS to exchange magnetization with the surrounding water molecules, reflecting damage to myelin or to the axonal membrane. As shown in (c), MS lesions have a variable range of MTR values.

of MTR values in MS-diseased tissues indicates severe structural damage, by showing strong correlations between MTR values from MS lesions and NAWM with the percentage of residual axons and the degree of demyelination. More recently, a strong inverse relationship between MTR values and myelin content in MS lesions and white matter has been demonstrated, whereas no association has been detected with the extent of gliosis[23,24].

The application of MT MRI to the study of individual MS lesions has allowed the demonstration, *in-vivo*, of the pathological heterogeneity of such lesions. In new enhancing lesions, higher MTR values have been shown in homogeneously enhancing lesions, which probably represent new lesions, than in ring-enhancing lesions, which may represent pre-existent, reactivated lesions[25]; in lesion enhancing on a single scan than in those enhancing on two or more serial scans[26]; and in lesion enhancing after the injection of a triple dose of Gd than in those enhancing after the injection of a standard dose[27]. Longitudinal studies have shown that, in new enhancing lesions, MTR drops dramatically when the lesions start to enhance and can show a partial or complete recovery in the subsequent one to six months[25–30]. Established MS lesions are also heterogeneous, as shown by the demonstration of lower MTR values in hypointense lesions than in lesions that are isointense to NAWM on T1-weighted scans[30]. MTR changes have also been detected in NAWM before lesion formation[29,31–33].

Average lesion MTR has been found to be lower in patients with relapsing-remitting (RR) MS than in those with clinically isolated syndromes (CIS) suggestive of MS[34], whereas no differences have been found in cross-sectional studies between patients with RRMS and those with secondary progressive (SP) MS[34] or between patients with SPMS and those with primary progressive (PP) MS[35]. However, longitudinal studies have shown a more severe and faster decline of average lesion MTR values in SPMS patients than in patients with other disease phenotypes[36,37], consistent with the unfavourable clinical evolution of these patients.

The pathological abnormalities observed in the NAWM of MS patients[12–14] also have the potential to modify the relative proportions of mobile and bound protons in the affected tissue and, as a consequence, the corresponding MTR values. Therefore, MT MRI can show normal-appearing brain tissue (NABT) microstructural abnormalities, which go undetected when using cMRI. MT MRI analysis of the NABT can be performed using either a region of interest (ROI) approach or a histogram analysis. More recently, with the development of new techniques which automatically segment the NAWM and the GM, it has become possible to study these two tissue compartments separately.

Using ROI analysis, a reduction of MTR values has been shown in the NAWM of MS patients with all the major MS phenotypes[38,39]. MTR changes, of a lower magnitude than those observed in T2-visible lesions, have been also detected in the dirty-appearing white matter of MS patients[40]. The application of histogram analysis[34,35,41–44] to the study of the NABT and of the NAWM, confirmed and extended the previous findings obtained with ROI analysis, by showing that these abnormalities can be detected even in patients with CIS suggestive of MS[41,44], are more pronounced in SPMS and PPMS patients than in patients with the other disease phenotypes[43], and are similar between patients with SPMS and those with PPMS[35]. The moderate correlation found between NABT MTR values and the extent of macroscopic lesions and the severity of intrinsic lesion damage[43] suggests that NABT pathology does not only reflect Wallerian degeneration of axons traversing large focal abnormalities, but it may represent small focal abnormalities beyond the resolution of conventional scanning and independent of larger lesions.

Several studies have shown moderate to strong correlations between various brain MTR histogram-derived metrics and the severity of physical disability[42,45–47]. These correlations have been found to be stronger in patients with RRMS and SPMS than in other disease phenotypes[42,46]. Subtle MTR changes in the NABT[48,49] and in the cortical/subcortical[50] brain tissue are well correlated with the presence of neuropsychological impairment in MS patients. In addition, a multivariate analysis of several cMRI and MT MRI variables has demonstrated that average NABT-MTR is more strongly associated to cognitive impairment in MS patients than the extent of T2-visible lesions and their intrinsic tissue damage[51]. MTR histogram parameters from specific brain structures, including the cerebellum and brainstem of MS patients, are significantly associated with impairment of these functional systems[45]. Longitudinal studies demonstrated that NABT-MTR values tend to decline over time in all MS phenotypes, even if these changes seem to be more pronounced in SPMS patients[37] and suggested that MT MRI metrics are useful markers to monitor disease evolution[41,52,53]. In patients at presentation with CIS, the extent of NABT changes has been found to be an independent predictor of subsequent evolution to clinically definite MS[41]; whereas in patients with established MS, NAWM-MTR reduction has been shown to predict the accumulation of clinical disability over the subsequent five years[52,53].

In agreement with pathological studies[15–17], using ROI[54] and histogram analysis[54–57], MT MRI abnormalities have also been shown in the GM of MS patients, including those with PPMS[57]. GM changes are more pronounced in patients with SPMS than in those with RRMS[56]. Using a voxel-based analysis, MTR abnormalities have also been shown in the cortical and deep GM of patients with CIS[58]. In patients with RR[55] and PP[57] MS, NAGM MTR metrics are correlated with the severity of clinical disability.

Reliable MTR measurements can be obtained from the optic nerve (ON)[59–62] and spinal cord[63–67]. Two ROI-based studies[59,60] reported abnormal MTR values in the ON after an episode of acute optic neuritis, independently of the presence of T2-visible abnormalities[60]. MTR of the ON has been found to be correlated with the visual evoked potential (VEP) latency[59] and with the degree of visual function recovery[61] after an acute episode of optic neuritis. In a one-year follow-up study of patients with acute optic neuritis, Hickman et al. (62) showed a progressive decline of average MTR of the affected ON, which reached a nadir after about eight months despite the rapid initial visual recovery.

Using ROI analysis, Silver et al. (63) found reduced MTR values in the cervical cord of 12 MS patients in comparison with healthy volunteers. However, no correlation was found between cord MTR and disability, probably due to the small number of subjects enrolled and the limited portion of the cord studied. These results have been partially confirmed by a subsequent study performed on 65 MS patients[64], where a weak correlation between the reduction of MTR values and the increase of clinical disability has been found. More recently, the use of histogram analysis has provided, as already demonstrated for the brain, a more global picture of cord pathology in patients with MS and different disease phenotypes. Histogram analysis has demonstrated the absence of cord MTR histogram metrics abnormalities in patients with RRMS[65], in those with early-onset MS[66], and in those at presentation with CIS suggestive of MS[67]. On the contrary, cord MTR metrics are markedly reduced in patients with SPMS and PPMS[35,68]. A recent study has compared cervical cord MTR histogram metrics of patients with PPMS and SPMS and found no significant difference between these two groups[35]. Average cervical cord MTR is lower in MS patients with locomotor disability than in those without[65]. In PPMS, a model including cord area and cord MTR histogram peak height was significantly, albeit modestly, associated with the degree of disability[35]. In patients with MS, cord MTR is only partially correlated with brain MTR[68], suggesting that MS pathology in the cord is not a mere reflection of brain pathology and, as a consequence, measuring cord pathology might be a rewarding exercise in terms of understanding MS pathophysiology.

2.2 DW MRI

Diffusion is the microscopic random translational motion of molecules in a fluid system. In the CNS, diffusion is influenced by the microstructural components of tissue, including cell membranes and organelles. The diffusion coefficient of biological tissues (which can be measured *in vivo* by MRI) is, therefore, lower than the diffusion coefficient in free water and, for this reason, is named apparent diffusion coefficient (ADC)[69]. Pathological processes which modify tissue integrity, thus resulting in a loss or increased permeability of 'restricting' barriers, can determine an increase of the ADC. Since some cellular structures are aligned on the scale of an image pixel, the measurement of diffusion is also dependent on the direction in which diffusion is measured. As a consequence, diffusion measurements can give information about the size, shape, integrity, and orientation of tissues[70]. A measure of diffusion independent of the orientation of structures is provided by the mean diffusivity (MD) — the average of the ADCs measured in three orthogonal directions. A full characterization of diffusion can be obtained in terms of a tensor[71] (a 3x3 matrix which accounts for the correlation existing between molecular displacement along orthogonal directions). From the tensor, it is possible to derive MD, equal to the one third of its trace, and some other dimensionless indexes of anisotropy. One of the most used of these indices is fractional anisotropy (FA)[72] (Fig. 11.3).

The pathological elements of MS have the potential to alter the permeability or geometry of structural barriers to water molecular diffusion in the CNS. The application of DW MRI technology to MS is, therefore, appealing to provide quantitative estimates of the degree of tissue damage and, as a consequence, to improve the understanding of the mechanisms leading to irreversible disability.

The application of DW MRI to the study of individual MS lesions has demonstrated that, consistent with their pathological heterogeneity, T2-visible lesions are characterized by highly variable ADC, MD, and FA values[54,73–80]. In particular, ADC and MD values

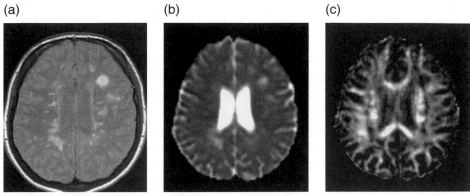

(a)   (b)   (c)

Fig. 11.3 Axial MR images from a patient with MS. The proton-density weighted scan (**a**) shows multiple lesions. On the mean diffusivity (MD) map (**b**), lesions appear as hyperintense areas. The degree of hyperintensity is related to an increase in MD and indicates a loss of structural barriers to water molecular motion. On the fractional anisotropy (FA) map (**c**), white matter pixels are bright because of the directionality of the white matter fibre tracts. Dark areas corresponding to macroscopic lesions indicate a loss of FA and suggest the presence of structural disorganization.

have been shown to be higher in T1-hypointense than in T1-isointense lesions[74,75,77,78]. While FA values are consistently lower in enhancing than in non-enhancing lesions[75,78], conflicting results have been achieved when comparing ADC or MD between these two lesion populations. While some studies reported higher ADC or MD values in non-enhancing than in enhancing lesions[74,75], others, based on larger samples of patients and lesions, did not report any significant difference between the two lesion populations[77,78]. The heterogeneity of enhancing lesions has been also underlined by the demonstration that water diffusivity is markedly increased in ring-enhancing lesions when compared to homogeneously enhancing lesions[81], or in the non-enhancing portions of enhancing lesions when compared with enhancing portions[81]. In agreement with MT MRI studies, DW MRI changes have also been shown in regions that will develop new lesions[76,80].

DW MRI technology has also been used to assess and quantify the presence and extent of damage of regions that appear as 'normal' on conventional imaging. In agreement with pathological observations[12–14], these studies have consistently shown increased ADC or MD values and decreased FA values in the NAWM and NABT of MS patients[54,73–80,82–86] independently of their disease phenotype. Such DT MRI changes in NAWM tend to be more severe in sites where macroscopic MS lesions are usually located and in periplaque regions and have also been shown in patients with CIS suggestive of MS[86]. The severity of MR-measured NAWM damage has been demonstrated to be associated with increased levels of disability and cognitive impairment and to evolve at different rates in the different patient groups, being more pronounced in patients with the progressive forms of the disease[54,78,82,87–89]. In addition, DW MRI metrics of specific brain structures, such as the pyramidal tracts[90,91] or the cerebellar peduncles[83], are strongly correlated with the impairment of these functional systems.

Consistent with post-mortem reports[15–17], several studies have shown increased MD values in the GM of MS patients[54,88,92,93]. These changes tend to be more pronounced in patients with the progressive forms of the disease, with no difference between PPMS and SPMS patients[88,92]. In patients with SPMS and PPMS[93], and also in those with RRMS[94], these changes worsen over time. This suggests a progressive accumulation of GM damage already in the RR phase of the disease, which was previously unrecognized and which might be one of the factors responsible for some of the clinical manifestations of the disease, such as neuropsychological impairment[95]. More recently, MD abnormalities have also been detected in the thalamus of patients with MS[96]. Recent studies have found a correlation between the severity of cognitive impairment and MD changes in the GM of patients with MS[97]. All of this fits with the notion that GM pathology might be an additional factor contributing to the worsening of clinical disability in patients with progressive MS, as a possible consequence of neuronal/axonal damage.

Although extremely technically demanding, successful DT MRI of the ON[98,99] has been obtained in healthy individuals[98,99] and MS patients[98]. Iwasawa *et al.*[98] assessed water diffusion in the ON of patients with optic neuritis, demonstrating significant different ON ADC values between controls and patients. In addition, this study demonstrated that ADC values are decreased in the acute (inflammatory) stage of optic neuritis and increased in the chronic phase. With increasing technical advances, it has also become possible to study cord MS pathology using DT MRI[100–105]. A preliminary study, which assessed water diffusion in seven cord lesions of three MS patients with locomotor disability[102], found increased MD values in MS cord lesions in comparison to the cord tissue from healthy volunteers. More recently, Valsasina *et al.*[104] used DW MRI histogram analysis to assess cervical cord damage in a cohort of 44 patients with either RRMS or SPMS and found reduced average cord FA in MS patients compared to controls. In MS patients, the reduction of cord FA was moderately correlated with the degree of disability. Altered MD and FA cord histogram derived metrics have also been found in patients with PPMS[105].

2.3 ¹H-MRS

Water suppressed, proton MR spectra of normal human brain at long echo times reveal four major resonances: one at 3.2 ppm from tetramethylamines (mainly from choline-containing phospholipids [Cho]), one at 3.0 ppm from creatine and phosphocreatine (Cr), one at 2.0 ppm from N-acetyl groups (mainly N-acetylaspartate [NAA]), and one at 1.3 ppm from the methyl resonance of lactate (Lac). NAA is a marker of axonal integrity, while Cho and Lac are considered as chemical correlates of acute inflammatory/demyelinating changes[106]. ¹H-MRS studies with shorter echo times can detect additional metabolites, such as lipids and myoinositol (mI), which are also regarded as markers of ongoing myelin damage. ¹H-MRS can complement conventional MRI in the assessment of MS patients, by defining, simultaneously, several chemical correlates of the pathological changes occurring within and outside T2-visible lesions. An immunopathological study[107] has shown that a decrease in NAA levels is correlated with axonal loss, while an increase in Cho correlates with the presence of active demyelination and gliosis.

The application of ^{1}H-MRS to the study of MS lesions has provided useful *in vivo* information concerning the heterogeneous pathological substrates of such lesions. In particular, increased Cho and Lac resonance intensities, which reflect the releasing of membrane phospholipids and the metabolism of inflammatory cells, respectively, have been shown in acute MS lesions[108,109]. In large, acute demyelinating lesions, decreases of Cr can also be seen[109]. Short echo time spectra can detect transient increases in visible lipids, released during myelin breakdown and of mI[110]. All these changes are usually associated with a decrease in NAA. After the acute phase and over a period of days to weeks, there is a progressive reduction of raised Lac resonance intensities to normal levels. Resonance intensities of Cr also return to normal within a few days. Cho, lipid, and mI resonance intensities return to normal over months. The signal intensity of NAA may remain decreased or show partial recovery, starting soon after the acute phase and lasting for several months[108,109,111]. These reversible decreases in NAA are strongly correlated with reversal of functional impairment[109]. Recovery of NAA may be related to resolution of oedema, increases in the diameter of previously shrunk axons secondary to remyelination and clearance of inflammatory factors, and reversible metabolic changes in neurons. Chronic MS lesions are characterized by markedly reduced NAA/Cr peaks. These changes are more pronounced in severely T1-hypointense MS lesions than in T1-iso- or mildly hypointense lesions[112,113] and in chronic lesions from patients with SPMS than in those from patients with benign MS[114]. Cho increase, probably reflecting an altered myelin chemistry or the presence of inflammation, and a decrease in NAA, have also been shown in pre-lesional NAWM[110,115,116].

Since changes in axonal viability may be important determinants of functional impairment in MS, one of the major contributions of ^{1}H-MRS to the understanding of MS is the possibility to quantify axonal pathology, by measuring NAA levels in lesions and NAWM. The application of ^{1}H-MRS imaging (MRSI) has enabled, on the one hand, spectra from large volumes of interest to be obtained and, on the other, to study, separately, brain pathology in T2-visible MS lesions and NAWM. Studies of limited and/or selected portions of the brain[113,115,117,118] have shown that NAA reduction is not restricted to MS lesions but also occurs in the NAWM. These changes are more severe in SPMS and PPMS patients than in those with RRMS[117,119]; however, such changes can also be detected in patients with no overt clinical disability[118] and in those in the early phase of the disease[120]. In patients with RRMS, longitudinal decrease over time of NAA/Cr in the NAWM correlates strongly with EDSS worsening[117,121]. More recently, it has been demonstrated that brain axonal damage begins in the early stages of MS, develops more rapidly in the earlier clinical stages of the disease, and correlates more strongly with disability in patients with mild, than in those with more severe, disease[120]. Diffusely elevated Cho and Cr concentrations have also been described in the NAWM of RRMS[122] and PPMS[119] patients, whereas elevated levels of Ins have been detected in the NAWM of patients with early RRMS[123] and in patients at presentation with CIS suggestive of MS[124].

Abnormalities of NAA levels in specific brain regions have been related to the impairment of the corresponding functional systems. Davie *et al.*[125] showed a significant reduction of NAA concentration in the cerebellar WM of patients with MS and severe ataxia compared with those having little or no cerebellar deficits. Lee *et al.*[126] demonstrated an association between reduction of NAA in the internal capsule and selective motor impairment. Pan *et al.*[127] found a relation between cognitive function and NAA levels in the periventricular WM. Gadea *et al.*[128] found a relationship between attentional dysfunction in early RRMS patients and NAA/Cr values in the locus coeruleus nuclei of the pontine ascending reticular activation system. The reduction of NAA/Cr ratio in MS patients NAWM has also been related to the presence of fatigue[129].

The recent development of an unlocalized ^{1}H-MRS sequence for measuring NAA levels in the whole brain (WBNAA)[130] has shown the presence of marked axonal pathology in clinically definite MS[131,132], in patients at the earliest clinical phase of MS[133], and in patients with PPMS[134]. No correlation has been found between WBNAA concentrations and T2-weighted lesion volumes in all these MS phenotypes[132–134], suggesting that T2-visible lesions represent just a small component of overall brain damage. This calls for an accurate assessment of NABT pathology for a better understanding of MS pathophysiology.

Metabolite abnormalities, including decrease of NAA, Cho, and glutamate, and increase of mI, have also been shown in the cortical GM of MS patients[123,135–137], since the early phases of established form of the disease[123], but not in CIS patients[138]. These changes are more pronounced in patients with SPMS than in those with RRMS[139]. NAA reduction has also been demonstrated in the thalamus of SPMS[140] and RRMS patients[141,142].

3. **Application of FMRI**

Although the resolution of acute inflammation, remyelination, redistribution of voltage-gated sodium channels in persistently demyelinated axons, and recovery from sublethal axonal injury are all factors likely to limit the clinical impact of damaging MS pathology[143,144], other mechanisms have been recently recognized as potential contributors to the recovery or to the maintenance of function in the presence of irreversible MS-related axonal damage. Plasticity is a well-known feature of the human brain which is likely to have several pathological substrates, including an increased axonal expression of sodium channels[145], synaptic changes, increased recruitment of parallel existing pathways or 'latent' connections, and reorganization of distant sites. All these changes might have a major adaptive role in limiting the functional consequences of axonal loss in MS. The basic principles of FMRI are explained in detail elsewhere in this book. Compared with other functional techniques, including electroencephalograpy (EEG) and magnetoencephalography (MEG), which allow mapping of the electrical activity of the brain and have high temporal resolution, FMRI is characterized by high spatial resolution.

Clinically, MS patients are characterized by the involvement of different functional systems. At present, however, FMRI studies in patients with MS have investigated selectively the patterns of cortical activations associated with the recruitment of the motor, visual, and cognitive systems. This is not only because these functional systems are those more frequently affected by the disease, but also because it is relatively easy to interrogate these three functional systems in healthy individuals and patients with different neurological conditions. Therefore, it is likely that future work in MS will focus on the development of FMRI paradigms aimed at testing the pattern of recruitment of other functional systems.

One of the main problems in the interpretation of clinical FMRI studies is that the observed changes might be influenced by differences in task performance between patients and controls. Clearly, this is a major issue in MS. To overcome this problem, FMRI studies of MS have either selected patients with no overt clinical symptomatology of the investigated functional systems[146–151] or, in case of motor impairments, passive movements[152] have been used as the experimental paradigm.

3.1 Visual system

For the investigation of the visual system, a 8 Hz photic stimulation is usually applied to one or both eyes[153–157].

A study of the visual system[153], in patients who had recovered from a single episode of acute optic neuritis, demonstrated that such patients had an extensive activation of the visual network (including the claustrum, lateral temporal and posterior parietal cortices, and thalamus, in addition to the primary visual cortex) compared to healthy volunteers (Fig. 11.4). Furthermore, the volume of the extra-occipital activation in patients with optic neuritis was found to be strongly correlated with VEP latency, suggesting that the functional reorganization of the cortex might represent an adaptive response to a persistently abnormal visual input. The results of this preliminary study have been confirmed and extended by two subsequent studies[154,155]. Toosy et al.[154] replicated the previous study[153], using a longer photic stimulation epoch to better elucidate the nature of the abnormal extra-occipital response observed. The results of this study confirmed the original findings, thus suggesting that cortical functional changes might have a role in compensating for a persistently disordered visual input. Russ et al.[155] used FMRI and VEP to monitor the functional recovery after an acute unilateral optic neuritis and found a strong relationship between FMRI and VEP latencies, suggesting that FMRI might contribute to the assessment of the temporal evolution of the visual deficits during MS recovery or therapy.

In patients with established MS and a RR course with a unilateral optic neuritis, a smaller activation of the visual cortex after stimulation of the affected and the unaffected eyes was found when compared to healthy subjects. On average, patients with optimal clinical recovery showed increased visual cortex activation than those with poor or no recovery, although activation remained reduced compared with controls[156]. A more recent study[157] performed in nine patients with previous optic neuritis, confirmed the results of the previous study[156] and showed that these patients not only have a reduced activation of the primary visual cortex but also a reduced FMRI percentage signal change of this region, suggesting an abnormality of its synaptic input.

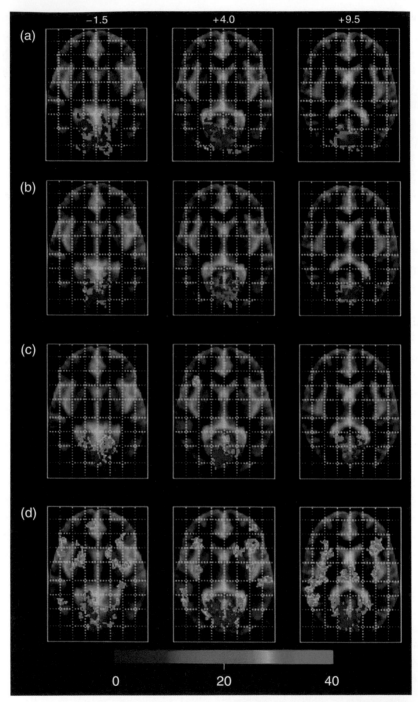

Fig. 11.4 Generic brain activation maps from seven control subjects and seven patients showing areas of significant response to monocular photic stimulation compared with binocular darkness. The one tailed probability of false positive activation p<0.0001 for each voxel; activated voxels are colour coded according to the delay (in seconds) of periodic response relative to the onset

3.2 Motor system

The investigation of the motor system in patients with MS has mainly focussed on the analysis of the performance of simple motor tasks with the dominant right upper limbs[146–152,158,159,164–173]. Such tasks were either self-paced or paced by a metronome. A few studies assessed the performance of simple motor tasks with the dominant right lower limbs[150,158,171], while even fewer studies have investigated the performance of more complex tasks, including phasic movements of dominant hand and foot[158,171] or object manipulation[173].

An altered brain pattern of movement-associated cortical activations, characterized by an increased recruitment of the contralateral primary sensorimotor cortex (SMC) during the performance of simple tasks[149,158] and by the recruitment of additional 'classical' and 'higher-order' sensorimotor areas during the performance of more complex tasks[158] (Fig. 11.5) has been demonstrated in patients with CIS. In these patients, the extent of functional cortical changes has been related to the severity of whole-brain axonal damage/dysfunction, measured using whole-brain ^{1}H-MRS[149]. The clinical and cMRI follow-up of the patients of these two studies has shown that, at disease onset, CIS patients with a subsequent evolution to definite MS tend to recruit a more widespread sensorimotor network than those without short-term disease evolution[159] (Fig. 11.6). These findings agree with the observation of an abnormal cortical activation in patients at high risk of developing Alzheimer's disease compared to healthy subjects[160,161]. This would suggest that, whereas increased recruitment of a widespread sensorimotor network contributes to limiting the impact of structural damage during the course of MS[162], its early activation might be counterproductive, as it might result in an early exhaustion of the adaptive properties of the brain. This hypothesis is also supported by studies on stroke patients, where a persistent overactivation and over-recruitment of a widespread cortical network has been related to an unfavourable clinical outcome[163].

An increased recruitment of several sensorimotor areas, mainly located in the cerebral hemisphere ipsilateral to the limb which performed the task, has also been demonstrated in patients with early MS and a previous episode of hemiparesis[164]. In patients with similar characteristics, but who presented with an episode of optic neuritis, this increased

---

of photic stimulation. The left side of each map represents the right side of the brain; z coordinates in standard space are given for each slice in mm. (a) In the control subject group (left eye), there is activation only in bilateral visual cortex, with a larger area of activation in the right compared with the left visual cortex. (b) The right eye response showed a similar pattern but with greater activation of the left visual cortex. (c) In the patient group (unaffected eye), there is an additional focus of activation in the right insula-claustrum. (d) In the patient group (affected eye), there is additional activation of a network of multimodal processing areas including the bilateral insula-claustrum, lateral temporal cortex, posterior parietal cortex, thalamus, and corpus striatum. Note that periodic response in extraoccipital areas is considerably delayed relative to the response in visual cortex. (Reproduced with permission from the BMJ Publishing Group[153].)

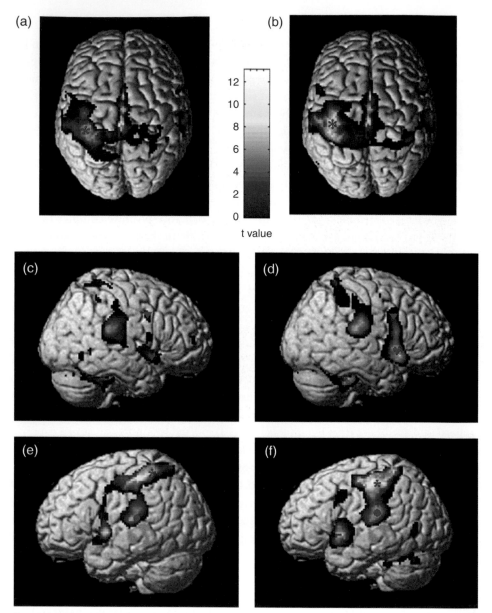

Fig. 11.5 Brain pattern of cortical activations on a rendered brain in right-handed healthy subjects (**a**), (**c**), and (**e**) and patients at presentation with clinically isolated syndromes (CIS) suggestive of MS (**b**), (**d**), and (**f**) during the performance of a complex motor task with their clinically unimpaired and fully normal functioning right limbs. Compared with healthy subjects, CIS patients had increased activations of the contralateral primary sensorimotor cortex (*), contralateral secondary sensorimotor cortex (•), ipsilateral middle frontal gyrus (∇), and ipsilateral inferior frontal gyrus (♥). Note that the activations are colour coded according to their t values.

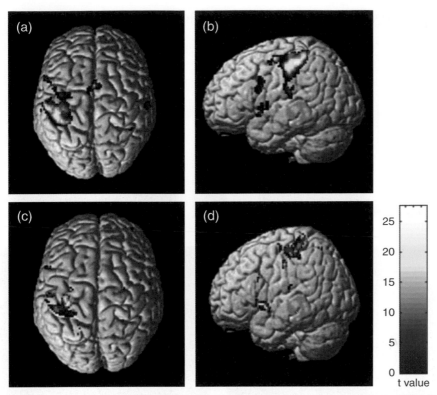

Fig. 11.6 Brain pattern of cortical activations on a rendered brain during a simple motor task with the dominant, functionally unaffected right hand in patients with clinically isolated syndromes suggestive of MS who evolved to definite MS over a short-term follow-up period (**a**), (**b**) compared to those who did not (**c**), **d**). Compared to (c) and (d), in (a) and (b), there is more extensive and widespread activation of several areas mainly located in the frontal lobes. Note that the activations are colour coded according to their t values.

recruitment involved sensorimotor areas which were mainly located in the contralateral cerebral hemisphere[165].

In patients with established MS and a RR course, functional cortical changes, mainly characterized by an increased activation of 'classical' motor areas, including the primary SMC, the supplementary motor area (SMA), and the secondary sensorimotor cortex, have been shown during the performance of motor tasks[146,148,166–168] and have been variously related not only to the extent of T2-visible lesions but also to the severity of intrinsic lesion damage, measured using T1-weighted images[165], MTR, and MD[148] and the severity of NABT damage, measured using ^{1}H-MRS[149,168], MT MRI or DW MRI[148,151]. More recently, the influence of lesion location in critical brain regions on the movement-associated brain pattern of cortical activations (i.e. in the pyramidal tract in case of motor tasks) has also been demonstrated[169] (Fig. 11.7). The impact of NABT damage, assessed using DT MRI, on movement-associated FMRI activations in patients with RRMS and non-specific

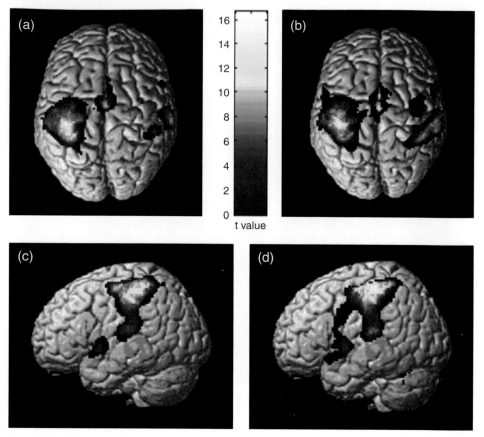

Fig. 11.7 Brain pattern of cortical activations on a rendered brain from MS patients without (**a**), (**c**) and with (**b**), (**d**) lesions in the left pyramidal tract, during the performance of a simple motor task with their clinically unimpaired, fully normal functioning and dominant right hands. In patients with pyramidal tract lesions, a more bilateral pattern of activations is visible. Note that the activations are colour coded according to their t values.

T2-weighted abnormalities on cMRI of the brain has also been investigated[151]. In these patients, an abnormal activation of several cortico-subcortical areas and an enhanced 'transcallosal inhibition' have been observed during the performance of a simple motor task. The role of the corpus callosum in interhemispheric connectivity has been underpinned by another FMRI study[170] in which, by measuring low-frequency BOLD fluctuations, reduced functional connectivity between the right and the left hemisphere primary motor cortices in MS patients was shown.

Movement-associated cortical changes, characterized by the activation of highly specialized cortical areas, have also been described in patients with SPMS[150] during the performance of a simple motor task. In this phenotype of the disease, such cortical changes have been related not only to the extent of T2-visible lesions, but also to

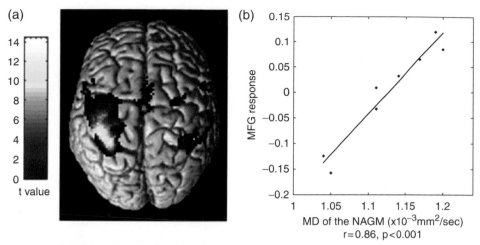

Fig. 11.8 (a) Cortical activations (colour coded according to their t values) from right-handed patients with secondary progressive MS during the performance of a simple motor task with their clinically unimpaired, fully normally functioning right hands are shown on a rendered brain. A widespread activation of several areas of the sensorimotor network (including the primary and secondary sensorimotor cortex, the supplementary motor area, and the middle frontal gyrus) is visible. The scatterplot of the correlation between the relative activation of the middle frontal gyrus and average mean diffusivity of the normal-appearing gray matter is shown in (**b**). Note that the values of some subjects are negative because they have been scaled to the mean value of the FMRI scans of each individual (i.e. values are mean centred).

the severity of NAWM and GM damage (Fig. 11.8). Two FMRI studies of the motor system[147,171] of patients with PPMS suggested a lack of 'classical' adaptive mechanisms as a potential additional factor contributing to the accumulation of disability. In particular, in these patients, during the performance of different motor tasks with non-impaired dominant limbs, a recruitment of a widespread movement-associated cortical network usually considered to function in motor, sensory, and multimodal integration processing (i.e. the frontal and temporal lobes, and the insula) was detected. The absence of a concomitant recruitment of the 'classical' motor areas, including the primary SMC, the SMA, the IPS, and the SII was interpreted as a failure of part of the adaptive capacity of the cerebral cortex in this severely disabling phenotype of the disease. To emphasize the possible adaptive role of such functional cortical changes, in this latter group of patients, FMRI measures have also been related (apart from T2-visible lesion loads and NABT damage) to the severity of spinal cord damage, measured using MT MRI[147]. The notion that brain functional cortical changes may be influenced by spinal cord damage has been underpinned by two other recent studies performed on patients with a previous episode of acute myelitis of probable demyelinating origin[172], and patients with Devic's neuromyelitis optica[173] (Fig. 11.9). In both these conditions, an increased activation of several cortical areas, mainly located in the ipsilateral hemisphere, was demonstrated

(a)

(b)

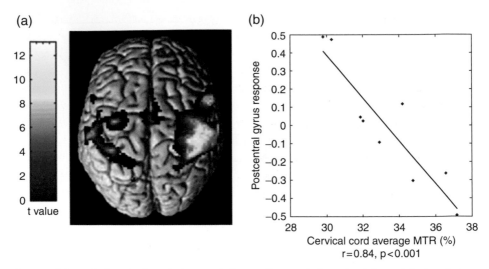

Fig. 11.9 (a) Cortical activations (colour coded according to their t values) from right-handed patients with Devic's neuromyelitis optica during the performance of a simple motor task with their clinically unimpaired and fully normally functioning left hands are shown on a rendered brain. Widespread activation of several areas of the sensorimotor network (including the primary sensorimotor cortex, the supplementary motor area, and the middle frontal gyrus) is visible. The scatterplot of the correlation between the relative activation of the postcentral gyrus and average magnetization transfer ratio of the cervical cord is shown in (**b**). Note that the values of some subjects are negative because they have been scaled to the mean value of the FMRI scans of each individual (i.e. values are mean centred).

during the investigation of a simple motor task performed with the clinically unaffected, upper limbs.

Two different studies, one conducted on patients with PPMS[171] and the other one on patients with RRMS[152], demonstrated that the severity of clinical disability might be among the factors influencing the pattern of cortical activations in MS patients. Whether an altered pattern of use might also modulate such cortical activation remains to be established.

The results of all these studies suggest that there might be a 'natural history' of the functional reorganization of the cerebral cortex in MS patients, which might be characterized at the beginning of the disease by an increased recruitment of those areas 'normally' devoted to the performance of a given task, such as the primary SMC and the supplementary motor area (SMA) in the case of a motor task. At a later stage, bilateral activation of these regions is first seen, followed by a widespread recruitment of additional areas, which are usually activated in normal people to perform novel/complex tasks. This notion has been supported by the results of a recent study[174] which has provided a direct demonstration that MS patients, during the performance of a simple motor task, activate some regions that are part of a fronto-parietal circuit, whose recruitment occurs typically in healthy subjects during object manipulation[174].

Although the actual role of cortical reorganization on the clinical manifestations of MS remains unclear, the demonstration that MS patients may have a normal level of performance despite the presence of diffuse tissue damage, suggests that cortical adaptive changes are likely to contribute to limiting the clinical consequences of MS-related structural damage[162]. The most compelling evidence that cortical reorganization may have a role in recovery from axonal damage derives from the study by Reddy *et al.*[167] who followed, with serial ^{1}H-MRS and FMRI scans, a patient after the onset of an acute hemiparesis and discovery of a new, large, demyelinating lesion located in the corticospinal tract. In this patient, clinical recovery preceded complete normalization of NAA and was accompanied by an increased recruitment of the ipsilateral primary SMC and SMA. In line with these findings, in a group of patients who complained of fatigue when compared to matched non-fatigued MS patients, a reduced activation of a complex movement-associated cortical/subcortical network, including the cerebellum, the rolandic operculum, the thalamus, and the middle frontal gyrus was found[146]. In these patients, a strong correlation between the reduction of thalamic activity and the clinical severity of fatigue was shown, indicating that a less marked cortical recruitment might be associated with the appearance of clinical symptomatology in MS.

A recent study[175] used FMRI to analyse how the motor network responds to motor training in MS patients with mild motor impairment of the right upper extremity. Before training, thumb movements elicited more prominent activation of the contralateral dorsal premotor cortex in MS patients than in healthy controls. After training, unlike the control group, MS patients did not exhibit task-specific reductions in activation in the contralateral primary SMC and adjacent parietal association corticex. These results indicate that patients engage the contralateral premotor cortex more than controls in order to perform movements before training. The absence of training-dependent reductions in activation is consistent with a decreased capacity to optimize recruitment of the motor network with practice. Further studies are now warranted to better understand training-dependent cortical plasticity in MS, which might help to optimize therapies and prolong preservation of motor function.

3.3 Cognition

The most common cognitive deficits in MS patients involve memory and attentional processes. Therefore, the majority of FMRI studies of cognition in these patients has investigated these cognitive fields.

In patients at presentation with CIS suggestive of MS, an altered pattern of cortical activations has been described during the performance of the Paced Auditory Serial Addition Test (PASAT)[176,177] and has been related to the extent of NAWM damage, measured using MT MRI[177]. These results confirm the presence of cortical reorganization at the earliest clinical stage of the disease and a role for such changes in limiting the functional consequences on cognitive performance of widespread tissue damage.

An increased recruitment of several cortical areas during the performance of a simple cognitive task has also been shown in patients with RRMS and mild clinical disability. Staffen *et al.*[178] found that, during the performance of the Paced Visual Serial Addition Task

(PVSAT), MS patients with intact task performance had an increased activation of several regions located in the frontal and parietal lobes, bilaterally, compared to healthy volunteers, suggesting the presence of functional compensatory mechanisms. An increased activation of regions exclusively located in the right cerebral hemisphere (in particular, in the frontal and temporal lobes) has also been found in MS patients when testing rehearsal within working memory[179]. The degree of right hemisphere recruitment was strongly related to patients' neuropsychological performance. In patients with RRMS and no cognitive deficits, using FMRI during a n-back test, a reduced activation of core area of working memory circuitry (including prefrontal and parietal regions) and a greater activation of other regions within and beyond the typical working memory circuitry (including areas in the frontal, parietal, temporal, and occipital lobes) have been found[180] (Fig. 11.10). This shift in activation in patients was most prominent when working memory demands were high. These findings suggest that, as shown for motor and visual tasks, dynamic alteration in brain activation patterns can occur in RRMS patients during cognitive tasks.

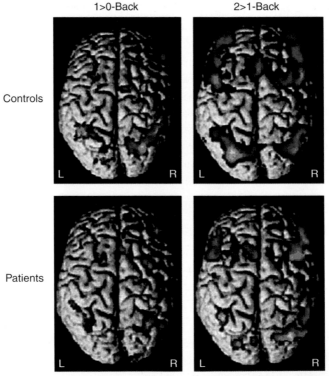

Fig. 11.10 Major cortical foci of activation as a function of increasing working memory demands are shown on surface-rendered projections for controls (top panel) and patients with multiple sclerosis (bottom panel). Overall, controls showed greater activation than patients in core regions of working memory circuitry, including parietal and frontal regions. (Reproduced with permission from Lippincott Williams and Wilkins[180].)

Two other studies[181,182], again investigating working memory performance in MS patients, demonstrated: (1) a greater activity in regions related to sensorimotor functions and anterior attentional/executive components of the working memory system in patients compared to healthy controls; and (2) a reduced recruitment of several regions in the right cerebellar hemisphere in patients compared with healthy individuals[182], thus suggesting that the cerebellum might play a role in the working memory impairment of MS.

The discrepancies between all these studies might be related either to the different clinical characteristics of the patients recruited or to the setting of the FMRI experiments and methods used for the analysis. Another confounder might be the presence and extent of macro- and microscopic tissue damage in these patients. This latter factor has been analysed by two recent studies[183,184]. Using an FMRI counting Stroop task, Parry et al.[183] showed, in cognitively intact MS patients, when contrasted to healthy subjects, an increased activation of a left prefrontal region that correlated with the normalized brain parenchymal volume. The activity of this region showed a relative normalization after the administration of rivastigmine, a central cholinsterase inhibitor. In RRMS patients, during the performance of attention and memory tasks, Mainero et al.[184] demonstrated an increased activation of specific brain areas that correlated with the extent of T2 lesions of the brain. Consistent with previous findings, these authors showed, in MS patients with preserved cognitive performance, an association of an increased activation of the regions normally devoted to the performance of a given task with the recruitment of additional brain areas. Task-related functional cortical changes were less pronounced in MS patients with low task performance. The concept that the exhaustion of the functional properties of the cortex might be among the factors leading to cognitive impairment in MS patients has also been underlined by another FMRI study[185] in which a 'poor' pattern of cortical activations was detected in cognitively impaired MS patients.

4. Future research work

The extensive application of FMRI to the assessment of patients with MS is improving our understanding of the factors associated with the accumulation of disability in this disease. The available FMRI data support the notion that cortical adaptive responses may have an important role in compensating for MS irreversible tissue damage, and that the rate of accumulation of disability in MS might not only be a function of tissue loss but also of the progressive failure of the adaptive capacity of the cortex. In particular, the results of all the previous studies seem to suggest that the increased and/or bilateral recruitment of areas devoted to the performance of a given task might help to preserve the function investigated with such a task. When this mechanism is exhausted, progressive recruitment of additional areas, involved at different levels in the performance of that given task, might contribute to limit the functional consequences of structural subcortical damage. When even this additional compensatory mechanism is inefficient, a pattern of erratic cortical activations, or the activation of areas not 'classically' devoted to the performance of that given task, might be among the factors contributing to the development of clinical deficits and, possibly, to disability accumulation.

There are at least two major issues, outlined below, which would warrant additional intensive research activity.

1) **The development and application of new FMRI paradigms and the need for studies on high-field scanners**

High field strengths lead to improved MRI resolution with the possibility to obtain detailed microneuroimaging. The development of diffusion-based tractography methods on these scanners would allow the determination of, with a reasonable degree of precision, the pathways connecting different CNS structures. If combined with FMRI findings, this approach should facilitate important *in vivo* structural-functional correlations, which might help define the substrates of specific neurological symptoms. In addition to an increased spatial resolution, another important advantage of high-field scanners is their ability to ameliorate the FMRI signal/noise ratio. With the development of appropriate analysis methodology, this might allow the design of sophisticated event-related procedures, with a temporal resolution closer to that of the haemodynamic response. This might also contribute to the development of FMRI paradigms to investigate 'deactivations' of given brain regions and to examine the functional relationships between different activated areas.

2) **The need for longitudinal studies**

Longitudinal FMRI studies in MS are, at present, lacking. Given the safety of the technique, especially when compared to that of other functional techniques such as positron emission tomography, and the possibility to obtain long activation sessions, FMRI is a promising tool to perform serial assessments. Therefore, longitudinal FMRI studies should aim to define the temporal evolution of functional cortical changes in the different phenotypes of the disease as well as their role in limiting the clinical consequence of increasing tissue damage. In addition, longitudinal FMRI studies would enable us to monitor the effect of motor and cognitive rehabilitation, as well as of pharmacological therapies, in enhancing any beneficial effect of cortical adaptive plasticity.

References

1. Confavreux C, Vukusic S, Adeleine P (2003). Early clinical predictors and progression of irreversible disability in multiple sclerosis: an amnesic process. *Brain* **126**, 770–82.
2. Trojano M, Liguori M, Bosco Zimatore G, *et al* (2002). Age-related disability in multiple sclerosis. *Ann Neurol* **51**, 475–80.
3. Rovaris M, Rocca MA, Filippi M (2003). Magnetic resonance-based techniques for the study and management of multiple sclerosis. *Br Med Bull* **65**, 133–44. Review.
4. Bakshi R, Hutton GJ, Miller JR, Radue EW (2004). The use of magnetic resonance imaging in the diagnosis and long-term management of multiple sclerosis. *Neurology* **14**, S3–11.
5. Rovaris M, Filippi M (1999). Magnetic resonance techniques to monitor disease evolution and treatment trial outcomes in multiple sclerosis. *Curr Opin Neurol* **12**, 337–44.
6. Molyneux PD, Barker GJ, Barkhof F, *et al* (2001). Clinical-MRI correlations in a European trial of interferon beta-1b in secondary progressive MS. *Neurology* **57**, 2191–7.

7. Ferguson B, Matyszak MK, Esiri MM, Perry VH (1997). Axonal damage in acute multiple sclerosis lesions. *Brain* **120**, 393–9.

8. Trapp BD, Peterson J, Ransohoff RM, Rudick R, Mork S, Bo L (1998). Axonal transection in the lesions of multiple sclerosis. *N Engl J Med* **338**, 278–85.

9. Kappos L, Moeri D, Radue EW, *et al* (1999). Predictive value of gadolinium-enhanced magnetic resonance imaging for relapse rate and changes in disability or impairment in multiple sclerosis: a meta-analysis. Gadolinium MRI Meta-analysis Group. *Lancet* **20**, 964–9.

10. Bjartmar C, Trapp BD (2001). Axonal and neuronal degeneration in multiple sclerosis: mechanisms and functional consequences. *Curr Opin Neurol* **14**, 271–8. Review.

11. Bjartmar C, Wujek JR, Trapp BD (2003). Axonal loss in the pathology of MS: consequences for understanding the progressive phase of the disease. *J Neurol Sci* **15**, 165–71. Review.

12. Allen IV, McKeown, SR (1979). A histological, histochemical and biochemical study of the macroscopically normal white matter in multiple sclerosis. *J Neurol Sci* **41**, 81–91.

13. Evangelou N, Esiri MM, Smith S, Palace J, Matthews PM (2000). Quantitative pathological evidence for axonal loss in normal appearing white matter in multiple sclerosis. *Ann Neurol* **47**, 391–5.

14. Bjartmar C, Kinkel RP, Kidd G, Rudick RA, Trapp BD (2001). Axonal loss in normal-appearing white matter in a patient with acute MS. *Neurology* **57**, 1248–52.

15. Lumdsen CE (1970). The neuropathology of multiple sclerosis. In: *Handbook of clinical neurology* (ed. PJ Vinken, GW Bruyn), Vol **9**, pp 217–309. North–Holland, Amsterdam.

16. Kidd D, Barkhof F, McConnell R, Algra PR, Allen IV, Revesz T (1999). Cortical lesions in multiple sclerosis. *Brain* **122**, 17–26.

17. Peterson JW, Bo L, Mork S, Chang A, Trapp BD (2001). Transected neurites, apoptotic neurons, and reduced inflammation in cortical multiple sclerosis lesions. *Ann Neurol* **50**, 389–400.

18. McDonald WI, Miller DH, Barnes D (1992). The pathological evolution of multiple sclerosis. *Neuropathol Appl Neurobiol* **18**, 319–34.

19. van Walderveen MAA, Kamphorst W, Scheltens P, *et al* (1998). Histopathologic correlate of hypointense lesions on T1-weighted spin-echo MRI in multiple sclerosis. *Neurology* **50**, 1282–8.

20. van Walderveen MA, Lycklama A Nijeholt GJ, Ader HJ, *et al* (2001). Hypointense lesions on T1-weighted spin-echo magnetic resonance imaging: relation to clinical characteristics in subgroups of patients with multiple sclerosis. *Arch Neurol* **58**, 76–81.

21. Filippi M, Rocca MA, Comi G (2003). The use of quantitative magnetic-resonance-based techniques to monitor the evolution of multiple sclerosis. *Lancet Neurol* **2**, 337–46. Review.

22. van Waesberghe JH, Kamphorst W, De Groot CJ, *et al* (1999). Axonal loss in multiple sclerosis lesions: magnetic resonance imaging insights into substrates of disability. *Ann Neurol* **46**, 747–54.

23. Barkhof F, Bruck W, De Groot CJ, *et al* (2003). Remyelinated lesions in multiple sclerosis: magnetic resonance image appearance. *Arch Neurol* **60**, 1073–81.

24. Schmierer K, Scaravilli F, Altmann DR, Barker GJ, Miller DH (2004). Magnetization transfer ratio and myelin in postmortem multiple sclerosis brain. *Ann Neurol* **56**, 407–15.

25. Silver NC, Lai M, Symms MR, Barker GJ, McDonald WI, Miller DH (1998). Serial magnetization transfer imaging to characterize the early evolution of new MS lesions. *Neurology* **51**, 758–64.

26. Filippi M, Rocca MA, Comi G (1998). Magnetization transfer ratios of multiple sclerosis lesions with variable durations of enhancement. *J Neurol Sci* **159**, 162–5.

27. Filippi M, Rocca MA, Rizzo G, *et al* (1998). Magnetization transfer ratios in multiple sclerosis lesions enhancing after different doses of gadolinium. *Neurology* **50**, 1289–93.

28. Dousset V, Gayou A, Brochet B, Caille JM (1998). Early structural changes in acute MS lesions assessed by serial magnetization transfer studies. *Neurology* **51**, 1150–5.

29. Goodkin DE, Rooney WD, Sloan R, *et al* (1998). A serial study of new MS lesions and the white matter from which they arise. *Neurology* **51**, 1689–97.

30. van Waesberghe JHTM, van Walderveen MA, Castelijns JA, *et al* (1998). Patterns of lesion development in multiple sclerosis: longitudinal observations with T1-weighted spin-echo and magnetization MR. *AJNR Am J Neuroradiol* **19**, 675–83.

31. Filippi M, Rocca MA, Martino G, Horsfield MA, Comi G (1998). Magnetization transfer changes in the normal appearing white matter precede the appearance of enhancing lesions in patients with multiple sclerosis. *Ann Neurol* **43**, 809–14.

32. Pike GB, De Stefano N, Narayanan S, *et al* (2000). Multiple sclerosis: magnetization transfer MR imaging of white matter before lesion appearance on T2-weighted images. *Radiology* **215**, 824–30.

33. Fazekas F, Ropele S, Enzinger C, Seifert T, Strasser–Fuchs S (2002). Quantitative magnetization transfer imaging of pre-lesional white-matter changes in multiple sclerosis. *Mult Scler* **8**, 479–84.

34. Filippi M, Iannucci G, Tortorella C, *et al* (1999). Comparison of MS clinical phenotypes using conventional and magnetization transfer MRI. *Neurology* **52**, 588–94.

35. Rovaris M, Bozzali M, Santuccio G, *et al* (2001). In vivo assessment of the brain and cervical cord pathology of patients with primary progressive multiple sclerosis. *Brain* **124**, 2540–9.

36. Rocca MA, Mastronardo G, Rodegher M, Comi G, Filippi M (1999). Long-term changes of magnetization transfer-derived measures from patients with relapsing-remitting and secondary progressive multiple sclerosis. *AJNR Am J Neuroradiol* **20**, 821–7.

37. Filippi M, Inglese M, Rovaris M, *et al* (2000). Magnetization transfer imaging to monitor the evolution of MS: a 1-year follow-up study. *Neurology* **55**, 940–946.

38. Filippi M, Campi A, Dousset V, *et al* (1995). A magnetization transfer imaging study of normal-appearing white matter in multiple sclerosis. *Neurology* **45**, 478–82.

39. Loevner LA, Grossman RI, Cohen JA, *et al* (1995). Microscopic disease in normal-appearing white matter on conventional MR images in patients with multiple sclerosis: assessment with magnetization-transfer measurements. *Radiology* **196**, 511–15.

40. Ge Y, Grossman RI, Babb JS, He J, Mannon LJ (2003). Dirty-appearing white matter in multiple sclerosis: volumetric MR imaging and magnetization transfer ratio histogram analysis. *AJNR Am J Neuroradiol* **24**, 1935–40.

41. Iannucci G, Tortorella C, Rovaris M, Sormani MP, Comi G, Filippi M (2000). Prognostic value of MR and magnetization transfer imaging findings in patients with clinically isolated syndromes suggestive of multiple sclerosis at presentation. *AJNR Am J Neuroradiol* **21**, 1034–8.

42. Kalkers NF, Hintzen RQ, van Waesberghe JH, *et al* (2001). Magnetization transfer histogram parameters reflect all dimensions of MS pathology, including atrophy. *J Neurol Sci* **184**, 155–62.

43. Tortorella C, Viti B, Bozzali M, *et al* (2000). A magnetization transfer histogram study of normal-appearing brain tissue in MS. *Neurology* **54**, 186–93.

44. Traboulsee A, Dehmeshki J, Brex PA, *et al* (2002). Normal-appearing brain tissue MTR histograms in clinically isolated syndromes suggestive of MS. *Neurology* **59**, 126–8.

45. Iannucci G, Minicucci L, Rodegher M, Sormani MP, Comi G, Filippi M (1999). Correlations between clinical and MRI involvement in multiple sclerosis: assessment using T1, T2 and MT histograms. *J Neurol Sci* **171**, 121–9.

46. Dehmeshki J, Ruto AC, Arridge S, Silver NC, Miller DH, Tofts PS (2001). Analysis of MTR histograms in multiple sclerosis using principal components and multiple discriminant analysis. *Magn Reson Med* **46**, 600–9.

47. Traboulsee A, Dehmeshki J, Peters KR, *et al* (2003). Disability in multiple sclerosis is related to normal appearing brain tissue MTR histogram abnormalities. *Mult Scler* **9**, 566–73.

48. Rovaris M, Filippi M, Falautano M, *et al* (1998). Relation between MR abnormalities and patterns of cognitive impairment in multiple sclerosis. *Neurology* **50**, 1601–8.

49. van Buchem MA, Grossman RI, Armstrong C, *et al* (1998). Correlation of volumetric magnetization transfer imaging with clinical data in MS. *Neurology* **50**, 1609–17.

50. Rovaris M, Filippi M, Minicucci L, *et al* (2000). Cortical/subcortical disease burden and cognitive impairment in multiple sclerosis. *AJNR Am J Neuroradiol* **21**, 402–8.

51. Filippi M, Tortorella C, Rovaris M, *et al* (2000). Changes in the normal appearing brain tissue and cognitive impairment in multiple sclerosis. *J Neurol Neurosurg Psychiatry* **68**, 157–61.

52. Santos AC, Narayanan S, De Stefano N, *et al* (2002). Magnetization transfer can predict clinical evolution in patients with multiple sclerosis. *J Neurol* **249**, 662–668.

53. Rovaris M, Agosta F, Sormani MP, *et al* (2003). Conventional and magnetization transfer MRI predictors of clinical multiple sclerosis evolution: a medium-term follow-up study. *Brain* **126**, 2323–2332.

54. Cercignani M, Bozzali M, Iannucci G, Comi G, Filippi M (2001). Magnetisation transfer ratio and mean diffusivity of normal-appearing white and gray matter from patients with multiple sclerosis. *J Neurol Neurosurg Psychiatry* **70**, 311–17.

55. Ge Y, Grossman RI, Udupa JK, Babb JS, Kolson DL, McGowan JC (2001). Magnetization transfer ratio histogram analysis of gray matter in relapsing-remitting multiple sclerosis. *AJNR Am J Neuroradiol* **22**, 470–5.

56. Ge Y, Grossman RI, Udupa JK, Babb JS, Mannon LJ, McGowan JC (2002). Magnetization transfer ratio histogram analysis of normal-appearing gray matter and normal-appearing white matter in multiple sclerosis. *J Comput Assist Tomogr* **26**, 62–8.

57. Dehmeshki J, Chard DT, Leary SM, *et al* (2003). The normal appearing grey matter in primary progressive multiple sclerosis: a magnetisation transfer imaging study. *J Neurol* **250**, 67–74.

58. Audoin B, Ranjeva JP, Duong MV, *et al* (2004). Voxel-based analysis of MTR images: a method to locate gray matter abnormalities in patients at the earliest stage of multiple sclerosis. *J Magn Reson Imaging* **20**, 765–71.

59. Thorpe JW, Barker GJ, Jones SJ, *et al* (1995). Magnetisation transfer ratios and transverse magnetisation decay curves in optic neuritis: correlation with clinical findings and electrophysiology. *J Neurol Neurosurg Psychiatry* **59**, 487–92.

60. Boorstein JM, Moonis G, Boorstein SM, *et al* (1997). Optic neuritis: imaging with magnetization transfer. *AJR Am J Roentgenol* **169**, 1709–12.

61. Inglese M, Ghezzi A, Bianchi S, *et al* (2002). Irreversible disability and tissue loss in multiple sclerosis: a conventional and magnetization transfer magnetic resonance imaging study of the optic nerves. *Arch Neurol* **59**, 250–5.

62. Hickman SJ, Toosy AT, Jones SJ, *et al* (2004). Serial magnetization transfer imaging in acute optic neuritis. *Brain* **127**, 692–700.

63. Silver NC, Barker GJ, Losseff NA, *et al* (1997). Magnetisation transfer ratio measurement in the cervical spinal cord: a preliminary study in multiple sclerosis. *Neuroradiology* **39**, 441–5.

64. Lycklama a Nijeholt GJ, Castelijns JA, Lazeron RH, *et al* (2000). Magnetization transfer ratio of the spinal cord in multiple sclerosis: relationship to atrophy and neurologic disability. *J Neuroimaging* **10**, 67–72.

65. Filippi M, Bozzali M, Horsfield MA, *et al* (2000). A conventional and magnetization transfer MRI study of the cervical cord in patients with MS. *Neurology* **54**, 207–13.

66. Mezzapesa DM, Rocca MA, Falini A, *et al* (2004). A preliminary diffusion tensor and magnetization transfer magnetic resonance imaging study of early-onset multiple sclerosis. *Arch Neurol* **61**, 366–8.

67. Rovaris M, Gallo A, Riva R, *et al* (2004). An MT MRI study of the cervical cord in clinically isolated syndromes suggestive of MS. *Neurology* **63**, 584–5.

68. Rovaris M, Bozzali M, Santuccio G, *et al* (2000). Relative contributions of brain and cervical cord pathology to multiple sclerosis disability: a study with magnetisation transfer ratio histogram analysis. *J Neurol Neurosurg Psychiatry* **69**, 723–7.

69. Le Bihan D, Breton E, Lallemand D, Grenier P, Cabanis E, Laval–Jeanter M (1986). MR imaging of intravoxel incoherent motions: application to diffusion and perfusion in neurologic disorders. *Radiology* **161**, 401–7.

70. Le Bihan D, Turner R, Pekar J, Moonen CTW (1991). Diffusion and perfusion imaging by gradient sensitization: design, strategy and significance. *J Magn Reson Imaging* **1**, 7–8.

71. Basser PJ, Mattiello J, Le Bihan D (1994). Estimation of the effective self-diffusion tensor from the NMR spin-echo. *J Magn Reson B* **103**, 247–254.

72. Pierpaoli C, Jezzard P, Basser PJ, Blarnett A, Di Chiro G (1996). Diffusion tensor MR imaging of the human brain. *Radiology* **201**, 637–48.

73. Horsfield MA, Lai M, Webb SL, *et al* (1996). Apparent diffusion coefficients in benign and secondary progressive multiple sclerosis by nuclear magnetic resonance. *Magn Reson Med* **36**, 393–400.

74. Droogan AG, Clark CA, Werring DJ, Barker GJ, McDonald WI, Miller DH (1999). Comparison of multiple sclerosis clinical subgroups using navigated spin echo diffusion-weighted imaging. *Magn Reson Imaging* **17**, 653–61.

75. Werring DJ, Clark CA, Barker GJ, Thompson AJ, Miller DH (1999). Diffusion tensor imaging of lesions and normal-appearing white matter in multiple sclerosis. *Neurology* **52**, 1626–32.

76. Werring DJ, Brassat D, Droogan AG, *et al* (2000). The pathogenesis of lesions and normal-appearing white matter changes in multiple sclerosis. A serial diffusion MRI study. *Brain* **123**, 1667–1676.

77. Filippi M, Iannucci G, Cercignani M, Rocca MA, Pratesi A, Comi G (2000). A quantitative study of water diffusion in multiple sclerosis lesions and normal-appearing white matter using echo-planar imaging. *Arch Neurol* **57**, 1017–21.

78. Filippi M, Cercignani M, Inglese M, Horsfield MA, Comi G (2001). Diffusion tensor magnetic resonance imaging in multiple sclerosis. *Neurology* **56**, 304–11.

79. Cercignani M, Iannucci G, Rocca MA, Comi G, Horsfield MA, Filippi M (2000). Pathologic damage in MS assessed by diffusion-weighted and magnetization transfer MRI. *Neurology* **54**, 1139–44.

80. Rocca MA, Cercignani M, Iannucci G, Comi G, Filippi M (2000). Weekly diffusion-weighted imaging of normal-appearing white matter in MS. *Neurology* **55**, 882–4.

81. Roychowdhury S, Maldijan JA, Grossman RI (2000). Multiple sclerosis: comparison of trace apparent diffusion coefficients with MR enhancement pattern of lesions. *AJNR Am J Neuroradiol* **21**, 869–74.

82. Nusbaum AO, Tang CY, Wei TC, Buchsbaum MS, Atlas SW (2000). Whole-brain diffusion MR histograms differ between MS subtypes. *Neurology* **54**, 1421–6.

83. Ciccarelli O, Werring DJ, Wheeler–Kingshott CA, *et al* (2001). Investigation of MS normal-appearing brain using diffusion tensor MRI with clinical correlations. *Neurology* **56**, 926–33.

84. Ge Y, Law M, Johnson G, *et al* (2004). Preferential occult injury of corpus callosum in multiple sclerosis measured by diffusion tensor imaging. *J Magn Reson Imaging* **20**, 1–7.

85. Rashid W, Hadjiprocopis A, Griffin CM, *et al* (2004). Diffusion tensor imaging of early relapsing-remitting multiple sclerosis with histogram analysis using automated segmentation and brain volume correction. *Mult Scler* **10**, 9–15.

86. Gallo A, Rovaris M, Riva R, *et al* (2005). Diffusion tensor magnetic resonance imaging detects normal-appearing white matter damage unrelated to short-term disease activity in patients at the earliest stage of multiple sclerosis. *Arch Neurol* **62**, 803–5.

87. Castriota Scanderbeg A, Tomaiuolo F, Sabatini U, Nocentini U, Grasso MG, Caltagirone C (2000). Demyelinating plaques in relapsing-remitting and secondary-progressive multiple sclerosis: assessment with diffusion MR imaging. *AJNR Am J Neuroradiol* **21**, 862–8.

88. Rovaris M, Bozzali M, Iannucci G, *et al* (2002). Assessment of normal-appearing white and gray matter in patients with primary progressive multiple sclerosis. *Arch Neurol* **59**, 1406–12.

89. Schmierer K, Altmann DR, Kassim N, *et al* (2004). Progressive change in primary progressive multiple sclerosis normal-appearing white matter: a serial diffusion magnetic resonance imaging study. *Mult Scler* **10**, 182–7.

90. Wilson M, Tench CR, Morgan PS, Blumhardt LD (2003). Pyramidal tract mapping by diffusion tensor magnetic resonance imaging in multiple sclerosis: improving correlations with disability. *J Neurol Neurosurg Psychiatry* **74**, 203–7.

91. Pagani E, Filippi M, Rocca MA, Horsfield MA (2005). A method for obtaining tract-specific diffusion tensor MRI measurements in the presence of disease: application to patients with clinically isolated syndromes suggestive of multiple sclerosis. *NeuroImage* **26**, 258–65.

92. Bozzali M, Cercignani M, Sormani MP, Comi G, Filippi M (2002). Quantification of brain gray matter damage in different MS phenotypes by use of diffusion tensor MR imaging. *AJNR Am J Neuroradiol* **23**, 985–8.

93. Rovaris M, Gallo A, Valsasina P, *et al* (2005). Short-term accrual of grey matter pathology in patients with progressive multiple sclerosis: an in vivo study using diffusion tensor MRI. *NeuroImage* **15**, 1139–46.

94. Oreja–Guevara C, Rovaris M, Iannucci G, *et al* (2005). Progressive grey matter damage in patients with relapsing remitting MS: a longitudinal diffusion tensor MRI study. *Arch Neurol* **62**, 578–84.

95. Rao SM, Leo GJ, Haughton VM, St Aubin-Faubert P, Bernardin L (1989). Correlation of magnetic resonance imaging with neuropsychological testing in multiple sclerosis. *Neurology* **39**, 161–6.

96. Fabiano AJ, Sharma J, Weinstock–Guttman B, *et al* (2003). Thalamic involvement in multiple sclerosis: a diffusion-weighted magnetic resonance imaging study. *J Neuroimaging* **13**, 307–14.

97. Rovaris M, Iannucci G, Falautano M, *et al* (2002). Cognitive dysfunction in patients with mildly disabling relapsing-remitting multiple sclerosis: an exploratory study with diffusion tensor MR imaging. *J Neurol Sci* **195**, 103–9.

98. Iwasawa T, Matoba H, Ogi A, *et al* (1997). Diffusion-weighted imaging of the human optic nerve: a new approach to evaluate optic neuritis in multiple sclerosis. *Magn Reson Med* **38**, 484–91.

99. Wheeler–Kingshott CA, Parker GJ, Symms MR, *et al* (2002). ADC mapping of the human optic nerve: increased resolution, coverage, and reliability with CSF-suppressed ZOOM-EPI. *Magn Reson Med* **47**, 24–31.

100. Wheeler–Kingshott CA, Hickman SJ, Parker GJ, *et al* (2002). Investigating cervical spinal cord structure using axial diffusion tensor imaging. *NeuroImage* **16**, 93–102.

101. Bammer R, Augustin M, Prokesch RW, *et al* (2002). Diffusion-weighted imaging of the spinal cord: interleaved echo-planar imaging is superior to fast spin-echo. *J Magn Reson Imaging* **15**, 364–73.

102. Clark CA, Werring DJ, Miller DH (2000). Diffusion imaging of the spinal cord in vivo: estimation of the principal diffusivities and application to multiple sclerosis. *Magn Reson Med* **43**, 133–8.

103. Cercignani M, Horsfield MA, Agosta F, Filippi M (2003). Sensitivity-encoded diffusion tensor MR imaging of the cervical cord. *AJNR Am J Neuroradiol* **24**, 1254–6.

104. Valsasina P, Rocca MA, Agosta F, *et al* (2005). Mean diffusivity and fractional anisotropy histogram analysis of the cervical cord in patients with multiple sclerosis. *Neuroimage* **26**, 822–8.

105. Agosta F, Benedetti B, Rocca MA, *et al* (2005). Quantification of cervical cord pathology in primary progressive MS using diffusion tensor MRI. *Neurology* **22**, 631–5.

106. Filippi M, Arnold DL, Comi G (eds) (2001). *Magnetic resonance spectroscopy in multiple sclerosis*. Springer–Verlag, Milan.

107. Bitsch A, Bruhn H, Vougioukas V, Stringaris A, *et al* (1999). Inflammatory CNS demyelination: histopathologic correlation with in vivo quantitative proton MR spectroscopy. *AJNR Am J Neuroradiol* **20**, 1619–27.

108. Davie CA, Hawkins CP, Barker GJ, *et al* (1994). Serial proton magnetic resonance spectroscopy in acute multiple sclerosis lesions. *Brain* **117**, 49–58.

109. De Stefano N, Matthews PM, Antel JP, Preul M, Francis G, Arnold DL (1995). Chemical pathology of acute demyelinating lesions and its correlation with disability. *Ann Neurol* **38**, 901–9.

110. Narayana PA, Doyle TJ, Lai D, Wolinsky JS (1998). Serial proton magnetic resonance spectroscopic imaging, contrast-enhanced magnetic resonance imaging, and quantitative lesion volumetry in multiple sclerosis. *Ann Neurol* **43**, 56–71.

111. Arnold DL, Matthews PM, Francis GS, O'Connor J, Antel JP (1992). Proton magnetic resonance spectroscopic imaging for metabolic characterization of demyelinating plaques. *Ann Neurol* **31**, 235–41.

112. van Walderveen MA, Barkhof F, Pouwels PJ, van Schijndel RA, Polman CH, Castelijns JA (1999). Neuronal damage in T1-hypointense multiple sclerosis lesions demonstrated in vivo using proton magnetic resonance spectroscopy. *Ann Neurol* **46**, 79–87.

113. He J, Inglese M, Li BS, Babb JS, Grossman RI, Gonen O (2005). Relapsing-remitting multiple sclerosis: metabolic abnormality in nonenhancing lesions and normal-appearing white matter at MR imaging: initial experience. *Radiology* **234**, 211–17.

114. Falini A, Calabrese G, Filippi M, *et al* (1998). Benign versus secondary progressive multiple sclerosis: the potential role of ^{1}H MR spectroscopy in defining the nature of disability. *AJNR Am J Neuroradiol* **19**, 223–9.

115. Sarchielli P, Presciutti O, Pelliccioli GP, *et al* (1999). Absolute quantification of brain metabolites by proton magnetic resonance spectroscopy in normal-appearing white matter of multiple sclerosis patients. *Brain* **122**, 513–21.

116. Tartaglia MC, Narayanan S, De Stefano N, *et al* (2002). Choline is increased in pre-lesional normal appearing white matter in multiple sclerosis. *J Neurol* **249**, 1382–90.

117. Fu L, Matthews PM, De Stefano N, *et al* (1998). Imaging axonal damage of normal-appearing white matter in multiple sclerosis. *Brain* **121**, 103–13.

118. De Stefano N, Narayanan S, Francis SJ, *et al* (2002). Diffuse axonal and tissue injury in patients with multiple sclerosis with low cerebral lesion load and no disability. *Arch Neurol* **59**, 1565–71.

119. Suhy J, Rooney WD, Goodkin DE, *et al* (2000). ^{1}H MRSI comparison of white matter and lesions in primary progressive and relapsing-remitting MS. *Mult Scler* **6**, 148–55.

120. De Stefano N, Narayanan S, Francis GS, *et al* (2001). Evidence of axonal damage in the early stages of multiple sclerosis and its relevance to disability. *Arch Neurol* **58**, 65–70.

121. De Stefano N, Matthews PM, Fu L, *et al* (1998). Axonal damage correlates with disability in patients with relapsing-remitting multiple sclerosis. Results of a longitudinal magnetic resonance spectroscopy study. *Brain* **121**, 1469–77.

122. Inglese M, Li BS, Rusinek H, Babb JS, Grossman RI, Gonen O (2003). Diffusely elevated cerebral choline and creatine in relapsing-remitting multiple sclerosis. *Magn Reson Med* **50**, 190–5.

123. Chard DT, Griffin CM, McLean MA, *et al* (2002). Brain metabolite changes in cortical grey and normal-appearing white matter in clinically early relapsing-remitting multiple sclerosis. *Brain* **125**, 2342–52.

124. Fernando KT, McLean MA, Chard DT, *et al* (2004). Elevated white matter myo-inositol in clinically isolated syndromes suggestive of multiple sclerosis. *Brain* **127**, 1361–1369.

125. Davie CA, Barker GJ, Webb S, *et al* (1995). Persistent functional deficit in multiple sclerosis and autosomal dominant cerebellar ataxia is associated with axon loss. *Brain* **118**, 1583–92.

126. Lee MA, Blamire AM, Pendlebury S, *et al* (2000). Axonal injury or loss in the internal capsule and motor impairment in multiple sclerosis. *Arch Neurol* **57**, 65–70.

127. Pan JW, Krupp LB, Elkins LE, Coyle PK (2001). Cognitive dysfunction lateralizes with NAA in multiple sclerosis. *Appl Neuropsychol* **8**, 155–60.

128. Gadea M, Martinez–Bisbal MC, Marti–Bonmati L, *et al* (2004). Spectroscopic axonal damage of the right locus coeruleus relates to selective attention impairment in early stage relapsing-remitting multiple sclerosis. *Brain* **127**, 89–98.

129. Tartaglia MC, Narayanan S, Francis SJ, *et al* (2004). The relationship between diffuse axonal damage and fatigue in multiple sclerosis. *Arch Neurol* **61**, 201–7.

130. Gonen O, Viswanathan AK, Catalaa I, Babb J, Udupa J, Grossman RI (1998). Total brain N-acetylaspartate concentration in normal, age-grouped females: quantitation with non-echo proton NMR spectroscopy. *Magn Reson Med* **40**, 684–9.

131. Gonen O, Catalaa I, Babb JS, *et al* (2000). Total brain N-acetylaspartate. A new measure of disease load in MS. *Neurology* **54**, 15–19.

132. Bonneville F, Moriarty DM, Li BS, Babb JS, Grossman RI, Gonen O (2002). Whole-brain N-acetylaspartate concentration: correlation with T2-weighted lesion volume and expanded disability status scale score in cases of relapsing-remitting multiple sclerosis. *AJNR Am J Neuroradiol* **23**, 371–5.

133. Filippi M, Bozzali M, Rovaris M, *et al* (2003). Evidence for widespread axonal damage at the earliest clinical stage of multiple sclerosis. *Brain* **126**, 433–7.

134. Rovaris M, Gallo A, Falini A, *et al* (2005). Axonal injury and overall tissue loss are not related in primary progressive MS. *Arch Neurol* **62**, 898–902.

135. Kapeller P, McLean MA, Griffin CM, *et al* (2001). Preliminary evidence for neuronal damage in cortical grey matter and normal appearing white matter in short duration relapsing-remitting multiple sclerosis: a quantitative MR spectroscopic imaging study. *J Neurol* **248**, 131–8.

136. Sarchielli P, Presciutti O, Tarducci R, *et al* (2002). Localized (1) H magnetic resonance spectroscopy in mainly cortical gray matter of patients with multiple sclerosis. *J Neurol* **249**, 902–10.

137. Sharma R, Narayana PA, Wolinsky JS (2001). Grey matter abnormalities in multiple sclerosis: proton magnetic resonance spectroscopic imaging. *Mult Scler* **7**, 221–6.

138. Kapeller P, Brex PA, Chard D, *et al* (2002). Quantitative^{1}H MRS imaging 14 years after presenting with a clinically isolated syndrome suggestive of multiple sclerosis. *Mult Scler* **8**, 207–10.

139. Adalsteinsson E, Langer–Gould A, Homer RJ, *et al* (2003). Gray matter N-acetyl aspartate deficits in secondary progressive but not relapsing-remitting multiple sclerosis. *AJNR Am J Neuroradiol* **24**, 1941–5.

140. Cifelli A, Arridge M, Jezzard P, Esiri MM, Palace J, Matthews PM (2002). Thalamic neurodegeneration in multiple sclerosis. *Ann Neurol* **52**, 650–3.

141. Wylezinska M, Cifelli A, Jezzard P, Palace J, Alecci M, Matthews PM (2003). Thalamic neurodegeneration in relapsing-remitting multiple sclerosis. *Neurology* **60**, 1949–54.

142. Inglese M, Liu S, Babb JS, Mannon LJ, Grossman RI, Gonen O (2004). Three-dimensional proton spectroscopy of deep gray matter nuclei in relapsing-remitting MS. *Neurology* **63**, 170–2.

143. Waxman SG, Ritchie JM (1993). Molecular dissection of the myelinated axon. *Ann Neurol* **33**, 121–36.

144. De Stefano N, Matthews PM, Arnold DL (1995). Reversible decreases in N-acetylaspartate after acute brain injury. *Magn Reson Med* **34**, 721–7.

145. Waxman SG (1998). Demyelinating diseases: New pathological insights, new therapeutic targets. *New Engl J Med* **338**, 323–6.

146. Filippi M, Rocca MA, Colombo B, *et al* (2002). Functional magnetic resonance imaging correlates of fatigue in multiple sclerosis. *NeuroImage* **15**, 559–67.

147. Filippi M, Rocca MA, Falini A, *et al* (2002). Correlations between structural CNS damage and functional MRI changes in primary progressive MS. *NeuroImage* **15**, 537–46.

148. Rocca MA, Falini A, Colombo B, Scotti G, Comi G, Filippi M (2002). Adaptive functional changes in the cerebral cortex of patients with non-disabling MS correlate with the extent of brain structural damage. *Ann Neurol* **51**, 330–9.

149. Rocca MA, Mezzapesa DM, Falini A, *et al* (2003). Evidence for axonal pathology and adaptive cortical reorganisation in patients at presentation with clinically isolated syndromes suggestive of MS. *NeuroImage* **18**, 847–55.

150. Rocca MA, Gavazzi C, Mezzapesa DM, *et al* (2003). A functional magnetic resonance imaging study of patients with secondary progressive multiple sclerosis. *NeuroImage* **19**, 1770–7.

151. Rocca MA, Pagani E, Ghezzi A, *et al* (2003). Functional cortical changes in patients with MS and non-specific conventional MRI scans of the brain. *NeuroImage* **19**, 826–36.

152. Reddy H, Narayanan S, Woolrich M, *et al* (2002). Functional brain reorganization for hand movement in patients with multiple sclerosis: defining distinct effects of injury and disability. *Brain* **125**, 2646–2657.

153. Werring DJ, Bullmore ET, Toosy AT, *et al* (2000) Recovery from optic neuritis is associated with a change in the distribution of cerebral response to visual stimulation: a functional magnetic resonance imaging study. *J Neurol Neurosurg Psychiatry* **68**, 441–9.

154. Toosy AT, Werring DJ, Bullmore ET, *et al* (2002). Functional magnetic resonance imaging of the cortical response to photic stimulation in humans following optic neuritis recovery. *Neurosci Lett* **330**, 255–9.

155. Russ MO, Cleff U, Lanfermann H, *et al* (2002). Functional magnetic resonance imaging in acute unilateral optic neuritis. *J Neuroimaging* **12**, 339–50.

156. Rombouts SA, Lazeron RH, Scheltens P, *et al* (1998). Visual activation patterns in patients with optic neuritis: an FMRI pilot study. *Neurology* **50**, 1896–9.

157. Langkilde AR, Frederiksen JL, Rostrup E, Larsson HB (2002). Functional MRI of the visual cortex and visual testing in patients with previous optic neuritis. *Eur J Neurol* **9**, 277–86.

158. Filippi M, Rocca MA, Mezzapesa DM, *et al* (2004). Simple and complex movement-associated functional MRI changes in patients at presentation with clinically isolated syndromes suggestive of MS. *Hum Brain Map* **21**, 108–17.

159. Rocca MA, Mezzapesa DM, Ghezzi A, *et al* (2005). A widespread pattern of cortical activations in patients at presentation with clinically isolated syndromes is associated with evolution to definite multiple sclerosis. *AJNR Am J Neuroradiol* **26**, 1136–9.

160. Bookheimer SY, Strojwas MH, Cohen MS, *et al* (2000). Patterns of brain activation in people at risk for Alzheimer's disease. *N Engl J Med* **343**, 450–6.

161. Smith CD, Andersen AH, Kryscio RJ, *et al* (2002). Women at risk for AD show increased parietal activation during a fluency task. *Neurology* **58**, 1197–202.

162. Filippi M, Rocca MA (2003). Disturbed function and plasticity in multiple sclerosis as gleaned from functional magnetic resonance imaging. *Curr Opin Neurol* **16**, 275–82. Review.

163. Calautti C, Baron JC (2003). Functional neuroimaging studies of motor recovery after stroke in adults: a review. *Stroke* **34**, 1553–66. Review.

164. Pantano P, Iannetti GD, Caramia F, *et al* (2002). Cortical motor reorganization after a single clinical attack of multiple sclerosis. *Brain* **125**, 1607–15.

165. Pantano P, Mainero C, Iannetti GD, *et al* (2002). Contribution of corticospinal tract damage to cortical motor reorganization after a single clinical attack of multiple sclerosis. *NeuroImage* **17**, 1837–43.

166. Lee M, Reddy H, Johansen–Berg H, *et al* (2000). The motor cortex shows adaptive functional changes to brain injury from multiple sclerosis. *Ann Neurol* **47**, 606–13.

167. Reddy H, Narayanan S, Matthews PM, *et al* (2000). Relating axonal injury to functional recovery in MS. *Neurology* **54**, 236–9.

168. Reddy H, Narayanan S, Arnoutelis R, *et al* (2000). Evidence for adaptive functional changes in the cerebral cortex with axonal injury from multiple sclerosis. *Brain* **123**, 2314–20.

169. Rocca MA, Gallo A, Colombo B, *et al* (2004). Pyramidal tract lesions and movement-associated cortical recruitment in patients with MS. *NeuroImage*, **23**, 141–7.

170. Lowe MJ, Phillips MD, Lurito JT, *et al* (2002). Multiple sclerosis: low-frequency temporal blood oxygen level-dependent fluctuations indicate reduced functional connectivity initial results. *Radiology* **224**, 184–92.

171. Rocca MA, Matthews PM, Caputo D, *et al* (2002). Evidence for widespread movement-associated functional MRI changes in patients with PPMS. *Neurology* **58**, 866–72.

172. Rocca MA, Mezzapesa DM, Ghezzi A, *et al* (2003). Cord damage elicits brain functional reorganization after a single episode of myelitis. *Neurology* **61**, 1078–85.

173. Rocca MA, Agosta F, Mezzapesa DM, *et al* (2004). A functional MRI study of movement-associated cortical changes in patients with Devic's neuromyelitis optica. *NeuroImage* **21**, 1061–8.

174. Filippi M, Rocca MA, Mezzapesa DM, *et al* (2004). A functional MRI study of cortical activations associated with object manipulation in patients with MS. *NeuroImage* **21**, 1147–54.

175. Morgen K, Kadom N, Sawaki L, *et al* (2004). Training-dependent plasticity in patients with multiple sclerosis. *Brain* **127**, 2506–17.

176. Audoin B, Ibarrola D, Ranjeva JP, *et al* (2003). Compensatory cortical activation observed by FMRI during a cognitive task at the earliest stage of MS. *Hum Brain Mapp* **20**, 51–8.

177. Audoin B, Van Au Duong M, Ranjeva JP, *et al* (2004). Magnetic resonance study of the influence of tissue damage and cortical reorganization on PASAT performance at the earliest stage of multiple sclerosis. *Hum Brain Mapp* **24**, 216–28.

178. Staffen W, Mair A, Zauner H, *et al* (2002). Cognitive function and FMRI in patients with multiple sclerosis: evidence for compensatory cortical activation during an attention task. *Brain* **156**, 1275–82.

179. Hillary FG, Chiaravalloti ND, Ricker JH, *et al* (2003). An investigation of working memory rehearsal in multiple sclerosis using FMRI. *J Clin Exp Neuropsychol* **25**, 965–78.

180. Wishart HA, Saykin AJ, McDonald BC, *et al* (2004). Brain activation patterns associated with working memory in relapsing-remitting MS. *Neurology* **62**, 234–8.

181. Sweet LH, Rao SM, Primeau M, Mayer AR, Cohen RA (2004). Functional magnetic resonance imaging of working memory among multiple sclerosis patients. *J Neuroimaging* **14**, 150–7.

182. Li Y, Chiaravalloti ND, Hillary FG, *et al* (2004). Differential cerebellar activation on functional magnetic resonance imaging during working memory performance in persons with multiple sclerosis. *Arch Phys Med Rehabil* **85**, 635–9.

183. Parry AM, Scott RB, Palace J, Smith S, Matthews PM (2003). Potentially adaptive functional changes in cognitive processing for patients with multiple sclerosis and their acute modulation by rivastigmine. *Brain* **126**, 2750–60.

184. Mainero C, Caramia F, Pozzilli C, *et al* (2004). FMRI evidence of brain reorganization during attention and memory tasks in multiple sclerosis. *NeuroImage* **21**, 858–67.

185. Penner IK, Rausch M, Kappos L, Opwis K, Radu EW (2003). Analysis of impairment related functional architecture in MS patients during performance of different attention tasks. *J Neurol* **250**, 461–72.

12

FMRI and pharmacology: what role in clinical practice?

Garry D. Honey and Edward T. Bullmore

1. Overview of the chapter

FMRI has had an enormous impact on cognitive neuroscience research. This technique, which allows us to investigate the functioning of the living human brain, has contributed significantly to the rapid progress witnessed in recent years in understanding the neural basis of human thought, action, and emotions. The technology is applied with increasing sophistication to address questions beyond experimental manipulation prior to its inception. The application of FMRI naturally turned toward psychiatric and neurological disease states, with optimistic early predictions of unprecedented advances in our understanding of cerebral dysfunction and radical breakthroughs in its treatment. It is now a little over a decade since the first studies involving FMRI in clinical populations were reported, and one might reasonably conclude that FMRI has yet to fulfil these initial, and with hindsight, perhaps unrealistic expectations. However, whilst clinical breakthroughs may not yet have emerged, considerable progress has been made in understanding the neurobiological basis of a number of diseases of the nervous system. A significant contribution to this progress has been via the combined application of FMRI with pharmacological manipulations, visualizing, albeit indirectly, the changes in brain function following exposure to both clinical pharmacotherapeutics and compounds in experimental medicine. Pharmacological imaging thereby offers a unique insight into disease pathology and its treatment. In this chapter, we consider the extent to which its application has contributed towards greater understanding in this area; for a related review of clinical applications of FMRI see Matthews et al.[71].

We begin by considering the methodological challenges in the use of FMRI in general and specifically those which pertain to the combined application of pharmacological challenge with FMRI, termed 'phMRI'. Whilst subsequent sections cover the clinical application of phMRI in patients with cerebral disorders, we begin our appraisal by reviewing the use of pharmacological probes in healthy subjects as a means to further understanding the transmitter basis of neurocognitive function. We believe this is directly relevant to evaluating the clinical impact of phMRI, since psychiatric and neurological conditions centrally involve disorders of neurocognition. In extending this to patient studies, we consider the role of phMRI in predicting treatment response and characterising transmitter dysfunction. The use of psychopharmacological models of psychiatric conditions is also presented as a complementary approach which may circumvent some of the difficulties encountered in patient studies. Finally, we consider the use of phMRI to investigate functional dysconnectivity as a pathophysiological disease mechanism. We conclude by suggesting that the translation from phMRI research to clinical management at the bedside may not yet have occurred, but that this field, still in its infancy, continues to hold considerable promise for future developments in drug discovery, disease prognosis, and characterising neurotransmitter (dys)function.

2. Methodological considerations

2.1 The blood–oxygen level dependent (BOLD) contrast: implications for pharmacological investigations

2.1.1 The BOLD signal

The BOLD contrast is the cerebrovascular mechanism by which neuronal activity can be indirectly indexed using magnetic resonance imaging (MRI). Functional MRI (FMRI) is based on the mismatch between oxygen consumption and blood supply. Neuronal activity leads to an initial transient (100–200ms) increase in oxygen consumption and concomitant increased deoxyhaemoglobin concentration. This is followed by increased local capillary blood flow and oxygen delivery to the activated region lasting several seconds. However, oxygen consumption does not increase proportionately with hyperoxemia. This causes a marked decrease in the ratio of deoxyhaemoglobin compared to oxyhaemoglobin concentration in that region and, consequently, produces an increase in the MR signal due to increased T2* relaxation time. The change in the local vasculature which is initiated by neuronal activity does not reach its peak instantaneously but takes several seconds to develop and decay. The BOLD response measured in FMRI, therefore, provides an indirect measure of the temporospatial pattern of neuronal activity, in the context of a haemodynamic lag, which smoothes and delays the signal. It is generally the underlying neuronal activity which is of interest in FMRI research and, thus, statistical procedures must be used to account for the haemodynamic delay.

2.1.2 Pharmacological modulation of neurovascular coupling

The experimental design used in phMRI involves introducing a centrally active pharmacological manipulation. Therefore, an important consideration is whether the compound itself interferes with the neurovascular coupling central to the BOLD response. Observed drug effects on the BOLD signal could potentially be mediated by cerebral vasoactivity rather than a direct neuronal effect. This confound can be mitigated, to some extent, given a region-specific pharmacological modulation of task-related activation in the absence of an effect in a related cognitive paradigm. This would be difficult to reconcile with a simple neurovascular explanation of the drug effect, since a non-specific (non-neuronal) mechanism would be expected to similarly perturb the BOLD response from a given region, regardless of the nature of the cognitive task.

More direct evidence awaits development of simultaneous acquisition of data from vascular-based technologies, such as FMRI, with that of direct neuronal-based measurements, such as electroencephalography (EEG). The combined application of these techniques promises to enhance functional imaging considerably, incorporating the temporal resolution of electrophysiology (in the order of milliseconds), and the spatial resolution of MR (in the order of millimetres). In lieu of this, acquisition of EEG and FMRI data in separate sessions within subjects under identical drug conditions has indicated that dopaminergic drug effects can be observed using phMRI. Arthurs *et al.* demonstrated that sulpiride has similar effects on the power law relationship observed between the objective intensity of somatosensory stimulation and both BOLD and evoked-potential responses, indicating that FMRI and electrophysiological data provide convergent indicators of drug effects on stimulus-response parameters[1]. Pharmacological manipulations are, therefore, potentially interpretable at a neuronal level using vascular-based functional imaging techniques such as FMRI. However, in the absence of direct simultaneous neuronal measurements, caution must be taken to exclude vascular confounds.

An alternative, though circumstantial approach frequently employed is to acquire data under several task conditions, with the aim to demonstrate regional specificity of the drug-related effect. Whilst this is indirectly consistent with a neural rather than vascular response, one must acknowledge that the spatial distribution of transmitter receptors throughout the brain is non-uniform, thus demonstrating, for example, that a dopaminergic compound is associated with a modulation of limbic but not occipital function could also be argued as a reflection of the discrepancy in dopaminergic receptors in these regions, which are known to interact with the cerebral vasculature. Perhaps more convincing is to demonstrate both task and regional specificity of the pharmacological effect. For example, the observation of a drug effect on the lateral frontal cortex during a working memory task may be more confidently related to the disruption of the process-dependent function of this region if it could also be demonstrated that the same regional response is unaffected during, for example, its involvement in a semantic categorization task. This would again provide circumstantial evidence in support of a primary neural effect of the drug response, though one would also need to interpret this cautiously, since the vascular decoupling could be dependent on the amplitude of the response, which may differ across tasks. Ultimately, whilst such indirect approaches provide important corroborative information, the definite ruling out of a vascular explanation would require non-vascular data, such as electrophysiological measures.

2.1.3 Behavioural and physiological levels of description

A related issue is how to interpret drug-related changes in BOLD response in the absence of behavioural changes. A nihilistic view might be that drug effects on BOLD in the absence of behavioural correlates are cerebrovascular in origin or otherwise epiphenomenal. However, there are strong grounds for suggesting that FMRI may be more informative than behaviour as an indicator of underlying neurocognitive function[2], and that FMRI may offer superior sensitivity as a pharmacodynamic assay.

Consider, for example, that a drug challenge administered during the performance of a cognitive task requiring verbal processing causes the subject to adopt an alternative (e.g. spatial) strategy in order to maintain task performance. If such drug-related adaptations in cognition are successful in maintaining task performance, these may not be evident using standard behavioural measures such as response accuracy or reaction time. However, one might expect that the adaptive use of a spatial strategy would lead to the recruitment of a different network of brain regions, engaging a primarily right-hemi-spheric spatial attention network, in contrast to a lateralized left- hemispheric response to the verbal task under placebo conditions.

Similarly, faced with a pharmacological challenge, the task may place greater demands on the subject's cognitive effort required to complete the task. If this increased demand remained within the subject's performance capacity, behavioural measurements may be insensitive to this change. Physiologically, the increased demand may be reflected by increases in local signal amplitude or increased functional connectivity between regions. Indeed, examples discussed later in the chapter demonstrate instances of 'physiological inefficiency' in patient groups (i.e. increased physiological activation is required to achieve the same level of cognitive performance). The directional effect of both increases and decreases in physiological response may, therefore, be informative under conditions in which the behavioural response is silent. Of course, one could conceivably design cognitive experiments to test hypotheses of drug-related changes in strategy modification or increased cognitive effort at a behavioural level. Indeed, functional imaging is most appropriately employed synergistically alongside behavioural experiments to guide psychological theory, with imaging data prompting the design of subsequent targeted behavioural experiments, and vice versa.

Neurophysiological and behavioural assessments are clearly different levels of description within cognitive psychology, and the absence of an observed effect of drug treatment at one level does not render an effect at the other any less meaningful. A comprehensive understanding of psychopharmacological effects will clearly require a multidisciplinary approach. Human studies cross-validating FMRI measures of drug action with behavioural, electrophysiological, and perfusion-weighted MRI measures, and non-human primate studies comparing drug effects on BOLD signal to local field potentials, axonal firing rates, and other direct indices of neuronal activity, will be invaluable in achieving this goal.

2.2 Task-dependent and task-independent measures

Psychopharmacological investigations using FMRI can be categorized into two distinct approaches. The first, and most frequently employed method, is to acquire FMRI data whilst the subject is performing a cognitive task, in the presence of both drug and placebo treatments, presented in randomized order to avoid order effects of repeated measures. Such experimental designs allow the observation of pharmacological modulation of task-related brain activation. The results are, therefore, potentially informative both about the pharmacodynamics of the drug, so-called 'neurocognitive profiling' of a novel compound, and the transmitter mechanisms normally underpinning neurocognitive systems. The second approach, more commonly used in anesthetized animals in which cognitive responses during imaging are precluded in non-primates, is to identify BOLD signal changes which follow the administration of a bolus. The pharmacodynamic and pharmacokinetic effects can thus be evaluated by observing changes in BOLD response which correlates with the fluctuations in arterial concentrations of the drug following administration.

2.3 phMRI in animal models

Psychopharmacological research depends, to a large extent, on the use of animal models for invasive procedures which are unfeasible in humans. The combination of psychopharmacological animal models and phMRI considerably increases the sensitivity of the technique: contrast agents can be introduced to increase the signal-to-noise ratio (SNR), and the use of high field strengths such as 9.4 Tesla (T) and 11.7T provide exquisite spatial resolution, up to an in-plane resolution of 300 micrometres in the rodent brain. The resolution afforded by these high field strength magnets is superior to that available in human studies. Field strength in human studies is limited by safety considerations and the size of the magnetic bore; human phMRI is typically performed using 1.5 and 3T magnets.

The combination of phMRI with more invasive techniques developed in animal research provides an unprecedented opportunity in neuroscience. For example, intra-cerebroventricular (ICV) administration of compounds with low penetration of the blood–brain barrier extends the use of phMRI to neuroactive substances, such as neuropeptides, for which systemic administration would result in insufficient brain concentration. Using this method, Gozzi et al.[3] reported a rapid onset and sustained increase in relative cerebral blood volume (rCBV) in the amygdala, basal ganglia, and cerebral cortex following administration of a potent neurokinin NK_1 receptor agonist (see Fig. 12.1). This extends the application of phMRI to a variety of clinical conditions in which dysfunction of neuropetides has been implicated, including eating disorders, hypothalamic disorders, and oncology.

The sensitivity and validity of phMRI for measuring metabolic activation resulting from direct dopaminergic stimulation has been confirmed by comparisons between phMRI and more conventional methods, including microdialysis and positron emission

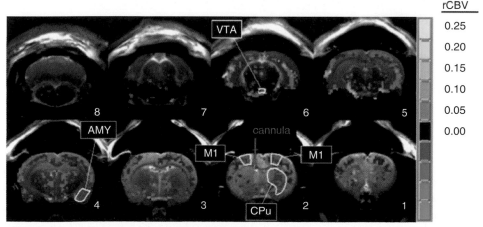

Fig. 12.1 Effects of intracerebroventricular administration of a NK1 receptor agonist (GR-73632) on regional cerebral volume in rats. (Reproduced with permission from Elsevier Publishers[3].)

tomography (PET). Chen *et al.*[4] showed that increasing dopamine levels following administration of D-amphetamine or a dopamine transporter antagonist, produced increased activation in dopamine-rich brain regions (frontal cortex, striatum, and cingulate cortex), which was ipsilaterally abolished following unilateral ablation using 6-hydroxydopamine (6-OHDA). The time-course of the BOLD signal for both compounds was observed to parallel changes observed using microdialysis, and correlated with receptor binding profiles obtained using PET and behavioural measurements of rotation in the lesioned animals.

The advantages of increased sensitivity afforded by the combined application of phMRI and animal models provides a powerful approach in clinical neuroscience. However, clinically oriented animal research is of course open to question on the basis of cross-species variations in structural and functional neuroanatomy, and species-specific responses to pharmacological challenge. Interpretation of animal-based phMRI research for the purposes of understanding human brain (dys)function, as with any other technique, must take these factors into account. Whilst some studies have investigated these issues and confirmed considerable functional homology (for example, for visually-guided saccades[5]), there are few comparative phMRI studies which have directly evaluated drug-induced metabolic activation across species within the same study.

A further consideration in the interpretation of animal phMRI is the concurrent use of general anaesthesia. Whilst non-human primates can be acclimatized to the scanning environment, studies involving rodents require the animal to be anaesthetized. This is frequently achieved using α-chloralose in preference to halothane (more commonly used for surgical procedures), due to its reduced propensity to depress the CNS, whilst achieving adequate anaesthesia. However, this raises the question of whether the anaesthetic agent itself may disrupt the neuronal-haemodynamic coupling underlying the BOLD response. Austin *et al.*[6] recently reported that the BOLD response to forepaw stimulation increased under α-chloralose compared to halothane anaesthesia, but that this occurred slowly over a six-hour period. As the authors point out, this could, therefore, bias physiological measurements which extend over a period of several hours. Whilst neuronal responses were observed to be stable under halothane anaesthesia, vascular reactivity may be reduced. In addition, the possibility of regional differences in the sensitivity to anaesthesia may also confound interpretation of these studies. The use of anaesthetic agents in FMRI studies therefore remains a contentious issue, and extrapolation of results to clinical research must be considered with caution at this stage.

2.4 Relative strengths and weaknesses of phMRI

There are a number of advantages of FMRI which primarily relate to its non-invasiveness, spatio-temporal resolution, and financial cost. These advantages have specific implications for phMRI. FMRI does not involve exposure to ionizing radiation. This is a critical advantage in relation to other imaging techniques, such as PET and SPECT, particularly given the parity of results obtained from direct comparisons of FMRI and PET. This is of special importance to phMRI studies in which repeated measures within-subject designs are crucial in confidently establishing pharmacological effects on physiological function, given that between-subject variability in BOLD response may seriously confound interpretation of between-group comparisons in phMRI. Similarly, the use of functional imaging to track disease-related changes over time, or treatment effects, necessarily requires a longitudinal design, thus the capability to perform repeated assessments on each subject, and the reduced financial cost of the procedure in relation to other techniques such as PET, is a critical consideration and represents a distinct advantage of phMRI for clinical applications.

The primary disadvantages of FMRI are the scanning environment and the vascular basis of the BOLD response. The scanning environment involves a narrow enclosure inside the bore of the magnet in which subjects lie. This can occasionally elicit feelings of anxiety and claustrophobia, which may confound anxiolytic or anxiogenic effects of a drug. From a safety perspective, the scanning environment also hinders observation of the patient, thus limiting the type of behavioural responses to drug manipulations that can be monitored in the scanner, the types of tasks that can be performed, and the types of drugs that can be administered where continuous patient observation can be safely waived. As discussed earlier (see 2.1.2), the primary disadvantage in applying FMRI to pharmacological questions is the problem of determining whether the drug response represents an effect at the neural level, or effects the nature of the indirect vascular index of neural activity. In addition, because phMRI involves a vascular-based measure, one has only indirect quantification of the level of drug at the effect site (e.g. drug plasma levels), in comparison to PET where it is possible to obtain an estimate of receptor occupancy. This is an important consideration as there is likely to be considerable inter-subject differences of drug availability at the effect site, as reflected in the wide variation in inter-subject pharmacokinetics.

2.5 Necessary and sufficient brain activation

A limitation of phMRI is that FMRI can reveal only the engagement of neural systems which are *correlated* with cognitive function, but cannot address the question of which regions are *necessary* or *sufficient* for the performance of a given function. As a cognitive process is experimentally manipulated, PET and FMRI provide a remarkable capability to visualize the brain regions which show task-related responsivity. By extension, phMRI identifies brain regions in which pharmacological modulation of task-related activity is observed. However, whilst the results of increasingly focussed experimental paradigms can be persuasively argued to represent a causal relationship, ultimately this cannot be demonstrated satisfactorily using these techniques in isolation. With regard to phMRI, this means that one cannot determine with certainty whether observed drug modulation of task-related activity is affecting a region which is actually *necessary* for performance of the task, only that which is *associated* with task performance.

The identification of regions which are *necessary* for task performance can only be determined conclusively using other methodological approaches which involve perturbed function, such as transcranial magnetic stimulation (TMS). TMS allows experimental manipulation of regional neuronal activity by applying a brief, high-amplitude pulse of current which temporarily interferes with the activity of local neurons. The observation of impaired cognitive performance following local disruption of neural activity in a given region indicates that the functional integrity of a region is *necessary* for performance of a task.

In summary, phMRI provides a unique window on the physiological effects of drug challenge. This has enormous potential for understanding the mechanisms of both disease processes and therapeutic interventions. However, appropriate interpretation of phMRI data requires an understanding of the nature of the measurement, the limitations of the scope of the technique, and an appreciation of information acquired from comparable and complementary approaches.

3. Pharmacological modulation of neurocognitive function in healthy subjects

3.1 Neuropsychopharmacological research and clinical practice

Whilst the emphasis of this chapter is on the impact that pharmacological applications of FMRI have made on clinical practice, and its future potential to do so, the increasingly influential role phMRI plays in understanding the neurobiological basis of neurocognitive functions is also an important factor in evaluating its clinical relevance. Pharmacological imaging studies have already contributed considerably to this endeavour, and given the increasing consensus that cognitive dysfunction is not epiphenomenal but central to a number of neuropsychiatric disorders, such research is likely to have a significant clinical impact. Below, we review pharmacological challenge studies in healthy volunteers using phMRI which have examined the neurophysiological effects of drug manipulations on cognitive function. These are grouped according to the primary neurotransmitter system targeted by the experimental design.

3.2 Dopamine

The dopaminergic system, centrally involved in the afferentation of key cortical and sub-cortical regions, has been implicated in motor and neurocognitive functions, as well as in a range of psychiatric and neurological conditions, including Parkinson's disease, schizophrenia, Huntington's disease, and substance addiction. Accordingly, the dopaminergic system has been the focus of a number of phMRI studies aimed at further understanding the role of dopamine in various aspects of cognition, using pharmacological agents to augment and deplete transmitter availability.

A powerful approach frequently employed in animal studies to determine the specific involvement of a transmitter system in a given cognitive function or physiological response is to incorporate pharmacological manipulations which have opposing effects on a neurotransmitter or receptor subtype. The observation of opposing cognitive/physiological effects in parallel with the contrasting pharmacological manipulations provides compelling evidence for the involvement of a transmitter system in a given functional response. This approach was first applied to phMRI data by Bullmore *et al.*[7] investigating the role of the dopaminergic system on the sensitivity of the fronto-striatal system to task repetition.

In a repeated measures, within-subject, placebo-controlled design, healthy elderly subjects were treated with placebo or one of two dopaminergic agents, which served to either increase (methylphenidate) or decrease (sulpiride) dopamine transmission. Subjects performed an objection-location learning paradigm in which both difficulty and practice were manipulated. In order to specify the involvement of the dopaminergic system in these cognitive manipulations, these subjects were compared to an independent group treated on separate occasions with placebo and two non-dopaminergic compounds (scopolamine and diazepam). Modulation of load-related activation of a spatial attention network, comprising premotor, cingulate, and parietal regions, was specific to the dopaminergic system, which showed increased activation during treatment with methylphenidate, reduced activation following sulpiride, and no significant modulation by the non-dopaminergic drugs (see Fig. 12.2).

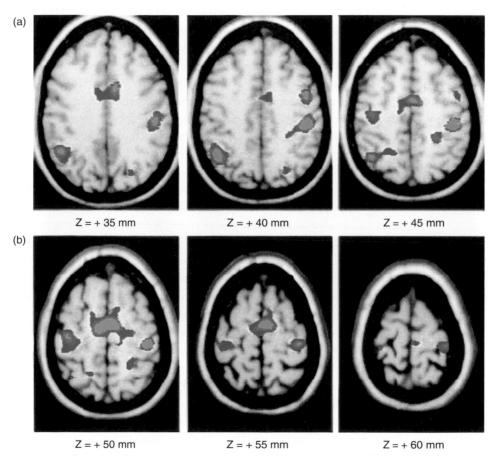

Fig. 12.2 Effects of various drug treatments on (**a**) load response and (**b**) response habituation. (**a**) Sulpiride, methylphenidate, and scopolamine (but not diazepam) attenuated the fronto-striatal response to cognitive load; (**b**) none of the compounds modulated the repetition-suppression effect. (Reproduced with permission from Oxford University Press[7].)

The process specificity of these findings is further supported by a previous study reporting no effect of methylphenidate on the BOLD response during a simple motor task[8], indicating that dopaminergic effects on task difficulty reported by Bullmore *et al.* are unlikely to be neurovascular in origin (however, see also 2.1.2). In addition, opposing effects of the dopaminergic treatments were observed on the inter-regional functional connectivity within the nigro-striatal pathway, between the caudate nucleus and ventral midbrain — increased by sulpiride and decreased by methylphenidate[9]. (This is discussed in greater detail in section 7.) The pharmacological specificity of these findings, in conjunction with the known neurochemistry of the functional pathways involved, persuasively demonstrates the process-dependent contribution of the dopaminergic system.

A similar approach was also recently employed using animal phMRI in which dopamine transmission was either increased using bromocriptine (a D_2 receptor agonist) or reduced using spiperone (a D_2 receptor antagonist)[10]. This study also exemplifies the advantages afforded by the application of phMRI to animal models; in this case, the use of transgenic animals in which a specific gene has been replaced with an inactive or mutated allele, creating 'knock-out' models in which the gene's function has been selectively inactivated. In this study, phMRI was conducted using transgenic mice lacking D_2 receptors, which were compared with wild-type mice with intact D_2 receptors. Consistent with the effects observed in humans, D_2 antagonism reduced activity in the basal ganglia, limbic system, and motor cortex in the wild-type mice, and the D_2 agonist increased activity in the hippocampus. The specificity of these findings in relation to the D_2 receptor were supported by the lack of effect in the knock-out mice.

Relating opposing pharmacological manipulations of a specific transmitter system, or receptor subtype, to cognitive processes or psychiatric phenomenon is likely to be of considerable importance to clinical research, in identifying the functional consequences of disease- or treatment-related effects on specific neurochemical systems. Another key development, using pharmacological imaging to explore the dopaminergic contribution to brain function, has been the advancement in understanding of how genetic mechanisms serve to influence central dopamine levels. The link between dopamine availability, individual cognitive capacity, and response to dopaminergic challenges, such as amphetamine, have led to clinical predictions regarding the efficacy of anti-psychotic treatments. This is discussed in greater detail in section 4.2.

3.3 Acetylcholine

Extensive disruption of the cholinergic system in Alzheimer's disease is thought to underlie the profound memory impairments associated with this illness. Accordingly, phMRI studies have utilized cholinergic pharmacological probes to further understanding of the cholinergic mechanisms which support learning and memory. Scopolamine, a selective muscarinic antagonist, has been proposed as a pharmacological model of Alzheimer's disease and its effects can be reversed by cholinergic agonists, such as the anticholinesterase inhibitor, physostigmine. Below, we consider phMRI studies which have utilized a number of cholinergic perturbations: physostigmine (cholinesterase inhibitor), scopolamine (muscarinic antagonist), and nicotine.

3.3.1 Physostigmine

The first phMRI study to investigate cholinergic modulation of memory systems exploited the temporal resolution of event-related FMRI, in the order of seconds, which allowed the investigators to distinguish drug effects on component processes engaged by task performance which would be technically intractable with other functional neuroimaging techniques. Furey et al.[11] reported that physostigmine increased activation of extrastriate cortex during a working memory paradigm, particularly during encoding, with reduced activation of the prefrontal cortex (see Fig. 12.3). These neurophysiological effects were also associated with improvements in memory performance. The authors interpreted these effects of cholinergic enhancement as augmenting perceptual 'bottom-up' processing of task-relevant stimuli during encoding, resulting in a reduced requirement for 'top-down' prefrontal involvement in the task.

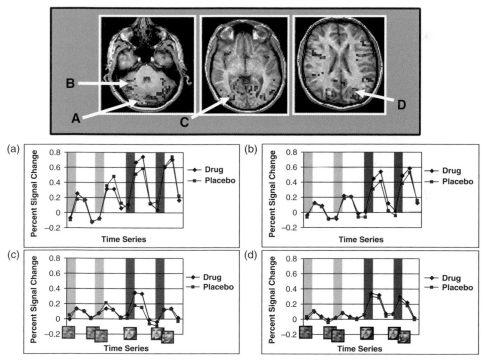

Fig. 12.3 (Upper panel) extrastriate activation during a face working memory task from a single subject; (lower panel) group-averaged time-series from (**a**) ventral occipital, (**b**) ventral temporal, (**c**) dorsal occipital, and (**d**) intraparietal across four conditions (illustrated from left to right at the bottom of the figure: scrambled face encoding; scrambled face working memory; face encoding; face working memory task). Results show regional and task-specific effects of physostigmine (blue) compared to placebo. (Reproduced with permission from the American Association for the Advancement of Science[11].)

Given this system 'tuning' effect of cholinergic enhancement, Thiel *et al.* predicted a facilitatory role for physostigmine in an operant conditioning paradigm, enhancing activation to behaviourally relevant stimuli (CS+) and decreasing response to behaviourally irrelevant stimuli (CS−)[12]. However, conditioning related activations were absent under physostigmine, due to augmented responses to the CS− trials. The suggestion that this discrepancy might reflect a region-specific sensitivity to the effects of cholinergic manipulation was supported in a subsequent study in which physostigmine was shown to enhance activity in the anterior fusiform gyrus in response to attended versus unattended faces, but suppressed the differential response in the posterolateral occipital cortex for attended compared to unattended images of houses[13]. Indeed, the same pattern was observed for null trials, when subjects were cued but no stimulus appeared. Thus, these studies demonstrated that the effect of cholinergic enhancement on selective attention is region-specific within the extrastriate cortex and serves to modify general responsiveness.

3.3.2 Scopolamine

Conversely, inhibition of cholinergic transmission using scopolamine, a potent muscarinic acetylecholine receptor antagonist, has been shown to impair memory processes and attenuate response in associated brain regions. Sperling *et al.*[14] reported that 0.4 mg i.v. scopolamine reduced frontal and hippocampal activation during a face–name associative encoding paradigm, and that the modulation of hippocampal function correlated with the degree of memory impairment associated with scopolamine. Interestingly, similar effects were also observed with the GABA agonist, lorazepam. Importantly, this study also confirmed the test–retest reliability of the cognitive task on functional activation under repeated placebo conditions, giving increased confidence in the interpretation of the effects of drug challenge. Additionally, the authors determined that the drug manipulations were not observed in the striate cortex, lending some support to the interpretation of a direct neural, rather than vascular effect of the drug, though one must treat this with some caution (see 2.1.2). An important question raised by this study is whether the phMRI response reflects transmitter-related modulation, since both cholinergic and GABAergic challenges resulted in similar physiological effects, or more simply reflect impaired behavioural performance. As discussed by the authors, it is possible that both drugs impacted both transmitter systems, given their close promixity and functional interaction in the hippocampus. However, it will be important in future studies to dissociate direct physiological effects of drug challenge from behavioural sequelae.

Another intriguing effect of cholinergic agents has been observed on the repeated presentation of stimuli which results in priming, a reaction time advantage for response to the second stimulus, and 'repetition suppression' of brain activation. Scopolamine has been shown to disrupt both priming of response latency and repetition suppression[15,16]. Intriguingly, in a group of elderly subjects with a mean age of 72 years, no effect of scopolamine on repetition adaptivity was observed, suggesting that functional changes in neurotransmitter systems associated with normal ageing may disrupt the cholinergic contribution to learning and memory[17].

3.3.3 Nicotine

Cholinergic stimulation using agonists such as nicotine has been shown to improve certain cognitive functions associated with the cholinergic system. These cognitive enhancing effects have been investigated in studies involving the administration of nicotine to healthy volunteers to study its effects on working memory[18] and attention[19,20]. Nicotine was found to increase parietal and basal ganglia activity in mildly abstinent smokers during performance of a sustained attention task, and was associated with improved target detection[19]. In non-smokers, Thiel *et al.* found that nicotine reduced parietal activity to non-attended stimuli, and speculated that this suggests a broader focus of attention under nicotine, which may explain the capacity for rapid target detection under the drug[20]. Effects of nicotine on attention and arousal systems may also underlie related improvements in working memory. This was supported by a phMRI study reported by Kumari *et al* in which improvements in accurancy and response latency as a consequence of nicotine exposure during a working memory task were observed in conjunction with modulation of fronto-parietal cortical activation[18]. These cognitive effects appear to be dissociable from the reinforcing properties of nicotine which stimulates the limbic reward system (see 5.4).

More generally, the implications of these effects of nicotine for phMRI studies serve as a reminder that one must carefully consider the characteristics of a selected sample and the impact that myriad factors may exert on the dependent measure. In this respect, phMRI is no different to any other scientific observation that might be made on a random sample of subjects ostensibly representative of a larger population. However, phMRI as a potentially more sensitive index, may reflect these confounds more readily than other measures such as behavioural performance, for example. Where prior evidence exists that commonly used substances may affect the measurement parameter (e.g. nicotine, caffeine, alcohol, marijuana), one should consider screening out these effects where possible, or quantifying them such that appropriate adjustments for their effects can be made. The corollary of this, of course, is the intriguing possibility that widely used substances such as caffeine and nicotine could potentially be used to enhance the sensitivity of FMRI. Mulderink *et al.*[21] suggested that it may be possible to capitalize on the vaso-constriction provided by caffeine, which results in a reduction of cerebral perfusion by 13.2% and a substantial (22–37%) increase in the BOLD contrast. This remains an interesting, though largely unexplored, possibility. However, one would need to firmly establish that such measures taken to enhance the BOLD contrast did not interact with other drug/disease manipulations more central to the experimental objective.

3.4 Gamma aminobutyric acid (GABA)

GABAergic mechanisms have been implicated in the adaptivity of brain systems to repeated presentation of the same task or stimulus. Benzodiazepines have amnestic effects, behaviourally, and can attenuate priming. Thiel *et al.*[16] used an event-related design to demonstrate attenuation by lorazepam of item-specific repetition suppression

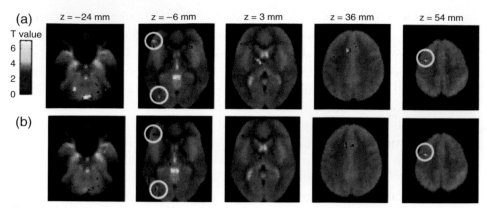

Fig. 12.4 (a) Regions demonstrating repetition-suppression under placebo treatment; **(b)** regions showing a repetition by drug interaction (lorazepam and scopolamine). (Reproduced with permission from the Society for Neuroscience[16].)

in the frontal and extrastriate cortex (see Fig. 12.4). Stephenson *et al.*[22] reported the similar observation that lorazepam abolished repetition adaptivity over a longer time period (minutes) in the context of a blocked periodic working memory experiment. This study also reported a comparable effect of flumazenil, an antagonist at the benzodiazepine binding site on the $GABA_A$ receptor, leading these authors to propose an inverted-U model for the relationship between GABAergic tone and repetition adaptivity. The hypothesis suggests that repetition adaptivity, both attenuation and enhancement of signal with repeated task presentation, and over a range of time scales, might be dependent on dynamic changes in GABAergic tone. Therefore, drugs which act tonically either to increase or decrease GABAergic tone outside the physiologically optimal range are expected to impair systems adaptivity to repeated task presentation. Important non-linear properties of other transmitter systems, notably dopamine, have been reported using a variety of approaches, with considerable clinical impact (see 4.2). It will therefore be important to further explore such non-linear relationships in other transmitter systems.

GABAergic mechanisms have also been strongly implicated in emotional processing, particularly negative affect, hence the clinical use of benzodiazepines in the treatment of anxiety. A phMRI study has suggested a possible neurophysiological mechanism underlying this effect. Northoff *et al.*[23] investigated the role of prefrontal function on affect processing in a double-blind, placebo-controlled study of lorazepam. They reported that the pattern of increased orbitofrontal activity to viewing positive emotional stimuli and decreased activity to negative emotional stimuli observed under placebo treatment was completely reversed under lorazepam. This effect was regionally specific, since the opposite relationship was found under placebo (increased activation to negative and decreased to positive stimuli), but this was unchanged by lorazepam. The authors suggested that this effect of lorazepam may be mediated via $GABA_A$ receptors involved in the projection from the basal nucleus of the amygdala and orbitofrontal cortex, and may contribute to the anxiolytic effect of benzodiazepines in disorders thought to involve the orbitofrontal cortex, such as obsessive compulsive disorder. The neural, as opposed to vascular basis of the effect in this study was supported by magnetoencephalography (MEG) investigations, which revealed a shift in the dipole underlying emotional processing from orbitofrontal to medial prefrontal cortex.

4. Predicting treatment response

4.1 Patient variability to pharmacological intervention

The variability in clinical response to neuropsychiatric therapeutic interventions is considerable, yet relatively little is known of the biological factors which contribute to this. These likely involve myriad sources, including physiological factors such as receptor density, transmitter availability, and drug metabolism; demographic factors such as age, current health status, tobacco use, alcohol intake, and concurrent medication; and psychosocial factors such as immediate support networks, treatment compliance, and insight. These are just a small number amongst many possibilities which may contribute to the variability in patients' response to treatment and explain why a proportion of patients remain refractory. An important challenge for pharmaceutical research is to develop more targeted treatments, identifying patients who are likely to respond to particular interventions. phMRI may play an important role in this endeavour since the physiological response may become apparent prior to the development of the clinical effect and, thereby, serve as a marker to predict outcome. Below we review some of the factors which have been identified in pharmacological imaging studies to be important in characterizing and predicting treatment response.

4.2 Pharmacological imaging and pharmacogenomics

Pharmacogenomics represents the intersection between an individual's genetic predisposition and response to pharmacological treatments. As noted earlier, there are numerous considerations which may influence a patient's treatment response, however it is thought that individual genetic make-up may be the single most important factor determining outcome. Pharmacogenomics aims for a greater understanding in this area and offers the potential for more targeted drug treatments with reduced side-effects, developed from a novel avenue of research in drug discovery. Pharmacogenetic research has already had an influence on clinical medicine, for example, in areas such as oncology, in which genetic screening is used to identify individuals with a deficiency in metabolizing thiopurines and to tailor subsequent chemotherapy.

The combination of pharmacogenetics and functional neuroimaging has produced some of the most important recent developments in neuropsychiatry. A series of landmark studies, reported from the National Institute of Mental Health (NIMH), have exploited the capacity of FMRI to examine inter-subject variability in brain physiology and relate this to variability in response to dopaminergic pharmacological challenge, cognitive

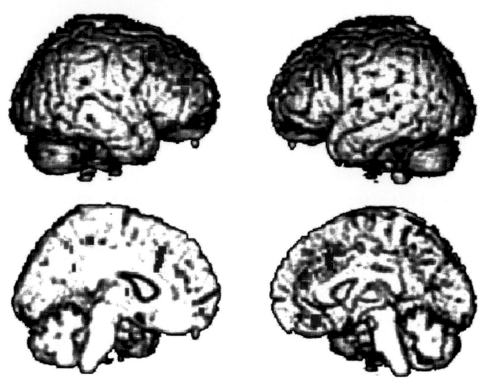

Fig. 12.5 Localization of physiological inefficiency (increased activation in the absence of concomitant increase in performance) in individuals with the Val/Val polymorphism of the COMT gene compared with subjects with the Val/Met allele. (Reproduced with permission from[26].)

capacity, and functional genomics (see Fig. 12.5)[24–29]. The authors investigated the role of dopamine in working memory: a construct in cognitive psychology which describes a limited capacity system for the short-term storage and manipulation of information, which is used to guide subsequent behaviour. Working memory deficits are reported in several clinical populations in which dopaminergic abnormalities are suspected, and disruptions of working memory performance have been reported in animal studies following pharmacological blockade of dopamine D_1 receptors. Mattay *et al.* administered dextroamphetamine, an indirect monaminergic agonist, to healthy volunteers, whilst subjects were scanned performing a working memory task. Intriguingly, the effect of dextroamphetamine varied across individuals: subjects with low working memory capacity prior to drug administration showed improved performance following drug exposure; conversely, subjects with high pre-drug working memory capacity showed performance impairment. Furthermore, the changes in behavioural performance correlated with changes in physiological response: signal change in the dorsolateral prefrontal cortex (DLPFC) was greatest in the subjects whose performance was impaired by the drug. As noted earlier, these results were consistent with an 'inverted-U' relationship between dopaminergic tone and both cognitive performance and BOLD activation, formally analogous to comparable relationships previously demonstrated between dopaminergic tone and single unit activity recorded from prefrontal neurons in non-human primates[30].

Given the relationship between working memory deficits, prefrontal function, and dopaminergic abnormalities in schizophrenia, subsequent investigations explored the possibility of a susceptibility to the illness involving genetic mechanisms regulating the functional recruitment of prefrontal dopamine during performance of working memory tasks. A common polymorphism [val (158)-met] in the catechol O-methyltransferase (COMT) gene, important for metabolism of synaptically released dopamine in the prefrontal cortex, was found to be related to cognitive performance and prefrontal cortical efficiency[26]. The low-activity Met allele predicted both enhanced cognitive performance and more efficient cortical response to the working memory task, whilst increased transmission of the Val allele, resulting in increased prefrontal dopamine catabolism, was observed with increased frequency in patients with schizophrenia.

Relating these findings to the earlier study with amphetamine, a further study demonstrated that the performance-dependent effects of amphetamine on prefrontal function were related to the COMT gene polymorphisms: individuals with the allele coding the more efficient form of the enzyme (Val) demonstrated relatively poor baseline working memory performance and more salient effects of d-amphetamine on prefrontal BOLD signal[28].

These seminal studies are collectively important in establishing the links between cognitive and FMRI measures of dopaminergic drug effects, and in linking both behavioural and physiological phenotypes to underlying allelic variation. There is clearly potential for phMRI to be used more widely in the emerging field of pharmacogenomics. With regard to the clinical implications of phMRI, these studies demonstrate that by using a combination of pharmacological imaging and pharmacogenomics, it is possible to explore the mechanisms by which treatment response is determined. Indeed, the relationship between these genetic variations and treatment outcome was recently investigated by Bertolino *et al.* COMT Val/Met genotyping was reported for 30 patients who had no previous exposure to neuroleptics. Consistent with previous work, loading of the Met allele predicted improvements in working memory, efficiency of prefrontal physiological response, and negative symptoms following eight weeks of treatment with the atypical anti-psychotic, olanzapine. These findings were subsequently replicated in a study incorporating a double-blind, on-off medication, within-subject, placebo-controlled design[29].

In these studies, phMRI data, demonstrating an inverted-U response in the prefrontal cortex to amphetamine challenge, led directly to the identification of the genetic mechanism underlying individual variability in the regulation of prefrontal dopamine levels and, ultimately, to an important contributory factor in determining response to anti-psychotic treatment.

It is possible that phMRI may also have a more direct clinical impact, as these studies raise the intriguing question of whether the physiological changes or the clinical effect occurs first, and whether a causal relationship can be demonstrated. There are strong grounds to suggest that the neurophysiological effect may precede and even predict the clinical effect in the genetically amenable subjects, which typically occurs at around 6–8 weeks post-treatment. Perhaps with more frequent scanning sessions using prospective treatment designs, it may be possible to identify subjects for which an early physiological change is apparent, perhaps in the first days/weeks following treatment, and which is predictive of subsequent remission of psychotic symptoms. This possibility would represent a remarkable breakthrough for clinical psychiatry, facilitating more targeted therapeutic strategies, more rapid assessment of treatment response, and more efficient clinical management. At present, these tantalizing possibilities are yet to be realised, but phMRI has clearly established itself as an important tool in monitoring and investigating treatment response.

5. Characterizing neurochemical changes associated with disease and its treatment

Pharmacological investigations involving healthy volunteers typically incorporate a single acute dosing regime, in which relatively selective compounds are used to target a particular transmitter system or receptor complex. In applying phMRI to clinical research, this experimental design is often not ethical or feasible, or indeed even desirable. In neuropsychiatric conditions, the clinical effects of most treatments emerge over a period of several weeks. Similarly, treatment side-effects, such as extrapyramidal symptoms, typically occur over an extended period of treatment. Whilst chronic dosing cannot be supported in experimental psychopharmacology studies in healthy volunteers on ethical grounds, acute dosing regimes are unlikely to fully characterize the neurobiological mechanisms involved in treatment response and side-effect profiles. Accordingly, careful manipulation of clinical management within a more naturalistic framework has, therefore, provided a productive approach in clinical phMRI studies, to explore the mechanisms of pharmacotherapeutic agents and disease pathophysiology. Below, we review some of the advances that have been made in the understanding of several disorders and associated treatments, using pharmacological imaging studies.

5.1 Schizophrenia: physiological mechanisms of improved efficacy of atypical anti-psychotics

5.1.1 Background

Schizophrenia is a profound mental illness which is chronic and disabling. It is associated with extreme phenomenology, such as hallucinations, delusions, and thought disorder, as well as severe cognitive deficits which encompass the whole spectrum of cognitive functioning, including memory, language, reasoning, attention, and learning. The illness affects 1% of the population and is relatively stable over time and across cultures. Our understanding of this illness is rudimentary; indeed, there is considerable debate as to exactly which symptoms constitute the illness and whether the cluster of symptoms associated with current diagnostic systems actually amount to a reliable and valid disease syndrome. Given this state of nosological disarray and conceptual uncertainty, it is perhaps unsurprising that our current understanding of the neurochemical basis of the disorder(s) and its treatment remains incomplete. There are numerous competing biochemical theories which span the whole range of neurotransmitter systems and their complex interactions, and none of these has yet led to the development of a treatment which is effective in all patients, prevents subsequent relapse, or in the majority of cases, enables patients to return to premorbid levels of social, occupational, or functional status. Pharmacological imaging involving FMRI arguably offers one of the foremost research tools in this area, facilitating *in vivo* clinical investigations of the effects of treatments in human patients. Indeed, it could conceivably lead to a re-definition of current disease taxonomy, based not on phenomenological but physiological criteria. This goal is some way off and there are considerable challenges which must be addressed before this potential may be realised (for review see[17,31]). However, phMRI will likely have a prominent role in this regard.

5.1.2 Potential confounds

A fundamental consideration in any functional imaging study involving psychiatric patients is the potentially confounding effect of anti-psychotic medication. However, the effects of pharmacotherapeutic interventions are frequently overlooked in experimental designs involving medicated psychiatric patients, and have been specifically investigated in relatively few studies. In such circumstances, it may be intractable to dissociate the effects of illness and treatment in the interpretation of any observed group difference. This is particularly problematic in functional imaging studies, in which drug treatment may affect outcome measures on several levels, including cognitive (anti-psychotics may induce cognitive impairment or exacerbate existing deficits associated with the illness), metabolic (anti-psychotics modulate regional cerebral metabolism in regions implicated in the illness), and neurovascular (dopaminergic terminals form synapses in close proximity to the cerebral vasculature and dopamine agonists have been shown to cause vasoconstriction and a global reduction in cerebral perfusion). Studies which aim to characterize the effects of anti-psychotic treatment are, therefore, critical in both advancing understanding of therapeutic mechanisms and also dissociating their effects from core disease processes.

5.1.3 Effects of treatment

The clinical management of patients with schizophrenia has evolved in recent years with the introduction of 'atypical' anti-psychotics. The neurobiological mechanisms which mediate the improved efficacy and reduced parkinsonism associated with these drugs remain unknown. phMRI offers the opportunity to study the effects of these compounds on neurocognitive systems in human patients *in vivo*, and holds considerable promise for future drug discovery and development.

The first phMRI study to investigate the effects of atypical anti-psychotics tested the hypothesis that improvement in negative and cognitive symptoms could reflect remediation of a hypodopaminergic state in the frontal cortex[32]. The authors hypothesized that substituting risperidone for typical anti-psychotics would enhance prefrontal function during performance of a working memory task, hypothetically via increased dopaminergic drive to the prefrontal cortex. This was predicted on the basis that patients with schizophrenia perform poorly on tests of working memory and typically exhibit a hypofrontal response to such tasks, which can be reversed by administration of dopamine agonists[33].

Furthermore, atypical anti-psychotics have been shown to increase prefrontal dopaminergic activity in animal models[34]. Patients treated with typical anti-psychotics were scanned during performance of a working memory task, and then switched to risperidone for six weeks' treatment, following which they were re-scanned. In comparison to patients treated with typical anti-psychotics for the duration of the study, treatment with risperidone was associated with increased activation of the prefrontal cortex, independent of symptomatic change, providing direct evidence of enhanced prefrontal function following atypical anti-psychotic treatment.

The suggestion that improved clinical and cognitive efficacy of atypical anti-psychotics may relate to the modulation of prefrontal function has been supported by subsequent studies which have investigated the physiological changes associated with response to anti-psychotic drug treatments. Quetiapine has a profile of receptor affinity which is broadly similar to that of clozapine and, like clozapine, has been shown to improve certain cognitive functions, including verbal fluency. Using a between-groups comparison, Jones *et al.*[35] reported that healthy volunteers and patients treated with quetiapine showed increased activation of the left inferior frontal cortex during verbal fluency performance compared to unmedicated patients. This is further supported by a similar study recently demonstrating that quetiapine also increased prefrontal response during affect processing, which correlated with improvement in blunted affect-related symptoms[36] (see Fig. 12.6). Nahas *et al.*[37] found that donepezil, an acetylecholinesterase

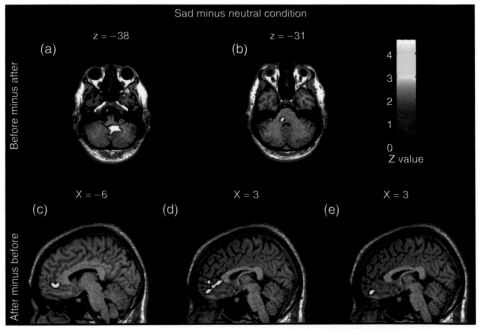

Fig. 12.6 Increased activation in patients with schizophrenia before quetiapine treatment ((**a**) and **b**)) and after treatment (**c**), (**d**), and (**e**). (Reproduced with permission from Elsevier Publishers[36].)

inhibitor which shows potential as a cognitive enhancing adjunctive treatment, produced increased left frontal and cingulate activity during verbal fluency performance after 12 weeks' treatment, compared to placebo. Interestingly, treatment of patients with Alzheimer's disease with donepezil also resulted in increased frontal activity during a working memory task[68] (see below).

Normalization of prefrontal function may, therefore, represent a potential mechanism by which cognitive deficits and symptoms of psychosis are improved following atypical treatment. However, other mechanisms are clearly possible and indeed likely. Using a double-blind, placebo-controlled design, Yurgelun–Todd et al.[38] found that combined D-cycloserine (a partial agonist at the glycine site of the NMDA receptor which improves cognitive function, including working memory) in conjunction with neuroleptic treatment enhanced temporal lobe activation during verbal fluency task performance, which correlated with reduced negative symptoms. It is likely that a regionally circumscribed account will be insufficient in explaining treatment response, and it is likely that the interaction between the prefrontal cortex and other brain regions will be critical. Modulation of inter-regional functional connectivity between regions, implicated in these studies, may suggest a mechanism for anti-psychotic efficacy. The integrative function associated with frontal, temporal, and cingulate regions may, therefore, be a potential target for novel therapeutics, and would be consistent with previous observations reported by Fletcher et al.[69] demonstrating abnormal cingulate modulation of inter-regional fronto-temporal functional connectivity. Effects of anti-psychotics and other pharmacological challenges on functional networks is discussed in greater detail later (see section 7). At present, these studies have identified physiological correlates of treatment response. It remains an appealing question as to whether normalization of frontal function, or its functional connections, represents a necessary prerequisite for cognitive/clinical response, or indeed may serve as an early predictive marker.

Finally, in tracking dynamic physiological changes over the course of treatment response, phMRI has been used in schizophrenia to identify pathophysiological changes which are state-related and resolve following symptom remission, compared to those which are trait-related, enduring beyond treatment response. Bertolino et al.[24,25] noted that following eight weeks of treatment with olanzapine, attenuated activation of the primary motor cortex resolved, in parallel with changes in patients' symptom profile. These findings are consistent with those of Braus et al.[39] who reported that patients treated with atypical anti-psychotics (primarily clozapine) showed normal motor cortex activation. However, Bertolino et al. also reported that the lateralization index of motor cortex response remained abnormal, suggesting a trait deficit in schizophrenia. This may relate to persistent abnormalities in the functional pathways from the cerebellum to motor projection areas (see section 7). The capability offered by using phMRI to perform longitudinal assessments across the disease course, tracking physiological changes which occur with the gradual resolution of psychotic symptoms, will increasingly provide a powerful methodology in neuropsychiatric and neurological disease research to identify and dissociate state- and trait-related pathophysiology.

5.2 Parkinson's disease: implications of dopaminergic transmission for cognitive function

Dopaminergic pathology is an established feature of Parkinson's disease (PD), with degeneration of the substantia nigra pars compacta resulting in disruption of cortico-striato-thalamic circuit function. phMRI offers the opportunity to explore the effects of hypodopaminergia and its therapeutic remediation. Mattay *et al.*[40] used phMRI to test two hypothesized mechanisms to explain frontal hypodopaminergia, thought to underlie the cognitive impairment observed in the illness. Reduced dopamine levels in the frontal cortex may result from impaired output from the caudate nucleus to the frontal cortex via the thalamus. Alternatively, frontal dopamine levels may be reduced resulting from reduced dopaminergic midbrain projections to the frontal cortex. PD patients were scanned during performance of a working memory task and a motor task on two occasions: during a dopamine-replete stage (following dopamimetic therapy) and during a hypodopaminergic phase (12 hours following treatment). They observed that frontal activation during the working memory task was increased in the hypodopaminergic state, which correlated with increased performance errors, indicating inefficiency of prefrontal function, consistent with a primary mesocortical deficit underlying cognitive dysfunction. However, motor cortical regions were more active during the dopamine-replete phase, and this correlated with improved motor function, consistent with increased nigrostriatal dopaminergic transmission following dopaminergic therapy supporting improved motor function. This study therefore confirmed predictions based on animal studies that dopamine supports working memory and motor function via two distinct mechanisms (mesocortical and nigrostriatal pathways respectively), and that these are functionally separable using phMRI. Furthermore, these findings show that neurodegenerative changes in dopaminergic nuclei associated with PD affect multiple, large-scale cortical-subcortical systems in the brain and might be partially restored following dopaminergic repletion.

The observed 'focussing' of prefrontal activity during working memory performance following dopaminergic treatment suggests that additional neural resources are recruited in the hypodopaminergic phase to compensate for the reduced dopaminergic prefrontal drive, and this compensatory response may fail as disease progression occurs. Using an identical design, this group also showed that during the hypodopaminergic stage, PD patients failed to show a normal amygdala response to affect processing which was observed in healthy controls and during the dopamine-replete stage (see Fig. 12.7). These findings suggest that abnormal amygdala function may underlie the occurrence of comorbid depression often seen in patients with PD[41]. However, this finding may be confounded by affective disorders and concurrent use of anti-depressants in the sample reported in this study, and studies involving larger sample sizes will be required to replicate these observations.

5.3 Unipolar depression: limbic pathology and disease prognosis

Patients with depression show enhanced response to negative, affectively valent images (e.g. sad or fearful images). This affective bias is likely to occur as a result of a functional abnormality within the limbic system and may be successfully treated with

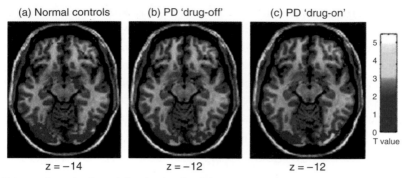

Fig. 12.7 Amygala activation whilst viewing fearful stimuli in healthy volunteers (**a**) and patients with Parkinson's disease before (**b**) and after (**c**) dopaminergic therapy. (Reproduced with permission from the Society for Neuroscience[41].)

anti-depressants. Davidson *et al.*[42] demonstrated that treatment with venlafaxine was associated with normalization of activation in the insular cortex after two weeks of treatment, with further improvement evident at eight weeks, showing normalization of anterior cingulate activity (see Fig. 12.8). The relationship between cingulate activity and treatment response was also replicated in a study involving treatment of depressed

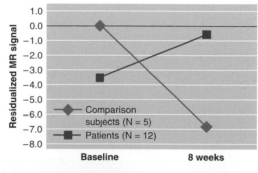

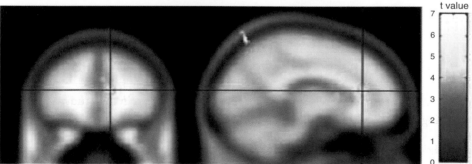

Fig. 12.8 Change over eight weeks in left anterior cingulate cortex activation after exposure to negative relative to neutral stimuli in healthy comparison subjects and depressed patients treated with venlafaxine. (Reproduced with permission from the American Psychiatric Association[42].)

patients with fluoxetine hydrochloride[43]. These changes correspond well to the time-scale of clinical efficacy of anti-depressants and indicate that phMRI is an appropriate tool for evaluating treatment mechanisms in depression. Moreover, phMRI might potentially be used to predict treatment response: consistent with data from other imaging modalities, baseline level of functional activation in the anterior cingulate was related to treatment response at eight weeks[42]. The prospect of tailoring therapy to patients based on an initial FMRI assessment will be of considerable clinical and economic benefit, and future studies are likely to place considerable emphasis on this possibility.

5.4 Substance addiction: physiological correlates of dependence

Animal studies have established that the reinforcing properties of addictive substances are linked to the involvement of the dopaminergic projection from the ventral tegmental area to the nucleus accumbens. phMRI enables research into the neurobiological basis of substance addiction to progress beyond animal models, which are not amenable to measures of subjective experience such as drug craving, 'rush' and 'high'. Breiter et al. demonstrated that regions with early- and short-duration signal maxima, including the ventral tegmentum, pons, basal forebrain, caudate, cingulate and lateral prefrontal cortex, correlated with subjective ratings of rush following cocaine[44]. Regions with early but sustained signal maxima were related to ratings of craving, including the nucleus accumbens, parahippocampal gyrus, and amygdala. Similar activation of reward-related circuitry was also reported for the effects of nicotine[45] and alcohol[46].

The potential translation of these observations to clinical practice was first indicated by Schneider et al.[47] who demonstrated that craving-related activation of subcortical limbic regions in alcoholics, in response to alcohol-related cues, resolved after three weeks of a cognitive-behavioural therapy programme that incorporated controlled abstinence. These findings are unlikely to be related to drug-induced global vascular changes, as reductions in cortical blood flow have been observed in the absence of effects of visual stimulation on the BOLD response following cocaine[48] and nicotine[49].

A further aspect of the abuse of narcotics is the detrimental effects these substances have on cognitive function, in particular memory. A number of studies have examined the physiological correlates of recreational use of 'ecstasy' (3,4-methylenedioxymethamphetamine; MDMA). Daumann et al.[50] found that subjects with extensive exposure to ecstasy (without exposure to other substances but abstinent from recreational use at the time of study) showed reduced activation in the inferior temporal, parietal, and striate cortex during a working memory task compared to polyvalent ecstasy users and subjects without a history of recreational drug use. However, the study did not control for the number of voxels tested, whilst a further study from this group which did correct for multiple comparisons, failed to show an effect of drug use[51]. In a preliminary study of six adolescent ecstasy users, Jacobsen et al.[52] reported that hippocampal deactivation during a working memory task observed in non-drug users was not observed in the ecstasy users, which correlated with the duration of abstinence. The authors suggest that this finding is consistent with the ablation of inhibitory serotonergic modulation of the hippocampus as observed in animal models. Moeller et al.[53] also reported abnormal hippocampal function during a working memory task in MDMA users (as well as in the medial frontal cortex and thalamus/putamen), though the association between duration of time since previous use was not supported in this study. Abnormal hippocampal activity has also been reported in ecstasy users during episodic memory retrieval[54]. However, a complication in this area is that individuals frequently use a variety of stimulants, and each of these studies did not control for the use of other substances and, therefore, cannot at present be specifically related to ecstasy use. Indeed, the only study to date to have reported data on subjects with an exclusive history of ecstasy use found no effect of the drug after appropriate correction[50]. The precise effects of ecstasy on phMRI response, therefore, remains to be determined.

5.5 Alzheimer's disease and mild cognitive impairment: developing early intervention strategies

Alzheimer's disease (AD) is a neurodegenerative illness which involves a progressive cortical atrophy and loss of cholinergic transmission resulting from degeneration of the basal forebrain nuclei. The impact of this is a devastating loss of short-term memory and learning. Current therapies aim to replace the loss of cholinergic function. Functional neuroimaging in this clinical population is technically challenging due to the extensive loss of gray matter tissue and difficulties in achieving satisfactory compliance with the procedure as a result of the confused nature of the patients. Despite this, considerable advances in understanding the functional implications associated with disease progression have been made using FMRI (for review see[70]). The first and to date, only phMRI study, to our knowledge, investigating *in vivo* physiological effects of cholinergic replacement therapy was reported by Rombouts *et al.*[55]. Rivastigmine, a cholinesterase inhibitor, was shown to increase task-related activity in the fusiform gyrus (face encoding task) and the prefrontal cortex (working memory task) in patients with mild AD. These effects may underlie the cognitive benefit of cholinergic replacement in this clinical population.

An alternative, though somewhat controversial approach in studying the progression of dementia is to identify high-risk populations, prior to the onset of the clinical disorder. Individuals with mild cognitive impairment (MCI) show abnormalities in cholinergic function, and whilst prognosis in this group is highly variable, these individuals, or perhaps a subgroup, may represent a precursor of dementia. Current research aims to characterize this further and to determine whether early pharmacological intervention to restore cholinergic levels in these individuals may prevent progression towards AD and other dementias. A further advantage in studying this population is that difficulties noted earlier in using imaging techniques to study patients with dementia are avoided. However, an important consideration in this population is that numerous mechanisms, including non-disease related such as healthy ageing, can result in deteriorating cognitive function. The concept of MCI, therefore, represents a heterogeneous group and the trajectory towards AD is currently uncertain.

Whilst acknowledging these limitations, a promising role for pharmacological imaging in this area is to identify physiological indicators of response to cholinergic treatments as an indicator of prognosis at the earliest possible phase of the illness, when behavioural indices may be too subtle to detect or may be masked by compensatory functional reorganization (as discussed earlier: see 2.1.3). Two phMRI studies have been reported to date in this area. Goekoop et al.[56] scanned MCI patients during performance of a working memory and face encoding task at baseline (prior to treatment), after a single acute dose of a cholinomimetic compound, galantamine, and at steady state after five days' treatment. No changes in FMRI response were observed after acute dosing. Increased frontal, hippocampal, and medial occipital activation was observed following steady-state treatment during the face encoding task, and increased activation of the frontal cortex and precuneus was seen during the working memory task. Saykin et al.[37] found that MCI patients showed reduced fronto-parietal activation during performance of a working memory task, and that after approximately five weeks' treatment with donepezil, increased frontal activation was observed compared to unmedicated controls, which correlated with improved task performance and baseline hippocampal volume.

It will be important to determine, in future studies, whether treatment results in a normalization of function. Saykin et al. found that the increase in fronto-parietal activation resulted in greater activity than observed in controls. Whilst this improved physiological function was clearly beneficial, in that it correlated with task improvement, it remained distinct from the control group, perhaps suggesting that although the MCI group were able to match control level performance after treatment, they were having to exert greater effort, reflected physiologically, in order to do so.

The broader implications of these studies lies in their potential to provide neurobiological support for the prognostic link between MCI and AD, if it can be identified that a pattern of physiological abnormality is predictive of disease progression. A further implication is the possibility that research may be able to identify high-risk subjects for whom early cholinergic therapy may be preventative against further cognitive decline and dementia.

5.6 Multiple sclerosis: understanding adaptive functional reorganization

As discussed earlier, behavioural responses may not be the most appropriate measure in a situation in which drug challenge produces physiological changes to which performance indices are insensitive (see 2.1.3). This is, of course, also true for the disease state, in which physiological abnormalities may cause the patient to modify cognitive performance in ways which are not easily detected using standard neuropsychological techniques. This point is illustrated clearly in the context of functional reorganization in patients with multiple sclerosis (MS).

Cognitive deficits are common in patients with MS but can be difficult to accurately measure due to the possibility of adaptive functional reorganization, and indeed may occur prior to overt clinical symptoms of the illness. This possibility was tested using an elegant design reported by Parry et al.[57]. The authors hypothesized that MS patients who showed intact performance on the Stroop task, likely achieved this via functional reorganization and recruitment of alternative brain regions, since patients with frontal lobe damage perform poorly on this task. They also tested whether this was influenced by cholinergic modulation, since cholinergic therapy has been shown to produce cognitive

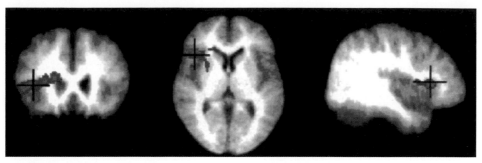

Fig. 12.9 Reduced activation of right inferior frontal cortex and right basal ganglia during performance of the Stroop task in patients with multiple sclerosis compared to healthy controls. (Reproduced with permission from Oxford University Press[57].)

benefit in this patient group. In accordance with the hypothesis, MS patients showed comparable performance but reduced activation of fronto-striatal regions and increased left medial frontal activation, indicating functional reorganization to limit performance impairment (see Fig. 12.9). Moreover, these deficits were normalized in all five subjects treated with rivastigmine, which had no effect in any of the five controls tested. This study provides a clear example of the complementarity of imaging and behavioural assays of disease processes. In addition, it demonstrates that by using phMRI, mean treatment effects observed at the group level can be quantified at the individual level, which is a critical consideration in terms of the clinical utility of the technique. Furthermore, the findings suggest a physiological mechanism which may mediate the clinical benefit of cholinergic therapy, involving facilitation of right prefrontal cortical activity, as observed in patients with AD[55] (see above), eliminating the requirement for functional recruitment of left medial prefrontal activation.

6. **Psychopharmacological modelling and drug discovery**

6.1 **Overview**

An increasingly popular approach in neuropsychiatric research involves the use of psychotomimetic compounds in healthy individuals, reproducing some of the phenomenological features of psychosis. Current research aims to determine the extent to which the neurobiological aspects of the illness are also reproduced by pharmacological disease models. The identification of a reliable and reversible neurobiological model of the psychotic state which can be used to evaluate putative anti-psychotic compounds would be of enormous benefit in neuropsychiatry, and has the potential to considerably expedite drug development. phMRI is likely to play an increasingly prominent role in this endeavour.

Exposure to psychedelic substances in non-psychotic individuals produces profound perceptual, sensorimotor, and cognitive disturbances. These effects vary considerably across drug categories such as psychomotor stimulants (e.g. cocaine and amphetamine), psychotomimetic indoleamines (e.g. lysergic acid diethylamide (LSD)), and dissociative anaesthetics (e.g. phencyclidine (PCP) and ketamine). The experiences produced by some of these compounds bear 'impressive similarity [to]... certain primary symptoms of the schizophrenic process'[58].

Whilst this approach introduces additional considerations, such as the effect of the drug on the dependent imaging measure (e.g. the blood oxygenation level dependent (BOLD) contrast), the primary advantage of this technique is that specific neurotransmitters can be experimentally augmented/inhibited in order to test hypotheses regarding their involvement in disease. This approach circumvents many of the interpretative problems of patient studies (such as disease/treatment chronicity, and interpretation of the significance of physiological deficits confounded by impaired cognitive performance). In contrast to the relatively static performance deficits in patient groups, dose administration can be graduated to establish a dose–response curve, up to and beyond cognitive capacity constraints. Furthermore, subjects serve as their own controls in double-blind, placebo-controlled, repeated measures designs, to some extent mitigating issues of group heterogeneity associated with between-group comparisons routinely reported in patient studies. The use of low-dose administration also offers the possibility of observing cognitive/physiological effects of the drug which are below the threshold at which psychotic phenomena are observed, thus facilitating a dissociation of these effects. For example, the presence of a hallucination may be sufficiently attentionally distracting to indirectly impair working memory performance, despite no specific effect on working memory processing per se. Eliciting cognitive disturbances at levels of drug exposure below that at which psychotic symptoms are evident thereby allows a more direct interpretation of the psychopharmacological manipulation. Before this approach can serve to clarify observations made on the basis of performance of schizophrenic patients, the validity of psychophar-macological models remains to be fully explored and validated at the cognitive and physiological level.

6.2 Ketamine and the NMDA hypofunction model

The proposed involvement of glutamate in schizophrenia stemmed from the observation that dissociative anaesthetics such as phencyclidine (PCP) and ketamine produce both positive and negative symptoms of psychosis in healthy volunteers[59], as well as exacerbating existing symptoms in patients[60], due to its affinity to the NMDA receptor[61]. Ketamine non-competitively blocks the NMDA receptor with affinity several times greater than its action at other sites, including the σ receptor, the μ opiate receptor, and acetyle-cholinesterase and monoamine transporter sites. Furthermore, blockade of non-NMDA mediated effects of ketamine does not block the psychotomimetic effects of the drug. Ketamine is, therefore, increasingly used as a human pharmacological model to investigate the hypothesis that schizophrenia is characterized by glutamatergic hypofunction.

Consistent with the use of ketamine as a model of schizophrenia, impairments in cognitive function are widely reported and show considerable overlap with those seen in patients with schizophrenia. phMRI studies are beginning to explore the physiological basis of these drug-induced cognitive impairments as a means to further understanding the pathophysiological mechanisms associated with the disturbances in schizophrenia.

On the basis of impaired episodic memory following ketamine administration[62], Honey *et al.* tested the hypothesis that this behavioural impairment, also consistently seen in patients with schizophrenia, is a consequence of frontal and hippocampal blockade of NMDA receptors, which may provide a model of the physiological basis of episodic memory impairment in schizophrenia[63]. The approach used in this study exploited the short half-life of ketamine (approximately 15 minutes), allowing assessments, pre- and post-drug administration, in order to isolate drug effects on specific components of episodic memory — encoding of information into memory stores and its retrieval from storage. Dissociation of the drug effects on encoding and retrieval processes was achieved using two study test cycles. In the first cycle, items were encoded prior to drug infusion and retrieval tested 'on drug' during FMRI scanning: drug-related effects on recognition are thereby attributed to a disruption of retrieval, since encoding occurred prior to drug infusion. In the second study cycle, encoding was scanned 'on drug', and retrieval tested once ketamine plasma levels had declined: drug-related effects on recognition are thus attributed to the encoding phase, since retrieval was performed in the relative absence of drug. This study illustrates how combining a pharmacological model with functional imaging offers an advantage in dissociating cognitive processes to identify pathophysiological mechanisms which would be inaccessible within the context of the disease itself, since the patient is, of course, subject to the influence of the disease process during both encoding and retrieval components of the task.

This was of particular advantage in this study, since it is proposed that deficits in episodic memory in schizophrenia may be principally related to an impairment of encoding processes, due to a failure of semantic strategies. In accordance with this, a prior cognitive study identified the deleterious effects of ketamine on behavioural performance to occur whilst encoding new information, rather than its retrieval from information stores[62,63]. phMRI data revealed that ketamine led to an increase in left frontal activation when elaborative semantic processing is required at encoding, which may underlie behavioural impairments observed when ketamine is administered at the encoding phase. In addition, successful encoding on ketamine, leading to correct item recognition at the retrieval stage, was predicted by increased right frontal activation compared to placebo, suggesting that verbal encoding may be compromised and is, therefore, supplemented by additional non-verbal processing. Interestingly, in contrast to previous cognitive studies which localized the behavioural deficit to an effect at the encoding stage, the phMRI study revealed fronto-hippocampal deficits consistent with impaired access to accompanying contextual features of studied items, even when overt behaviour is unimpaired. This therefore provides a further example of how phMRI studies may identify effects of disease/drug processes to which behavioural measures may be insufficiently sensitive due to compensatory performance strategies (as discussed previously; see 5.6).

Given the theoretical and clinical importance of working memory deficits in schizophrenia, a further study aimed to identify the physiological basis of working memory impairment following ketamine administration[64]. This study demonstrated that ketamine augments fronto-parietal activation in response to manipulation of information held in working memory, compared to simply maintaining information in storage[64].

The extent to which this provides a valid model of the pathophysiological mechanisms in schizophrenia requires further studies using similar tasks in schizophrenic patients.

These studies also indicated a further advantage of the pharmacological modelling approach, which is the possibility to separate physiological mechanisms underlying cognitive deficits from psychotic effects. The doses used in these studies (50 and 100 ng/ml plasma) were targeted to be sufficient to replicate specific cognitive deficits seen in schizophrenia, but sufficiently low as to induce only very mild levels of experiential phenomena.

6.3 Other transmitter systems

Pharmacological models of schizophrenia also incorporate other transmitter systems, for example, using psilocybin (the 5-HT2A receptor agonist), delta9-tetrahydrocannabinol (CB1 antagonist which is the psychoactive component in cannabis), and amphetamine (indirect dopamine agonist). phMRI studies have yet to be reported relating the psychotic effects of these compounds to the physiological effects observed using FMRI. An intriguing possibility is that phMRI studies using these drugs may identify a final common pathway which is likely to be of fundamental importance to understanding the pathophysiological basis of psychosis.

7. Pharmacological modulation of inter-regional functional integration

7.1 Functional specialization and functional integration

The preceding review of pharmacological imaging is largely focussed on the localization of drug/disease to discrete brain regions. This provides a useful starting point in understanding disease mechanisms and the effects of treatment. However, a more complete account requires a systems-level description: the evaluation of the adaptivity and inter-dependency of large-scale neurocognitive networks to pathological and pharmacological challenge. These approaches are sometimes referred to as functional specialization and function integration, respectively.

Multivariate analysis of FMRI time-series data, such as path analysis and structural equation modelling, provide an opportunity to evaluate perturbations of inter-regional functional integration. This approach aims to quantify the contribution a given region makes to the activity in functionally and anatomically connected regions, and is termed 'effective connectivity'. In practice, this involves comparing the fit of a theoretically predicted model of inter-regional coefficients relative to the observed data. Currently, modelling of FMRI time-series is, therefore, somewhat limited to a confirmatory approach where there is substantial prior knowledge of the anatomical and functional connections between regional nodes, based on evidence from other sources (e.g. electrophysiological and autoradiographic techniques in non-human primates, lesion data from neuropsychological patients, and post-mortem tissue analysis). The predicted model can, therefore, be supported or refuted on the basis of the observed FMRI data.

In the absence of extensive prior knowledge to constrain the theoretical model, exploratory model-free assessments of simple inter-regional task-dependent correlations can be informative in assessing inter-regional functional dependencies. This is based on the assumption that a task-dependent correlation between activity observed in two or more distinct brain regions likely indicates a functional relationship. In contrast to measures of 'effective connectivity', or model-based assessments, the inter-regional functional integration quantified by correlational analyses is termed 'functional connectivity'. This distinction aims to reflect the fact that correlational analyses do not, by themselves, provide a causal hierarchy of cerebral functional organization: they are neutral with respect to the directionality of functional influences between regions, and do not address the extent to which an observed covariance between two regions may be mediated by a third.

7.2 Pharmacological challenge in healthy volunteers

In a study comparing opposing dopaminergic pharmacological manipulations on fronto-striatal function (as described earlier, see 3.2), Honey *et al.*[9] reported both functional and effective connectivity analyses which were convergent in suggesting a modulation of the nigrostriatal pathway, which was not observed with two non-dopaminergic compounds. The study capitalized on the rich prior knowledge of the anatomy and neurochemistry of the cortico-striatal-thalamic feedback loops in order to construct a theoretically constrained model of the functional organization of the network, and make testable predictions regarding the localization of dopaminergic manipulations on functional pathways. Functional connectivity analysis revealed opposing effects on the correlation between activity in the caudate nucleus and ventral midbrain following drug challenge which served to increase (methylphenidate) or decrease (sulpiride) dopaminergic transmission. This was supported by a path model of the circuit, which demonstrated a significant fit to the data in two independent samples under placebo. The additional information revealed by model-based path analysis indicated the directionality of the pharmacological effect, which was to modulate the connection from the ventral midbrain to the caudate and is known to be a dopaminergic projection (see Fig. 12.10).

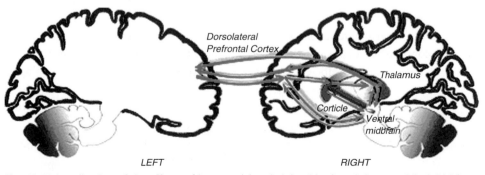

Fig. 12.10 Localization of the effects of increased (methylphenidate) and decreased (sulpiride) dopaminergic transmission on the functional connection of the nigrostriatal pathway between the ventral midbrain and caudate nucleus. (Reproduced with permission from Oxford University Press[9].)

This study demonstrated that multivariate analyses of phMRI data enables the evaluation of pharmacological effects on integrative brain function. Since even discrete focal lesions have fundamental implications for the neurocognitive network that each brain region participates in, such techniques are likely to be critical in understanding complex psychiatric and neurological disorders in which the integrity of neurobiological circuits is central to the pathophysiological basis of disease and its treatment.

7.3 Treatment effects in schizophrenia

Schizophrenia is increasingly viewed as a disconnection syndrome, in which the inter-regional communication in the brain is compromised, as opposed to a localized deficit in any one region. Accordingly, the mechanism of action of anti-psychotic treatments presumably involves the modulation of inter-regional functional connectivity. Recent studies have begun to characterize the effects of pharmacological treatment on integrative brain function.

Stephan et al.[65] evaluated the effects of the atypical anti-psychotic, olanzapine, on functional connectivity within the motor system. In comparison to the drug-free state, olanzapine treatment modulated functional connections of the cerebellum, including projections to the thalamus and prefrontal cortex. Interestingly, correlational patterns were normalized by drug treatment for the right, but not the left cerebellum. This may provide a systems-level explanation of a previous regional analysis which reported that signal intensity was normalized by olanzapine within the primary motor cortex, but fails to resolve abnormal lateralization of motor function[24]. Schlosser et al.[66] reported the first implementation of effective connectivity data analysis to study dysconnectivity in schizophrenia. Patients treated with typical and atypical anti-psychotics showed reduced pre-fronto-cerebellar and cerebellar-thalamic connectivity during performance of a working memory task, and enhanced thalamo-cortical connectivity. Patients treated with atypical anti-psychotics showed increased inter-hemispheric connectivity. This is consistent with a previous effectivity connectivity study of working memory in healthy volunteers, showing that increased inter-hemispheric connection strengths between prefrontal regions is observed as working memory load is increased[67]. The use of analytical techniques which address the functional relationships between remote brain regions will clearly be central to increased understanding of the pathophysiological basis of schizophrenia and other disorders, and the efficacy of pharmacological therapeutic agents.

8. Conclusions

In the decade since its application to psychiatric and neurological disorders, a nihilistic view of the contribution of FMRI research might be that it has not yet identified a pattern of brain activation which would serve as a diagnostic marker of any disease condition. FMRI has not characterized disease subtypes to the extent that phenomenological classification is no longer necessary, and it has not identified a fundamental pathophysiological mechanism. Similarly, phMRI is not, at present, used to determine treatment options in individual patients; it has not led directly to drug treatments with greater efficacy or generated novel pathways for drug discovery. In short, functional imaging is yet to translate to a routine clinical investigation which would aid clinicians' diagnosis or guide treatment options. There are suggestions that this may be in sight, but does this mean that FMRI and phMRI have failed to make a clinical impact?

We suggest that the role of phMRI in clinical practice, so far, has been to further our understanding of the disease mechanisms and drug treatments presently available. We believe this is an important and considerable contribution in the short period in which the technology has been available to the scientific community. phMRI is currently a research tool in the infancy of its development. It is testament to the potential implications of this technique that, in the short time it has been available to neuroscientists (only the past five years), one legitimately asks whether a clinical impact has yet been observed at the bedside. However, a meaningful answer to this question is somewhat premature and the clinical potential is yet to be realised. The translation from neuroscience research to clinical medicine is a complex, expensive, and time-consuming process, and it will be some time before the knowledge gained from phMRI research can be exploited for direct clinical benefit. However, the possibility that phMRI, particularly in combination with other techniques such as genotyping, electrophysiology, and the identification of high-risk populations, may be used to predict treatment response appears to be a realistic medium-term goal, and considerable advances have been made towards this end. In the meantime, the scientific community will continue to learn from the unique insights phMRI reveals about the transmitter basis of normal and dysfunctional cognitive states.

References

1. Arthurs, O. J., Stephenson, C. M. E., Rice, K., Lupson, V. C., Spiegelhalter, D. J., Boniface, S. J. *et al.* 2004, Dopaminergic effects on electrophysiological and functional MRI measures of human cortical stimulus-response power laws, *Neuroimage* **21**, 540–46.

2. Wilkinson, D. and Halligan, P. 2004, Opinion: the relevance of behavioural measures for functional-imaging studies of cognition, *Nat Rev Neurosci*, **5**, 1, 67–73.

3. Gozzi, A., Schwarz, A. J., Reese, T., Crestan, V., Bertani, S., Turrini, G., *et al.* 2005, Functional magnetic resonance mapping of intracerebroventricular infusion of a neuroactive peptide in the anaesthetised rat, *J Neurosci Methods*, **142**, 1, 115–24.

4. Chen, Y. C., Galpern, W. R., Brownell, A. L., Matthews, R. T., Bogdanov, M., Isacson, O., *et al.* 1997, Detection of dopaminergic neurotransmitter activity using pharmacologic MRI: correlation with PET, microdialysis, and behavioral data, *Magn Reson Med*, **38**, 3, 389–98.

5. Koyama, M., Hasegawa, I., Osada, T., Adachi, Y., Nakahara, K., and Miyashita, Y. 2004, Functional magnetic resonance imaging of macaque monkeys performing visually guided saccade tasks: comparison of cortical eye fields with humans, *Neuron*, **41**, 5, 795–807.

6. Austin, V. C., Blamire, A. M., Allers, K. A., Sharp, T., Styles, P., Matthews, P. M. *et al.* 2005, Confounding effects of anesthesia on functional activation in rodent brain: a study of halothane and alpha-chloralose anesthesia, *Neuroimage*, **24**, 1, 92–100.

7. Bullmore, E., Suckling, J., Zelaya, F., Long, C., Honey, G., Reed, L., *et al.* 2003, Practice and difficulty evoke anatomically and pharmacologically dissociable brain activation dynamics, *Cereb Cortex*, **13**, 2, 144–54.

8. Rao, S. M., Salmeron, B. J., Durgerian, S., Janowiak, J. A., Fischer, M., Risinger, R. C., *et al.* 2000, Effects of methylphenidate on functional MRI blood-oxygen-level-dependent contrast, *Am J Psychiatry*, **157**, 10, 1697–9.

9. Honey, G. D., Suckling, J., Zelaya, F., Long, C., Routledge, C., Jackson, S., *et al.* 2003, Dopaminergic drug effects on physiological connectivity in a human cortico-striato-thalamic system, *Brain*, **126**, Pt 8, 1767–81.

10. Kuriwaki, J., Nishijo, H., Kondoh, T., Uwano, T., Torii, K., Katsuki, M. *et al.* 2004, Comparison of brain activity between dopamine D2 receptor-knockout and wild mice in response to dopamine agonist and antagonist assessed by FMRI, *Neurosignals*, **13**, 5, 227–40.

11. Furey, M. L., Pietrini, P., and Haxby, J. V. 2000, Cholinergic enhancement and increased selectivity of perceptual processing during working memory, *Science*, **290**, 5500, 2315–9.

12. Thiel, C. M., Bentley, P., and Dolan, R. J. 2002, Effects of cholinergic enhancement on conditioning-related responses in human auditory cortex, *Eur J Neurosci*, **16**, 11, 2199–206.

13. Bentley, P., Vuilleumier, P., Thiel, C. M., Driver, J., and Dolan, R. J. 2003, Cholinergic enhancement modulates neural correlates of selective attention and emotional processing, *Neuroimage*, **20**, 1, 58–70.

14. Sperling, R., Greve, D., Dale, A., Killiany, R., Holmes, J., Rosas, H. D., *et al.* 2002, Functional MRI detection of pharmacologically induced memory impairment, *Proc Natl Acad Sci USA*, **99**, 455–60.

15. Thiel, C. M., Henson, R. N., and Dolan, R. J. 2002, Scopolamine but not lorazepam modulates face repetition priming: a psychopharmacological FMRI study, *Neuropsychopharmacology*, **27**, 2, 282–92.

16. Thiel, C. M., Henson, R. N., Morris, J. S., Friston, K. J., and Dolan, R. J. 2001, Pharmacological modulation of behavioral and neuronal correlates of repetition priming, *J Neurosci*, **21**, 17, 6846–52.

17. Bullmore, E. and Fletcher, P. 2003, The eye's mind: brain mapping and psychiatry, *Br J Psychiatry*, **182**, 381–4.

18. Kumari, V., Gray, J. A., Ffytche, D. H., Mitterschiffthaler, M. T., Das, M., Zachariah, E., *et al.* 2003, Cognitive effects of nicotine in humans: an FMRI study, *Neuroimage*, **19**, 3, 1002–13.

19. Lawrence, N. S., Ross, T. J., and Stein, E. A. 2002, Cognitive mechanisms of nicotine on visual attention, *Neuron*, **36**, 3, 539–48.

20. Thiel, C. M., Zilles, K., and Fink, G. R. 2005, Nicotine modulates reorienting of visuospatial attention and neural activity in human parietal cortex', *Neuropsychopharmacology*.

21. Mulderink, T. A., Gitelman D. R., Mesulam M. M., and Parrish T. B. (2002) On the use of caffeine as a contrast booster for BOLD FMRI studies. *Neuroimage*, **15**, 37–44.

22. Stephenson, C. M., Suckling, J., Dirckx, S. G., Ooi, C., McKenna, P. J., Bisbrown–Chippendale, R., *et al.* 2003, GABAergic inhibitory mechanisms for repetition-adaptivity in large-scale brain systems, *Neuroimage*, **19**, 4, 1578–88.

23. Northoff, G., Witzel, T., Richter, A., Gessner, M., Schlagenhauf, F., Fell, J., *et al.* 2002, GABA-ergic modulation of prefrontal spatio-temporal activation pattern during emotional processing: a combined FMRI/MEG study with placebo and lorazepam, *J Cogn Neurosci*, **14**(3), 348–70.

24. Bertolino, A., Blasi, G., Caforio, G., Latorre, V., De Candia, M., Rubino, V., *et al.* 2004, Functional lateralization of the sensorimotor cortex in patients with schizophrenia: effects of treatment with olanzapine, *Biol Psychiatry*, **56**, 3, 190–7.

25. Bertolino, A., Caforio, G., Blasi, G., De Candia, M., Latorre, V., Petruzzella, V., *et al.* 2004, Interaction of COMT (Val(108/158)Met) genotype and olanzapine treatment on prefrontal cortical function in patients with schizophrenia, *Am J Psychiatry*, **161**, 10, 1798–805.

26. Egan, M. F., Goldberg, T. E., Kolachana, B. S., Callicott, J. H., Mazzanti, C. M., Straub, R. E., *et al.* 2001, Effect of COMT Val108/158 Met genotype on frontal lobe function and risk for schizophrenia, *Proc Natl Acad Sci USA*, **98**, 12, 6917–22.

27. Mattay, V. S., Callicott, J. H., Bertolino, A., Heaton, I., Frank, J. A., Coppola, R., *et al.* 2000, Effects of dextroamphetamine on cognitive performance and cortical activation, *Neuroimage*, **12**, 3, 268–75.

28. Mattay, V. S., Goldberg, T. E., Fera, F., Hariri, A. R., Tessitore, A., Egan, M. F., *et al.* 2003, Catechol O-methyltransferase va1158-met genotype and individual variation in the brain response to amphetamine, *Proc Natl Acad Sci USA*, **100**, 10, 6186–91.

29. Weickert, T. W., Goldberg, T. E., Mishara, A., Apud, J. A., Kolachana, B. S., Egan, M. F. *et al.* 2004, Catechol-O-methyltransferase va1108/158met genotype predicts working memory response to antipsychotic medications, *Biol Psychiatry*, **56**, 9, 677–82.

30. Williams, G. V. and Goldman–Rakic, P. S. 1995, Modulation of memory fields by dopamine D1 receptors in prefrontal cortex, *Nature*, **376**, 6541, 572–5.

31. Honey, G. D., Fletcher, P. C., and Bullmore, E. T. 2002, Functional brain mapping of psychopathology, *J Neurol Neurosurg Psychiatry*, **72**, 4, 432–9.

32. Honey, G. D., Bullmore, E. T., Soni, W., Varatheesan, M., Williams, S. C., and Sharma, T. 1999, Differences in frontal cortical activation by a working memory task after substitution of risperidone for typical antipsychotic drugs in patients with schizophrenia, *Proc Natl Acad Sci USA*, **96**, 23, 13432–7.

33. Daniel, D. G., Berman, K. F., and Weinberger, D. R. 1989, The effect of apomorphine on regional cerebral blood flow in schizophrenia, *J Neuropsychiatry Clin Neurosci*, **1**, 4, 377–84.

34. Hertel, P., Nomikos, G. G., Iurlo, M., and Svensson, T. H. 1996, Risperidone: regional effects in vivo on release and metabolism of dopamine and serotonin in the rat brain, *Psychopharmacology (Berl)*, **124**, 1–2, 74–86.

35. Jones, H. M., Brammer, M. J., O'Toole, M., Taylor, T., Ohlsen, R. I., Brown, R. G., *et al.* 2004, Cortical effects of quetiapine in first-episode schizophrenia: a preliminary functional magnetic resonance imaging study, *Biol Psychiatry*, **56**, 12, 938–42.

36. Stip, E., Fahim, C., Mancini–Marie, A., Bentaleb, L. A., Mensour, B., Mendrek, A. *et al.* 2005, Restoration of frontal activation during a treatment with quetiapine: an FMRI study of blunted affect in schizophrenia, *Prog Neuropsychopharmacol Biol Psychiatry*, **29**, 1, 21–6.

37. Nahas, Z., George, M. S., Horner, M. D., Markowitz, J. S., Li, X., Lorberbaum, J. P., *et al.* 2003, Augmenting atypical antipsychotics with a cognitive enhancer (donepezil) improves regional brain activity in schizophrenia patients: a pilot double-blind placebo controlled BOLD FMRI study, *Neurocase*, **9**, 3, 274–82.

38. Yurgelun–Todd, D. A., Coyle, J. T., Gruber, S. A., Renshaw, P. F., Silveri, M. M., Amico, E., *et al.* 2005, Functional magnetic resonance imaging studies of schizophrenic patients during word production: effects of d-cycloserine, *Psychiatry Res*, **138**, 1, 23–31.

39. Braus, D. F., Ende, G., Weber–Fahr, W., Sartorius, A., Krier, A., Hubrich–Ungureanu, P., *et al.* 1999, Antipsychotic drug effects on motor activation measured by functional magnetic resonance imaging in schizophrenic patients, *Schizophr Res*, **39**, 1, 19–29.

40. Mattay, V. S., Tessitore, A., Callicott, J. H., Bertolino, A., Goldberg, T. E., Chase, T. N., *et al.* 2002, Dopaminergic modulation of cortical function in patients with Parkinson's disease, *Ann Neurol*, **51**, 2, 156–64.

41. Tessitore, A., Hariri, A. R., Fera, F., Smith, W. G., Chase, T. N., Hyde, T. M., *et al.* 2002, Dopamine modulates the response of the human amygdala: a study in Parkinson's disease, *J Neurosci*, **22**, 20, 9099–103.

42. Davidson, R. J., Irwin, W., Anderle, M. J., and Kalin, N. H. 2003, The neural substrates of affective processing in depressed patients treated with venlafaxine, *Am J Psychiatry*, **160**, 1, 64–75.

43. Fu, C. H., Williams, S. C., Cleare, A. J., Brammer, M. J., Walsh, N. D., Kim, J., *et al.* 2004, Attenuation of the neural response to sad faces in major depression by antidepressant treatment: a prospective, event-related functional magnetic resonance imaging study, *Arch Gen Psychiatry*, **61**, 9, 877–89.

44. Breiter, H. C., Gollub, R. L., Weisskoff, R. M., Kennedy, D. N., Makris, N., Berke, J. D., *et al.* 1997, Acute effects of cocaine on human brain activity and emotion, *Neuron*, **19**, 3, 591–611.

45. Stein, E. A., Pankiewicz, J., Harsch, H. H., Cho, J. K., Fuller, S. A., Hoffmann, R. G., *et al.* 1998, Nicotine-induced limbic cortical activation in the human brain: a functional MRI study, *Am J Psychiatry*, **155**, 8, 1009–15.

46. Wrase, J., Grusser, S. M., Klein, S., Diener, C., Hermann, D., Flor, H., *et al.* 2002, Development of alcohol-associated cues and cue-induced brain activation in alcoholics, *Eur Psychiatry*, **17**, 5, 287–91.

47. Schneider, F., Habel, U., Wagner, M., Franke, P., Salloum, J. B., Shah, N. J., *et al.* 2001, Subcortical correlates of craving in recently abstinent alcoholic patients, *Am J Psychiatry*, **158**, 7, 1075–83.

48. Gollub, R. L., Breiter, H. C., Kantor, H., Kennedy, D., Gastfriend, D., Mathew, R. T., *et al.* 1998, Cocaine decreases cortical cerebral blood flow but does not obscure regional activation in functional magnetic resonance imaging in human subjects, *J Cereb Blood Flow Metab*, **18**, 7, 724–34.

49. Jacobsen, L. K., Gore, J. C., Skudlarski, P., Lacadie, C. M., Jatlow, P., and Krystal, J. H. 2002, Impact of intravenous nicotine on BOLD signal response to photic stimulation, *Magn Reson Imaging*, **20**, 2, 141–5.

50. Daumann, J., Schnitker, R., Weidemann, J., Schnell, K., Thron, A., Gouzoulis–Mayfrank, E. 2003, Neural correlates of working memory in pure and polyvalent ecstasy (MDMA) users, *Neuroreport*, **14**(15), 1983–7.

51. Daumann, J., Schnitker, R., Weidemann, J., Schnell, K., Thron, A., Gouzoulis–Mayfrank, E. 2003, Neural correlates of working memory in pure and polyvalent ecstasy (MDMA) users, *Neuroreport*, **14**, 1983–7.

52. Jacobsen, L. K., Mencl, W. E., Pugh, K. R., Skudlarski, P., and Krystal, J. H. 2004, Preliminary evidence of hippocampal dysfunction in adolescent MDMA ('ecstasy') users: possible relationship to neurotoxic effects, *Psychopharmacology (Berl)*, **173**(3–4), 383–90.

53. Moeller, F. G., Steinberg, J.L., Dougherty, D. M., Narayana, P.A., Kramer, L. A., Renshaw, P. F. 2004, Functional MRI study of working memory in MDMA users, *Psychopharmacology (Berl)*, **177**(1–2), 185–94.

54. Daumann, J., Fischermann, T., Heekeren, K., Henke, K., Thron, A., Gouzoulis–Mayfrank, E. 2004, Memory-related hippocampal dysfunction in poly-drug ecstasy (3,4-methylenedioxymethamphetamine) users, *Psychopharmacology (Berl)*, Sep 15 (Epub ahead of print).

55. Rombouts, S. A., Barkhof, F., Van Meel, C. S., and Scheltens, P. 2002, Alterations in brain activation during cholinergic enhancement with rivastigmine in Alzheimer's disease, *J Neurol Neurosurg Psychiatry*, **73**, 6, 665–71.

56. Goekoop, R., Rombouts, S. A., Jonker, C., Hibbel, A., Knol, D. L., Truyen, L., *et al.* 2004, Challenging the cholinergic system in mild cognitive impairment: a pharmacological FMRI study, *Neuroimage*, **23**, 4, 1450–9.

57. Parry, A. M., Scott, R. B., Palace, J., Smith, S., and Matthews, P. M. 2003, Potentially adaptive functional changes in cognitive processing for patients with multiple sclerosis and their acute modulation by rivastigmine, *Brain*, **126**, 12, 2750–60.

58. Luby, E. D., Cohen, B. D., Rosenbaum, G., Gottlieb, J. S., and Kelley, R. 1959, Study of a new schizophrenicomimetic drug: serenyl, *Archives of Neurology and Psychiatry*, **71**, 363–369.

59. Krystal, J. H., Karper, L. P., Seibyl, J. P., Freeman, G. K., Delaney, R., Bremner, J. D., *et al.* 1994, Subanesthetic effects of the noncompetitive NMDA antagonist, ketamine, in humans. Psychotomimetic, perceptual, cognitive, and neuroendocrine responses, *Arch Gen Psychiatry*, **51**, 3, 199–214.

60. Lahti, A. C., Koffel, B., LaPorte, D., and Tamminga, C. A. 1995, Subanesthetic doses of ketamine stimulate psychosis in schizophrenia, *Neuropsychopharmacology*, **13**, 1, 9–19.

61. Javitt, D. C. and Zukin, S. R. 1991, Recent advances in the phencyclidine model of schizophrenia, *Am J Psychiatry*, **148**, 10, 1301–8.

62. Honey, G. D., Honey, R. A. E., Sharar, S. R., Turner, D. C., Pomarol–Clotet, E., Kumaran, D., *et al.*, 2005, Impairment of specific episodic memory processes by sub-psychotic doses of ketamine: the effects of levels of processing at encoding and of the subsequent retrieval task, *Psychopharmacology* Jun 28, 1–13 (Epub ahead of print).

63. Honey, G. D., Honey, R. A. E., Sharar, S. R., Kumaran, D., O'Loughlin, C., Suckling, J., *et al.* 2005, Ketamine disrupts fronto-hippocampal function during the encoding and retrieval of episodic memory, *Cerebral Cortex*, **15**(6), 749–59.

64. Honey, R. A., Honey, G. D., O'Loughlin, C., Sharar, S. R., Kumaran, D., Bullmore, E. T., *et al.* 2004, Acute ketamine administration alters the brain responses to executive demands in a verbal working memory task: an FMRI study, *Neuropsychopharmacology*, **29**, 6, 1203–14.

65. Stephan, K. E., Magnotta, V. A., White, T., Arndt, S., Flaum, M., O'Leary, D. S., *et al.* 2001, Effects of olanzapine on cerebellar functional connectivity in schizophrenia measured by FMRI during a simple motor task, *Psychol Med*, **31**, 6, 1065–78.

66. Schlosser, R., Gesierich, T., Kaufmann, B., Vucurevic, G., Hunsche, S., Gawehn, J. *et al.* 2003, Altered effective connectivity during working memory performance in schizophrenia: a study with FMRI and structural equation modeling, *Neuroimage*, **19**, 3, 751–63.

67. Honey, G. D., Fu, C. H., Kim, J., Brammer, M. J., Croudace, T. J., Suckling, J., *et al.* 2002, Effects of verbal working memory load on corticocortical connectivity modeled by path analysis of functional magnetic resonance imaging data, *Neuroimage*, **17**, 2, 573–82.

68. Saykin, A. J., Wishart, H. A., Rabin, L. A., Flashman, L. A., McHugh, T. L., Mamourian, A. C. *et al.* 2004, Cholinergic enhancement of frontal lobe activity in mild cognitive impairment, *Brain*, **127**, 7, 1574–83.

69. Fletcher, P., McKenna, P. J., Friston, K. J., Frith, C. D., and Dolan, R. J. 1999, Abnormal cingulate modulation of fronto-temporal connectivity in schizophrenia, *Neuroimage*, **9**, 3, 337–42.

70. Matthews, B., Siemers, E. R., and Mozley, P. D. 2003, Imaging-based measures of disease progression in clinical trials of disease-modifying drugs for Alzheimer disease, *Am J Geriatr Psychiatry*, **11**, 2, 146–59.

71. Matthews, P. M., Honey, G. D., Bullmore, E. T. 2006, Applications of fMRI in translational medicine and clinical practice. *Nature Reviews Neuroscience*, **7**, 739–44.

Index

acquisition paradigms 7–10
addiction 366–7
AFNI 56
ageing
  FMRI activations 60, 141–2
  memory 115–48
alcoholics 366
Alzheimer's disease
  apolipoprotein E 153, 162–4
  attention 155
  cell-death 173
  cell-sickness 173–4, 179–82
  cholinesterase inhibitors 165
  cingulate cortex 153, 155
  clinical dementia rating 160
  'default mode' network 155, 159
  diagnosis 149
  differential diagnosis 164
  donepezil 165
  early stage 23
  entorhinal cortex 150, 153, 162, 163,
      173, 179–82
  functional imaging 152–66
  functional MRI 154–67
  functional signature 153
  galanthamine 165
  genetic risk 153, 162–4, 267
  hippocampus 150, 155, 156, 173
  language 155
  medial temporal lobe 150, 156, 162
  memory 115, 155–7
  molecular imaging of pathology 152
  MRS 151–2
  parahippocampus 155
  parietal cortex 155
  PET 153
  phMRI 164–5, 367–8
  prefrontal recruitment 138, 155
  presymptomatic 149
  prodromal 149, 162, 166
  SPECT 153
  structural MRI 150–1
  synaptic function 150
amobarbital test 19, 27, 72, 83–9
amygdala 214, 215, 216–18, 229, 364
angular gyrus 74
anisotropy 28
anterior cingulate 194, 196, 213,
    215, 218, 219–20
antihistamines 5
anxiety disorders 209, 222–47
apathy 290
aphasia 72
apolipoprotein E 153, 162–4

apparent diffusion coefficient 300–1, 316
application accuracy 60
arterial disease 60
arterial spin labelling 54, 164, 179, 302
arteriovenous malformations 20–1, 79, 81–2, 97
associative deficit theory 116, 137
attention 60, 117, 155, 187, 329, 331
auditory cortex 8, 21
auditory queues 60
auditory stimuli 8
auditory verbal hallucinations 187
automatic processing 194–5

basal ganglia 74, 120, 213, 287
behavioural therapy 21, 23
benzodiazepines 355–7
binding 116, 118–19
bite-bars 14
blindness 21
block designs 7–9, 55, 56, 156
blood oxygen level dependent (BOLD) contrast
  basal metabolic rate 178
  brain pathology 4–5, 59, 97
  in-line 17
  language studies 97
  pharmacological effects 5, 344–6
  principles 2–4, 54, 344
bracket sign 44
brain
  activations 2, 60, 141–2
  age-related atrophy 120–1
  bionics 23
  essential/expendable regions 10–11, 26–8
  physiological motion 12
  plasticity 20 1, 77, 320
  shift 61
  tumours 4–5, 28–30, 46–61, 92–3, 98
brain boundary shift integral approach 151
brain-derived neurotrophic factor (BDNF) 198
Brain Voyager 17, 56
Broca's area 71, 73

caffeine 5, 355
carbon dioxide challenge 240
cell-sickness 173–4, 175–82
central executive 116
central sulcus 43–6, 52, 59
centres of gravity 60
centres of the masses 60
cerebral blood flow 2, 175, 302
cerebral blood volume 2, 175–6, 181–2
cholecystokinin 240–1
choline 151–2
cholinergic system 226, 352–5

cholinesterase inhibitors 165
cingulate cortex 153, 155;
    see also anterior cingulate
cingulate motor area 42
clinical FMRI
  applications 18–26
  challenges 4–18
  difficulty 1–2
  essential/expendable brain regions 10–11, 26–8
  future directions 26–30
  limitations 57–61
  methodology 7–11, 53–7, 94–103, 210–12
  post-processing 11–18, 56–7, 60
  task design 7–10, 54–6, 94–6, 139
clinical status 57–8
clonidine 241–2
cognition 72–3, 218–22, 230–3, 288–90, 298, 300,
    305, 329–31, 349–50, 368–9
cognitive resources 116, 136–7
coherence 195–6
compliance 60
computed tomography (CT) 293
COMT gene 197–8, 359
conjunction approach 96
connectivity 196
controlled processing 194–5
corpus callosum 326
cravings 366
critical language area 75

data presentation 57
deafness 21
deep brain stimulation 292
'default mode' network 155, 159
deoxyhaemoglobin 3
depression 209, 212–22
  activation studies 215–22
  amygdala 214, 215, 216–18
  anterior cingulate 213, 215, 218, 219–20
  antidepressants 212
  basal ganglia 213
  biochemistry 214
  brain abnormalities 213–14
  cognition 218–22
  differential diagnosis 23, 164
  dorsolateral prefrontal cortex 218–19, 221
  frontal cortex 215
  hippocampus 213–14, 215, 222
  limbic system 215, 247, 364–5
  medial temporal lobe 213, 218
  mood induction 215
  MRS 214
  neurotransmitters 214
  orbitofrontal cortex 213, 218, 220
  Parkinson's disease 290, 364
  phMRI 364–5
  prefrontal cortex 213, 215, 218
  resting state studies 215
  serotonergic transmission 214
  stimulus appraisal 247
  striatum 215
  thalamus 215
  TMS 212
  treatment 212
  tryptophan depletion 215
dextroamphetamine 26
diaschisis 276
diffusion tensor imaging 28–30, 102–3
diffusion-weighted imaging 300–1, 316–18
divided attention 117
donepezil 165
dopaminergic system 121, 194, 196, 225,
    293–6, 350–2, 359, 364
dorsolateral prefrontal cortex 76, 123, 124, 191,
    192–4, 196, 197, 218–19, 221, 230–1
draining veins 5–7, 59–60, 100–1
drug discovery 369–72

early response 2
echo-planar imaging (EPI) 4, 54, 100
ecstasy 366–7
effective connectivity 196, 372
electrocortical stimulation mapping 27, 48–50, 51,
    52, 53, 72, 75, 90–4
electroencephalography 20, 50, 210
eloquent cortex mapping 18–19
embryonic tissue implants 293, 295
emotional processing 10
endophenotype approach 197–9
energy metabolism 174
entorhinal cortex 150, 153, 162, 163,
    173, 179–82
epilepsy 12, 19–20, 23, 79, 103
episodic memory 115, 118–19, 123,
    125–30, 132–6
event-related designs 7, 10, 55, 141, 142
executive function 187–8, 191, 289–90
experience-induced adaptation 194

face–name association 155–7
false negatives/positives 17, 57
familiarity 119
fear 10, 247
fenfluramine challenge 242
fibre tractography 28
FLASH 54
fractional anisotropy 316
frontal lobe 76, 188–9, 190–1, 215
fronto-temporal dementia 164
FSL 17, 56
functional connectivity 196, 373, 374
functional integration 372–3
functional magnetic resonance
    imaging (FMRI)
  3T 26
  absence of activity 5
  basic principles 2–4
  intrinsic influencing factors 60
  see also clinical FMRI
functional specialization 372–3
function of interest 95–6

GABA 355–7
galanthamine 165

gender 60
glial tumours 4, 59, 98
glutamate 226, 370
gradient echo 54, 179
gray matter 120, 186, 311, 315, 318, 320

haemoglobin 3–4
haemorrhages 4, 5
hallucinations 187
hand knob 44, 46, 52
head fixation 14
head movement 12–16, 57–8, 97
Hemispheric Asymmetry Reduction in
    Older Adults (HAROLD) 122, 124,
    125–6, 127, 128, 129, 130, 136, 137
hippocampus
    ageing and memory 120–1, 130–2,
        133, 134, 135, 136, 137, 138
    Alzheimer's disease 150, 155, 156, 173
    depression 213–14, 215, 222
    mild cognitive impairment 157, 160, 162
    panic disorder 239, 240
    PTSD 234, 246
    schizophrenia 194
HIV 267
hypertension 120, 140

image registration and transformation 56
implantable stimulators 23
independent component analysis 56
information processing 185, 187, 188–99
in-line BOLD 17
insula 75
inter-image motion 12
intermediate approach 197–9
intra-image motion 12
intraoperative electrical corticography 27,
    48–50, 51, 52, 53, 72, 75, 90–4

ketamine 370–2

lactate infusion 240
language
    Alzheimer's disease 155
    children 103
    cognition 72–3
    continuum 82–3
    critical language area 75
    functional neuroimaging 75–6
    lateralization 19, 21, 76, 77–89
    lesion studies 73–4, 76–7
    localization 89–94
    mapping paradigms 8–9
    models and theories 71–2, 73–6
    modularity 75
    neural networks 74–5
    neuropsychology 74–5
    Parkinson's disease 289
    plasticity 77
    preoperative assessment 77–94, 103–4
    schizophrenia 187
lateralization index 82

late response 2
levodopa 286–7, 292, 295
Lewy bodies 285
limbic system 10, 215, 247, 364–5
lorazepam 355–6
lying 10

magnetic resonance spectroscopy (MRS) 151–2,
    210, 214, 225–6, 301, 318–20
magnetization transfer imaging 301–2, 313–16
magneto-encephalography (MEG) 7, 50, 210
major depressive disorder, see depression
MDMA 366–7
mean diffusivity 316
medial temporal lobe 115, 120, 122, 123, 130–6,
    137–8, 150, 156, 157, 160–2, 213, 218
MEDx 56
memory 19–20, 115–48, 155–7, 289, 329–31;
    see also working memory
microhaemorrhages 5
mild cognitive impairment (MCI) 149, 150, 151,
    153, 157–62, 166, 367–8
mood induction 215
motion correction algorithm 14–15
motor cortex 7, 46–53, 178, 187
motor foot area 46
motor hand area 44, 46, 52
motor homunculus 46
motor system 39–43, 287–8, 299–300,
    302–5, 323–9
motor tongue area 46
motor training 329
movement artefacts 12–16, 57–8, 97
multiple sclerosis 311–41
    attention 329, 331
    axonal damage 311, 319, 320
    cognition 329–31, 368–9
    cord pathology 315–16, 318
    corpus callosum 326
    cortical reorganization 325–9
    demyelination 311
    diffusion-weighted imaging 316–18
    FMRI 320–31, 332
    gray matter 311, 315, 318, 320
    heterogeneity 314
    longitudinal FMRI 332
    magnetization transfer imaging 313–16
    memory 329–31
    motor system 323–9
    motor training 329
    MRI 311–12
    MRS 318–20
    normal-appearing brain tissue 314–15, 317
    normal-appearing white matter 311, 314, 317, 319
    optic neuritis 315, 318, 321
    phMRI 368–9
    sensorimotor cortex recruitment 323–5
    visual system 321–2
    working memory 330–1
multiple system atrophy 291
myoinositol 151–2

N-acetyl aspartate 151–2, 226, 234–5, 301
naloxone 26
narcotic abuse 366
near infrared spectroscopy 59
neural networks 74–5
neurocognitive profiling 346
neurodegeneration, preclinical 23
neuronavigation 60–1, 100
neurophysiological FMRI 1
neuroprotection 292, 294
neurorehabilitation 21
neurostimulation 23
neurosurgery 18–19; *see also* preoperative
    assessment
neurovascular coupling 2, 5, 59, 166, 344–5
nicotine 355
nitric oxide 4, 59

obsessive compulsive disorder 209, 222–33
  activation studies 228–33
  amygdala 229
  biochemistry 225–6
  brain abnormalities 223–4
  cholinergic dysfunction 226
  cognition 230–3
  comorbidity 223
  compensatory posterior brain activity 231
  dopamine system 225
  dorsolateral prefrontal cortex 230–1
  frontal-striatal circuits 223, 225, 226–7, 229
  glutamatergic system 226
  heterogeneity 229
  implantable stimulators 23
  implicit learning 230
  MRS 225–6
  neurodevelopmental disorder 224
  PET 225
  prevalence 222
  pruning defect 224, 246
  relapse 222–3
  resting-state studies 226–8
  serotonergic system 225, 226
  SPECT 225
  striatum 223
  symptom dimensions 229
  symptom provocation 228–30
  treatment 222
  working memory 231–2
oedema 4–5, 58–9, 97
optic neuritis 315, 318, 321
orbitofrontal cortex 213, 218, 220
oxyhaemoglobin 4

pain 23, 103
panic disorder 209, 237–43
  activation studies 240–3
  biochemistry 238–9
  brain abnormalities 237–8
  brain stem 237
  carbon dioxide challenge 240
  cholecystokinin 240–1
  clonidine 241–2

fenfluramine challenge 242
functional MRI 242–3
GABA-benzodiazepine receptor 238–9
hippocampus 239, 240
lactate infusion 240
noradrenergic dysregulation 241
parahippocampus 239, 240
patho-genetic models 237
pentagastrin 240, 241
prefrontal cortex 239–40
resting state studies 239–40
serotonergic agonists 242
serotonergic system 239
yohimbine 241–2
parahippocampus 132, 133, 134, 136,
    137, 138, 155, 160, 239, 240
parallel imaging 26
paresis 57
parietal cortex 115, 155, 194
parkinsonism 285, 291
Parkinson's disease 285–310
  amygdala 364
  apathy 290
  arterial spin labelling 302
  bilateral disease 286
  cognition 288–90, 298, 300, 305
  combined medication 292
  COMT inhibitors 292
  CT 293
  DATATOP study 292
  DDC inhibitors 292
  deep brain stimulation 292
  dementia 288–9
  depression 290, 364
  diagnostic criteria 291
  differential diagnosis 291, 295–6, 298–9, 301
  diffusion-weighted imaging 300–1
  dopamine agonists 292
  dopaminergic system 121, 293–6, 364
  drug honeymoon 287
  embryonic tissue implants 293, 295
  executive function 289–90
  FMRI 302–6
  functional imaging 293–302
  genetics 290–1
  glucose metabolism 296–9
  implantable stimulators 23
  language 289
  levodopa treatment 286–7, 292, 295
  Lewy bodies 285
  magnetic resonance tomography 300–2
  magnetization transfer imaging 301–2
  memory 289
  mood 290, 298
  motor system 287–8, 299–300, 302–5
  MRI 293
  MRS 301
  neuropathology 285–6
  neuroprotection 292, 294
  Parkinson's disease-related pattern 296–7
  perfusion MRI 302
  PET 293–6, 300

Parkinson's disease (*cont.*)
  phMRI 364
  prognosis 286
  progression 286–7
  selegiline 292
  SPECT 293–6, 299
  speech 289
  stages of disease 285–6
  stereotactic ablation 287, 292–3
  structural imaging 293
  substantia nigra 285
  supplementary motor area 299–300
  therapy 286–7, 292–3
  ultrasound 293
  unilateral symptoms 286
  visuospatial skills 289
pentagastrin 240, 241
perceived oldness scale 134
performance measures 140–1
perfusion MRI 54, 175, 302
phantom limb 21
pharmacogenomics 357–60
pharmacological MRI (phMRI) 23, 25–6, 343–79
  acetylcholine 352–5
  advantages 348–9
  Alzheimer's medication 164–5, 367–8
  anaesthetic agents 348
  animal models 347–8, 352
  benzodiazepines 355–7
  BOLD contrast 5, 344–6
  caffeine 355
  cholinergic system 352–5
  cognition 349–50
  depression 364–5
  dextroamphetamine 26
  disadvantages 349
  dopaminergic drugs 345
  dopaminergic system 350–2
  drug discovery 369–72
  GABA 355–7
  inter-regional functional integration 372–4
  lorazepam 355–6
  mild cognitive impairment 367–8
  multiple sclerosis 368–9
  naloxone 26
  neurocognitive profiling 346
  neurovascular coupling 344–5
  nicotine 355
  Parkinson's disease 364
  pharmacogenomics 357–60
  physostigmine 353–4
  psychopharmacological modelling 369–72
  schizophrenia 359, 360–3
  scopolamine 354
  substance addiction 366–7
  task-dependent/-independent measures 346
  treatment response prediction 357–60
phobic disorders 209, 243–5, 246, 247
phonological loop 116
physostigmine 353–4
plasticity 20–1, 77, 320
positional shift 60–1

positron emission tomography
  (PET) 50, 51, 75, 153, 164, 189,
  210, 211, 212, 225, 293–300
post-processing 11–18, 56–7, 60
post-traumatic stress disorder 209, 233–6, 246, 247
practice 195
precentral gyrus 52
preclinical disease 23
prefrontal cortex 42, 115, 120, 122–30, 136–7, 155,
  187, 191, 213, 215, 218, 239–40
premotor area 42
preoperative assessment
  diffusion tensor imaging 28–30, 103
  language 77–94, 103–4
  motor cortex 46–53
  Type I/II errors 17
PRESTO technique 100
pre-supplementary motor area 42
primary motor cortex 39, 43–6
proactive interference 117
progressive supranuclear palsy 291
prosody 74
pruning defect 224, 246
psychiatry 23, 210–12
psychopharmacological modelling 369–72
pure insertion 96

reaction time 140, 141
real-time statistical post-processing 16–18
recognition memory 119
recruitment 137, 166, 270–2, 323–5
reliability 60, 101–2
resource deficit theory 116, 136–7
resting metabolism 175
rhinal cortex 120, 134, 138
Rolandic sulcus, *see* central sulcus
Rolandic tumours 46–61

schizophrenia 185–208
  anterior cingulate cortex 194, 196
  attention 187
  atypical anti-psychotics 360–3
  auditory verbal hallucinations 187
  brain abnormalities 186
  COMT gene 197–8, 359
  disconnection 196, 374
  dopaminergic system 194, 196, 359
  dorsolateral prefrontal cortex 191,
    192–4, 196, 197
  executive function 187–8, 191
  frontal lobe function 188–9, 190–1
  fronto-temporal connectivity 196
  functional connectivity 374
  genetic predisposition 196–9, 200
  glutamate 370
  gray matter 186
  hippocampus 194
  information processing 185, 187, 188–99
  ketamine model 370–2
  language 187
  motor cortex 187
  network-based theories 195–6

schizophrenia (*cont.*)
parietal cortex 194
PET 189
pharmacological models 370–2
phMRI 359, 360–3
practice effects 195
prefrontal cortex 187, 191
visual cortex 187
working memory 188, 190–1, 192, 194, 195
scopolamine 354
seizures 178
sensitivity 96–9
serotonergic system 214, 225, 226, 239
signal of pathology 152
single photon emission computed tomography
(SPECT) 50, 153, 210, 225, 293–6, 299
smoothing 56, 99
social phobia 243–5
software packages 17, 56
somatotopy 43, 46
spatial accuracy 6–7, 99–101
specific phobias 243–5, 247
spike-triggered approach 20
spin echo 54
spin history 12
SPM 17, 56
spontaneous ictal activity 20
statistics 16, 56–7
stereotactic ablation 287, 292–3
stimulation paradigms 7–10
stimulus appraisal 247
stress 60
striatum 215, 223, 287
stroke 265–83
activation site shift 272–3
activation size 273–4
behavioural changes 274–5
bilateral hemispheric recruitment 270–2
brain function 270–6
diaschisis 276
heterogeneity 268–9
infarct rim 276
infarct volume 266
laterality 270–2
network changes 270
primary cortex 275

recovery 20, 21, 265–6
secondary motor areas 275
therapeutic use of FMRI 268
structural equation modelling 142
subcortical areas 102
substance addiction 366–7
subtraction method 95–6, 139
sudden unmasking 53
supplementary motor area 41–2, 75, 299–300
surgery 18–19; *see also* preoperative assessment
symptom provocation 211–12, 228–30
synaptic activation/strength 176–8

task designs 7–10, 54–6, 94–6, 139
temporal lobe epilepsy 19–20
test–retest effect 194
thalamus 75, 120, 215
therapeutic development 21, 23
tinnitus 23
tissue pH 4, 5
transcranial magnetic stimulation
(TMS) 27–8, 50, 51, 212, 349–50
tryptophan depletion 215
T statistics 16
Type I/II errors 17

ultrasound 293

validity 102
vascular disease 269–70
vascular steal 5
ventrolateral prefrontal cortex 123, 124
visual cortex 21, 178, 187
visuospatial sketchpad 116
VoxBo 56
voxel-based morphometry 223–4

Wada test 19, 27, 72, 83–9
wash-out effect 178
Wernicke's area 71, 74
white matter 28–30, 102, 120
whole body scanners 26
working memory 115, 116–117, 122–5, 130–2, 188,
190–1, 192, 194, 195, 197, 231–2, 330–1

yohimbine 241–2